Human Physiology and Health

and Health

DAVID WRIGHT

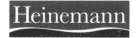

Heinemann

Contents

Heinemann Educational Publishers
Halley Court, Jordan Hill, Oxford, OX2 8EJ
a division of Reed Educational & Professional Publishing Ltd
Heinemann is a registered trademark of Reed Educational & Professional Publishing Ltd

OXFORD MELBOURNE AUCKLAND
JOHANNESBURG BLANTYRE GABARONE
IBADAN PORTSMOUTH NH (USA) CHICAGO

First published 2000

ISBN 0 435 63304 X

04 03 02
10 9 8 7 6 5 4 3

Edited by Alexandra Clayton

Designed by Ken Vail Graphic Design and produced by Cambridge Publishing Management

Cover design by JPH Design and Illustration

Printed and bound in Spain by Edelvives

Acknowledgements
The author and publishers would like to thank the following for permission to use photographs:

Cover photo by Science Photo Library

p2 fig.1: SPL; **p3 fig.2:** SPL/GCa/CNRI; **p3 fig.3:** SPL/CNRI; **p4 fig.1:** SPL/Claude Nuridsany & Marie Perennou;
p5 fig.2: Biophoto Associates; **p7 fig.2:** SPL/BSIP VEM; **p 17 fig.1:** Wellcome Photo Library; **p17 fig.2:** SPL/Dr P Marazzi; **p20 fig.1:** Wellcome Photo Library; SPL/Biophoto Associates; **p23 fig.1:** Science 2000 Booklet; **p27 fig.1:** Tony Stone Images; **p31 fig.1:** SPL/Biophoto Associates; **p55 fig.1:** SPL; **p57 fig.1:** SPL/St Bartholomew's Hospital; **p61 fig.2:** SPL/Brad Nelson Custom Medical Stock Photo; **p65 fig.2:** Biophoto Associates; **p86 fig.1:** SPL/Volker Steger; **p95 fig.1:** SPL/Bettina Cirone; **p99 fig.2:** SPL/Mark Clarke; **p109 fig.1:** SPL/Sheila Terry; **p115 fig.2:** SPL/Dr Tony Brain; **p117. fig.3:** SPL/Dr Tony Brain; **p119 fig.2:** SPL/P.Motta/Dept of Anatomy/University "La Sapienza" Rome; **p127 fig.3:** (Biophotos Associates); **p142 fig.1:** Bubbles/Loisjoy Thurston; **p151 fig.1:** SPL/Dr Karl Lounatmaa; **p153 fig.3:** SPL/Biophoto Associates; **p157 fig.2:** Geoscience Features; **p163 fig.3:** Camera Press; **p165 fig.1:** Wellcome Photo Library; **p165 fig.4:** SPL/Biophoto Associates; **p173 fig.5:** Roger Scruton; **p175 fig.2:** SPL; **p175 fig.3:** Dental Health Unit, Manchester University; **p195 fig.3:** SPL/Eye of Science; **p197 fig.3:** SPL; **p197 fig.4:** SPL; **p199 fig.1:** SPL/Eye of Science; **p199 fig.1:** SPL/David Scharf; **p199 fig.1:** SPL/Cath Wadforth; **p203 fig.2:** SPL/Dr P. Marazzi; **p209 fig.2:** SPL/John Durham; **p215 fig.2:** SPL/Martin Bond; **p217 fig.1:** SPL/Linda Stannard; **p217 fig.2:** SPL/Barry Dowsett; **p217 fig.2:** SPL/Juergen Berger, Max Planck Institute; **p217 fig.2:** SPL/Michael Abbey; **p231 fig.2:** Roger Scruton; **p241 fig.1:** OSF; **p241 fig.2:** Holt Studios International; **p248 fig.3:** OSF; **p253 fig.1:** OSF; **p257 fig.3:** Bruce Coleman; **p261 fig.3:** SPL/Peter Menzel; **p261 fig.3:** OSF; **p263 fig.2:** OSF; **p267 fig.4:** W. Eugene Smith/Magnam Photos; **p269 fig.2:** OSF.

The author and publisher would like to thank the following for permission to use tables and figures:

p19 table 1: Tesco 'Tesco Guide to Nutrition Information'; **p23 table 1, fig.1,2,3:** Crown copyright is reproduced with the permission of the Controller of Her Majesty's Stationery Office; **p51 table 1, fig.3:** Crown copyright is reproduced with the permission of Her Majesty's Stationery Office; **p57 table 1:** ASH Crown copyright is reproduced with the permission of the Controller of Her Majesty's Stationery Office; **p129 table 1:** Blackwell Science Ltd "Clinical Physiology in Obstetrics" by Chamberlain; **p169 table 1, fig.1:** ASH Crown copyright is reproduced with the permission of the Controller of Her Majesty's Stationery Office; **p171 fig.4:** ONS 'Cancer Statistics' National Statistics © Crown Copyright 2000; **p177 fig.2,3,4:** WHO (1994–1997); **p193 fig.1,3,4:** WHO (1994–1997); **p195 fig.4:** National Meningitus Trust 1999; **p201 table 1:** WHO (1994–1997); **p201 fig.1:** Health Education Authority; **p203 table 2:** ONS; p207 table 1: WHO; **p211 fig.2:** Health Education Authority; **p255 fig.2,3,4:** ONS; **p257 fig.1:** Greenpeace 'Fight for the Forests'.

The publishers have made every effort to trace the copyright holders, but if they have inadvertently overlooked any, they will be pleased to make the necessary arrangements at the first opportunity.

Picture research by Thelma Gilbert

Tel: 01865 888058   www.heinemann.co.uk

Introduction

This book has been written to give you a thorough introduction to all aspects of human biology. It covers the material you will require to pass a course in *Human Physiology and Health* or *Health Studies* at level 2 (GCSE or equivalent). It will also be a valuable resource to support anyone studying a *GNVQ Health* or *Science* course at intermediate level. I also hope it will be a worthwhile and stimulating book for anyone simply interested in the human body or how we relate to our environment.

The book breaks the major topics down into easily managed units, each presented as a double page spread. In the text, I have explained the facts and concepts using clear and simple language. Important words are highlighted in bold type, which will help you to build up your own glossary.

The text is also backed up by full colour diagrams which contain additional information to help clarify it. Colour photographs are used to bring the subject to life. The diagram pages also contain lots of data presented in easily accessible tables, charts or graphs.

Each chapter starts with a synopsis and broad learning targets based on the GCSE syllabus requirements. These learning targets are expanded on each double page in the chapter. If you are using this book as part of a course of study at a school or college, your teacher will be able to supply you with a worksheet for most double page spreads, to help you achieve the learning targets.

When you have completed a topic, you can take a short test to check how many of the facts you have managed to learn and test your understanding of the concepts.

The book also contains some past examinations questions so that your can practise your answers and start developing your examination technique.

Every chapter in the book starts with an extension topic related to human biology. These topics emphasise the personal, social, environmental, economic or technological aspects of human biology. Some are related to the content of the chapter, others are included for interest. Your teacher will have some resource material which will help you access and build on this information.

Finally I would like to mention several people who have helped make this book possible:

Ann Carlin for the selfless way she supported me throughout

Colin Clegg for believing in me during difficult times, and encouraging me to write again

The nursing, ancillary staff and doctors on the Leukaemia and Lymphoma Ward at Leeds General Infirmary.

You may be interested to know that a percentage of the royalties from this book will go to support the Leukaemia and Lymphoma Ward at the Leeds General Infirmary.

I wish you every success in your course of study and hope that this book helps you enjoy it that much more.

David B. Wright

The organisation of the body

We look at the human body and see hair, eyes, skin, arms, legs and so on. We can even see some of the internal structures, such as the teeth and tonsils, and can imagine others. We can do this for other animals, too. What is hard to imagine is that all animals, including ourselves, are made from the same tiny building 'bricks' called cells. In this chapter, you will find out about cells; the substances that form them and the processes going on inside them. You will discover how they are organised into the comparatively larger and more complex human body.

After you have worked through this chapter, you should be able to:

- Describe the basic structure of an animal cell.
- Identify some of the different types of cell.
- Explain how cells form tissues and list the main tissues in the human body.
- Describe how tissues work together in organs.
- Name and assign functions to the main organs in the human body.
- List and outline the functions of the main organ systems in the human body.

- Explain the term metabolism and outline the difference between anabolism and catabolism.
- Explain the principles of enzyme action and describe how changes in temperature and pH affect enzyme action.
- Explain how substances can enter and leave a cell by diffusion, osmosis, active transport and phagocytosis.

Looking inside a body

Not so long ago, the only way a doctor could look inside your body was by cutting it open. Technology has now given the medical profession a range of less invasive methods, some of which not only show structure, but can also be used to show function.

The oldest of these is the **X-ray**. X-rays are high energy forms of electromagnetic radiation. As they pass through a body, they are absorbed by dense tissues much more than less dense tissues, so different amounts penetrate the tissues. The rays which pass through can be used to produce a radiograph, the most dense structures showing as white and the least dense as black. The biggest problem with X-rays is that they may damage DNA and therefore the patient dose must be as low as possible. The eye, thyroid gland and reproductive organs are particularly vulnerable and their exposure should be kept to a minimum. The doctors and radiographers using X-rays also need to protect themselves.

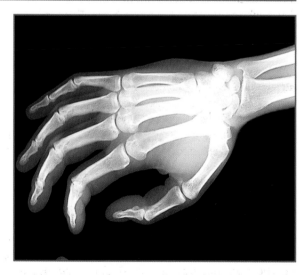

Figure 1 X-rays can be used to 'see' structures inside the body, like bones.

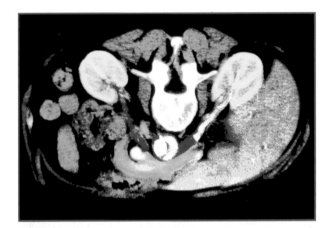

Figure 2 *A coloured CT scan of the upper abdomen.*

imaging techniques because it can penetrate all tissues (even bone) and as yet, there is no evidence to suggest that it causes any damage. The only limitation is that it can not be used on people who have metal implants or a pacemaker.

Nuclear medicine is used to look for damage or to study the functioning of an organ. For example, bone damage from the spread of tumour cells, or how well the kidneys are working. A **radioactive tracer** which emits gamma radiation is injected into the patient and its movement is followed using a special camera. The tracer selected depends on the organ being studied. To look at bones isotopes of calcium or technetium are used. These will accumulate more rapidly in damaged or diseased bone and show up after a short time as **'hot spots'** (see figure 3).

The **CT scanner** (computed tomography) combines an X-ray machine with a computer. X-rays are taken around a section of the body and the computer combines these to produce a cross-sectional image.

Modern CT scanners can even produce 3D images of organs like the brain, spine and blood vessels.

Sometimes artificial contrast mediums are used to highlight soft tissues. A **barium meal** (solution of barium salts which absorb X-rays) for example, taken before an X-ray, can be used to look for signs of ulcers in the stomach. Blood vessels can also be injected with a dense substance before taking an X-ray. This kind of X-ray is called an **angiogram** and is used to detect diseased or blocked arteries.

Another much used method of looking at soft tissues is **ultrasound**. High frequency sound waves are reflected differently by different tissues. The pattern of reflection can be used to form an image. Ultrasound is especially useful for studying the development of a foetus because it does not damage living tissue (chapter 9.7). When linked to a computer, the images can be used to create a 3D-image of the foetus and even show movements.

MRI (magnetic resonance imaging) uses a very strong fluctuating magnetic field to produce very detailed images of the inside of the body. Because it uses data at the atomic level, it can also provide biochemical details, e.g. chemical composition and pH. This allows doctors to study, for example, how a drug is metabolised in a tissue. MRI is probably the most useful of all the

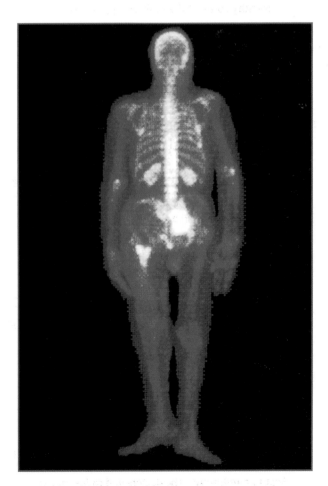

Figure 3 *This skeleton has a 'hot spot' because of a tumour in the pelvic region.*

1.1 Cell structure

What are you made of?

The human body is made of millions of small units called **cells**. These cells contain living material. Compare this to a house that is made of clay bricks. Cells are the building 'bricks' of your body.

What does a cell look like?

Cells are very small. They are so small that we measure them in **micrometres (μm)**. One micrometre is equal to one thousandth of a millimetre (1 mm = 1000 μm). Most of the cells in your body are between 10 and 300 μm in diameter. Because cells are so small you have to use a **microscope** to see them (see figure 1).

Although animal cells vary in shape and size, they all have three things in common: an outer covering called the **cell membrane**; surrounding two distinct areas, the **nucleus** and the **cytoplasm**. The nucleus is separated from the cytoplasm by a nuclear membrane. The functions of these parts are described in figure 2.

Powerful microscopes called **electron microscopes** reveal a complex organisation within the cell. For example, within the nucleus are thread like structures called **chromosomes** (chapter 11.1), and the cytoplasm contains many small structures called **organelles**. Some of these organelles are also bounded by their own membranes which separate them from the rest of the cytoplasm. One very important organelle is the **mitochondrion**. It is inside a mitochondrion that energy is released from food (chapter 4.1). Several hundred mitochondria may be present in a cell. The more energy a cell requires, the more mitochondria it has. Another important organelle is the **ribosome**. Proteins are assembled in ribosomes (chapter 11.2).

Cells contain many more different types of organelle, each carrying out a specific job within the cytoplasm. The full structure of a typical animal cell is shown in figure 2.

Are all the cells in your body the same?

Cells are designed to do all sorts of different jobs. All cells are made from protoplasm surrounded by a membrane, but once formed they grow differently and become specialised for a particular job. For example, skin cells are designed for protection and muscle cells are designed for moving. Figure 2 in chapter 1.2 shows some of the different types of cells that make up your body.

What are plants made of?

Plants are also made of cells but these differ from animal cells in the following ways:

- The whole cell is bounded by a **cell wall** made from a rigid material called **cellulose**. This gives the cell a fixed shape.

- Most plant cells have a large central **vacuole** usually containing a sugary solution called **cell sap**. This vacuole with its cell sap and the cell wall are very important in providing support for the plant.

- Plant cells, which are exposed to light contain several small green organelles called **chloroplasts**. These are green because they contain a green pigment called **chlorophyll**. Chlorophyll can absorb light energy, which the plant can then use to make food by a process called photosynthesis.

- The cytoplasm often contains starch grains. This is how most plants store the food they have made by photosynthesis.

The full structure of a typical plant cell is shown in figure 3.

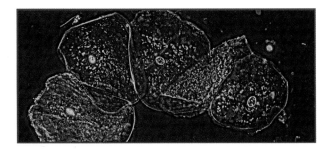

Figure 1 *Human cheek cells seen through a light microscope.*

What do **you** know?

You should now be able to:

- Draw a generalised animal cell. Label the cell membrane, cytoplasm, nucleus and mitochondria. Identify these on a photograph of a cell.
- Describe the role (function) of each of these structures.
- Calculate the size of a cell from a photograph or drawing. State the size in micrometers (μm).
- Work out the magnification of a cell from a photograph or drawing.
- List the 4 structures a plant cell has in common with an animal cell.
- List the 4 structural differences between a plant cell and an animal cell.

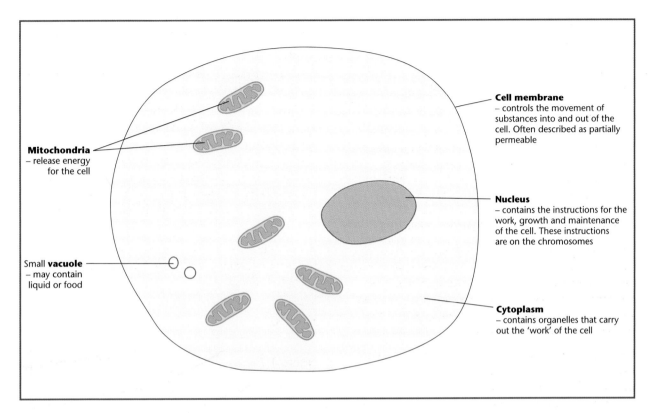

Figure 2 *Some of the structures inside a typical animal cell.*

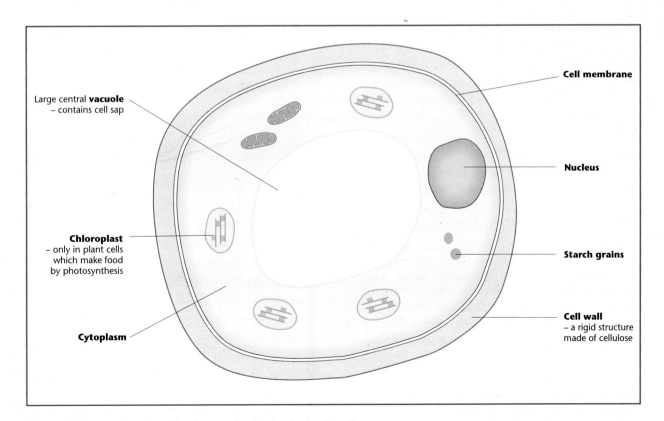

Figure 3 *Some structural features of a typical plant cell.*

1.2 Cells into bodies

Cells and more cells

We all start off as one cell. This is the cell which results from the fertilisation of a human egg by a human sperm (chapter 9.4). By the time you are ready to be born, your body will contain millions of cells. These cells have been produced from existing cells by **cell division** (chapter 11.3). The production of more cells results in **growth**.

Even when you are fully grown, your body goes on making new cells to replace worn out and damaged ones.

How are cells organised into a body?

The cells in your body are of many different types. These cells do not float around, but are organised in a very fixed way. This organisation can be understood in three stages:

1 Cells form tissues

Different kinds of cell in your body do different jobs. For example, all **muscle cells** help you to move and **nerve cells** carry messages. Cells which have a similar structure and do the same job in a body, group together to form a **tissue**.

There are many kinds of tissue in your body. The main ones are **muscle tissue**, made of muscle cells; **nervous tissue**, made of nerve cells, and **epithelial tissue** made of cells which line surfaces. Skin is epithelial tissue, which is made of skin cells. The tissue may also contain a non-cellular material called a **matrix**.

You will come across these tissues and many more as you read through this book.

2 Tissues form organs

Most tissues do not work independently, but join forces to do a particular job. For example, your heart pumps blood around your body. To do this the heart needs muscle tissue so that it can contract, nervous tissue to tell it how fast to contract and epithelial tissue to provide a smooth surface for the blood to flow over.

How are these tissues held together? The answer is, with another tissue suitably called **connective tissue**. Connective tissue is made from several different types of cell and a matrix, usually containing protein fibres. Connective tissue does more than just bind tissues together. It also provides a structural framework, support and protection.

A structure which contains several tissues, all working to perform one function, is called an **organ**. Figure 2 shows the three types of tissue found in the small intestine. The positions of some of the main organs in your body are also shown in figure 2.

3 Organs work in systems

For you to see anything, you need your eyes and brain. To hear anything, you need your ears and brain. For almost any action carried out by your body, several organs are used. When organs work together like this, they are called an **organ system**. For example, the kidneys, bladder, ureters and urethra make up the **excretory** (urinary) **system** (see figure 1).

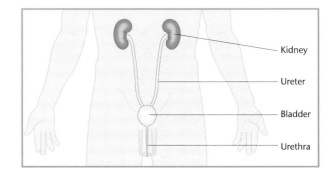

Figure 1 *The excretory system.*

Other organ systems found in your body are the **respiratory** system, **muscular** system, **skeletal** system, **digestive** system, **reproductive** system, **circulatory** system, **endocrine** system, **nervous** system and **sensory** system.

Many organs have a function in more than one system, for example the male urethra acts as a duct for both urine and sperm, and the pancreas produces a digestive juice and hormones.

What do **you** know?

You should now be able to:

- Draw diagrams of the following types of cell: ciliated epithelial, nerve, striated muscle, blood and sex.
- Assign a function to each of these cells within a tissue or organ.
- List the 4 main tissues in the human body and assign a function to each.
- State one place in the human body where each of these can be found.
- Identify the main organs in the human body.
- List the main organ systems in the human body and state their functions.

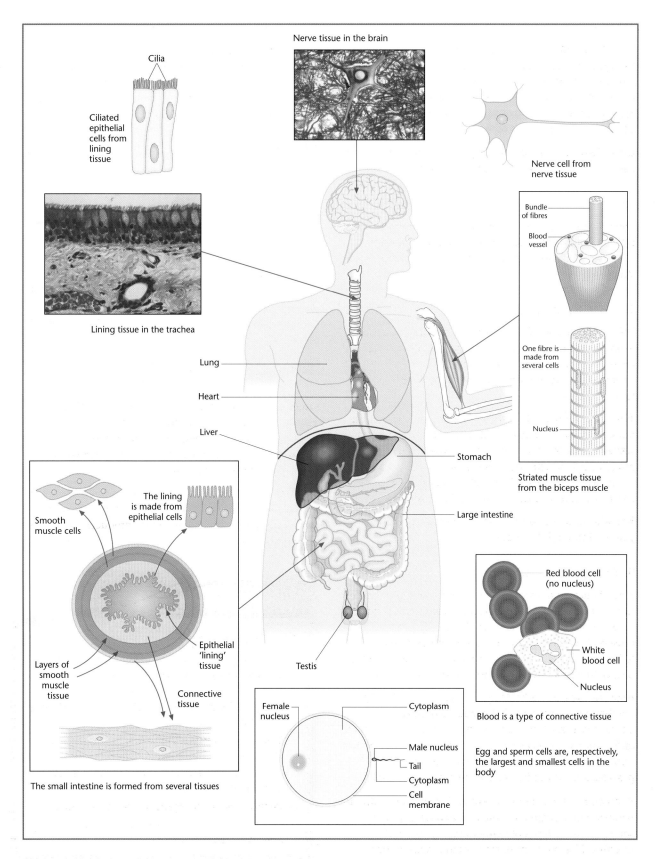

Figure 2 *Cells form tissues which form organs. Organs work in systems.*

1.3 Metabolism

What goes on inside a cell?

Even though cells are tiny in size a lot goes on in each individual cell. Each cell is like a chemical factory. Within the cytoplasm hundreds of life-giving chemical reactions are taking place. This chemical activity is usually referred to as the cell **metabolism**. Metabolism involves two main kinds of reaction (see figure 1):

- When raw materials are used to build more complex substances, this is called **anabolism**. For example, using amino acids to build proteins, or glucose molecules to build starch. Anabolic reactions usually require some **energy**.

- This energy is supplied from catabolic reactions. **Catabolism** is the breaking down of complex substances, such as carbohydrates and fats, into smaller simpler substances, such as carbon dioxide and water. This is always accompanied by the release of some energy. All living things obtain the energy they need for their cellular activities from a type of catabolism called **respiration** (chapter 4.1).

The speed at which these reactions take place is called the **metabolic rate**. The metabolic rate can speed up or slow down to meet the needs of your body. At its slowest rate, it is called the **basal metabolic rate** (BMR). Basal metabolism will only just keep you alive.

Can a cell control its metabolism?

Most anabolic and catabolic processes do not take place as single reactions, but as a series of reactions. This chain of reactions is called a **metabolic pathway**. Respiration is a metabolic pathway involving over 30 separate chemical reactions before the final products are produced. Each of these reactions is controlled by an enzyme.

Enzymes are very special chemicals produced by the cells to speed up their chemical reactions. They are organic '**catalysts**'. Without these, metabolism would be too slow to maintain living cells.

An enzyme will also only speed up one particular type of reaction. By carefully producing the correct enzymes, a cell can therefore organise its metabolism, i.e. only those reactions for which enzymes are present will take place.

Why will enzymes only catalyse one type of reaction?

The equation below can be used to summarise an enzyme-controlled reaction.

$$\text{Substrate molecules} \xrightarrow{\text{enzyme}} \text{product molecules}$$

Enzymes are large proteins with a complex three-dimensional (3D) structure. A small but important part of this structure is the **active site**. This is the place where the substrate molecule must bind for the enzyme to work. The active site has a fixed shape which is different on each type of enzyme. The enzyme can only work on a substrate molecule that will fit into its active site. This is often compared to a key fitting a lock and is called the **lock and key hypothesis** of enzyme action. A full explanation is shown in figure 2.

How fast do enzymes work?

We measure how fast an enzyme is working by the speed, or **rate** at which it does something. This can be *the amount of product formed in a fixed time, the amount of substrate used in a fixed time*, or even *the total time for a fixed amount of the substrate to be used up and converted to product*. For example, the waste substance hydrogen peroxide is produced during metabolism. It is dangerous if too much hydrogen peroxide builds up in your body so the cells produce an enzyme called **catalase** to speed up its breakdown, i.e.

$$\text{Hydrogen peroxide} \xrightarrow{\text{catalase}} \text{water} + \text{oxygen}$$

The rate at which catalase is working can be expressed as *the amount of oxygen produced per minute, the amount of hydrogen peroxide used per minute*, or *the time taken for all the hydrogen peroxide to be broken down into water and oxygen*.

Catalase is one of the fastest acting enzymes in the human body. Just one molecule of it will breakdown 40 000 molecules of hydrogen peroxide per second.

What do **you** know?

You should now be able to:

- Describe metabolism.
- Give examples of anabolism and catabolism and show how these are linked together.
- Outline the importance of enzymes in the control of metabolism.
- Explain the terms: substrate, enzyme and product.
- Write an equation which links these.
- Describe and explain the 'lock and key hypothesis' of enzyme action.
- Suggest with an example how you could measure the rate of an enzyme controlled reaction.
- Write an equation to show the function of catalase.

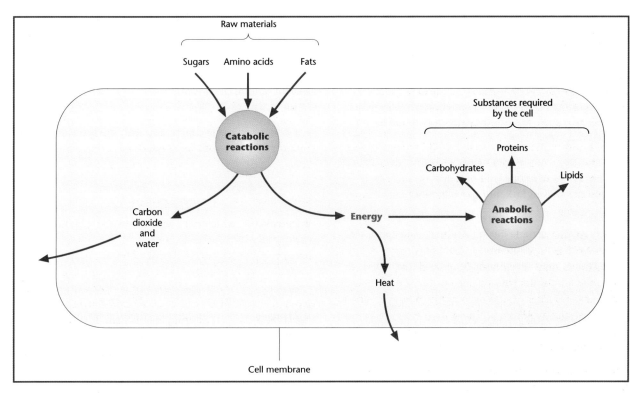

Figure 1 *Metabolism is the name given to all the chemical reactions that take place in a cell. These can be building up (anabolic) or breaking down (catabolic) reactions.*

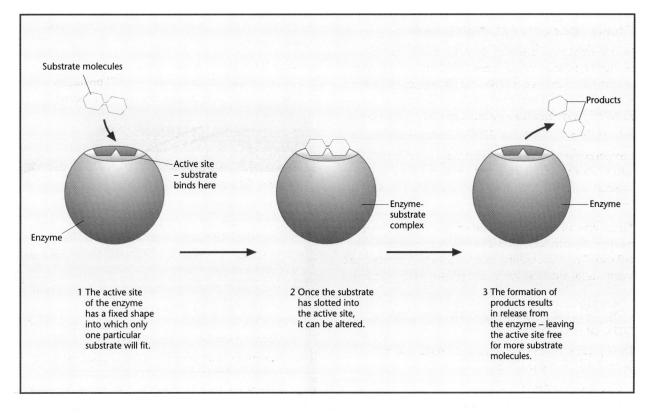

1 The active site of the enzyme has a fixed shape into which only one particular substrate will fit.

2 Once the substrate has slotted into the active site, it can be altered.

3 The formation of products results in release from the enzyme – leaving the active site free for more substrate molecules.

Figure 2 *The lock and key hypothesis of enzyme action.*

1.4 Enzymes

The features of enzymes

The following summarises the main characteristics of enzymes:

- Enzymes are only produced in living cells.

- Enzymes are not changed in reactions and therefore can be re-used. As such, they are only required in small amounts.

- Enzymes are very specific, that is a particular enzyme will only catalyse one type of reaction. This can be explained by the lock and key hypothesis.

- Enzymes are complex three-dimensional (3D) proteins. Each type of enzyme has a fixed shape. Keeping this shape is crucial to the working of the enzyme. Altering the shape can affect the shape of the active site and the function of the enzyme.

- Enzymes are affected by heat. They each have a temperature at which they work best, called the **optimum** temperature. The enzymes in your body work best at temperatures around 37 °C (body temperature). At temperatures above this, the shape of the enzyme starts to be altered, thereby altering the shape of the active site. The enzyme is said to be **denatured** and stops working. At temperatures below the optimum, the enzyme holds its shape, but works more slowly.

  This is explained by the kinetic theory. For enzymes to work, they need to collide with the substrate. The higher the temperature the more energy the molecules have and the faster they will move around and collide with one another. Lower temperatures reduce the number of collisions.

- Enzymes are affected by **pH** (i.e. acidity or alkalinity). Most enzymes have an optimum pH but will also work more slowly within a narrow range around this (see figure 1). Extremes of pH can denature the enzyme and stop it working altogether.

- Enzymes are affected by some chemicals. These chemicals, called **inhibitors** (see figure 2), interfere with the activity of the enzyme by either binding to its active site or changing the shape of the enzyme. This will either slow the enzyme down or stop it working. Many drugs and poisons work like this. For example, cyanide inhibits an enzyme involved in respiration.

Some important enzymes

Enzymes can only be produced by living cells. If they are produced to work inside a cell, for example to control metabolism, they are known as **intracellular** enzymes.

Catalase and **phosphatase** are examples of intracellular enzymes.

The enzymes involved in the digestion of food are called **extracellular** enzymes. These are produced inside special glandular cells and are then secreted into the alimentary canal. Digestive enzymes are of three types:

- **Carbohydrases**, which help with the breakdown of carbohydrates such as starch.
  e.g.

  Starch $\xrightarrow{\text{amylase}}$ maltose $\xrightarrow{\text{maltase}}$ glucose

- **Proteases**, which help with the breakdown of proteins.
  e.g.

  Protein $\xrightarrow{\text{pepsin}}$ polypeptides $\xrightarrow{\text{trypsin}}$ dipeptides

- **Lipases**, which catalyse reactions involving lipids.
  e.g.

  Lipids $\xrightarrow{\text{lipase}}$ fatty acids + glycerol

All these enzymes work best at 37 °C, but have different pH requirements (see table 1).

What do **you** know?

You should now be able to:

- List the main characteristics of enzymes.
- Describe how and why enzymes are affected by heat.
- Draw a graph to show how pH affects the activity of the enzymes involved in digestion.
- Explain why inhibitors affect enzymes.
- Distinguish between intracellular and extracellular enzymes.
- Name two intracellular enzymes.
- Outline what carbohydrases, proteases and lipases do in digestion.
- State named examples of these extracellular enzymes.

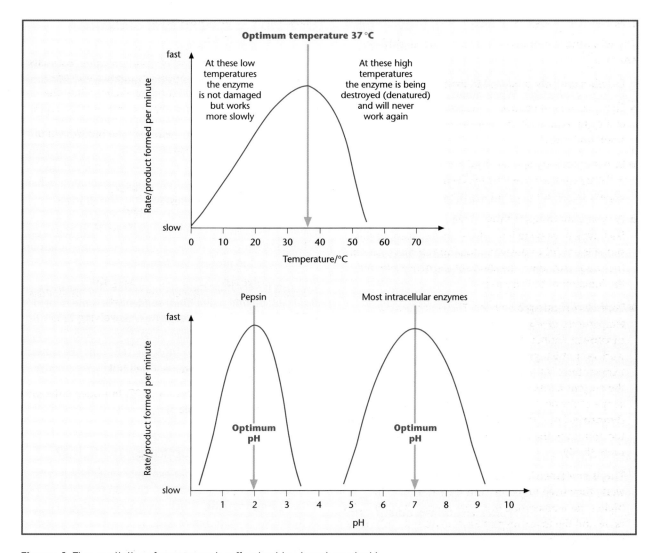

Figure 1 *The activity of enzymes is affected by heat and pH.*

Table 1 *The optimum pH for some enzymes.*

Enzyme	Optimum pH
Catalase	7
Amylase	7
Pepsin	2
Trypsin	8–9
Lipase	8–9
Most intracellular	7

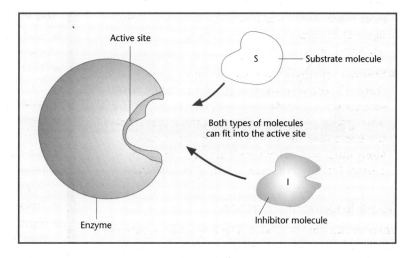

Figure 2 *The activity of an enzyme can be affected by inhibitors.*

1.5 Movement in and out of cells

How do substances enter and leave cells?

Substances pass in and out of cells as tiny particles. These can be molecules or ions. **Atoms** are the smallest and simplest forms of matter. When atoms join together they form **molecules**. When atoms or molecules lose or gain an electron to become electrically charged, they are referred to as **ions**.

To get in or out of a cell, these particles have to pass through the cell membrane. The cell membrane allows some substances to pass through, but not others. For this reason it is referred to as **partially permeable** (or sometimes described as **selectively permeable**).

The four main processes by which substances pass through the cell membrane are **diffusion**, **active transport**, **osmosis** and **phagocytosis**.

What is diffusion?

All particles possess a kind of energy, called **kinetic energy**. They use this to move around. They move randomly in all directions, but the net movement will always be from an area where there are a lot of the same particles to an area where there are very few, or none at all. By doing so particles of the same kind spread themselves out. This net movement of particles from an area where they are in high concentration to an area where they are in a lower concentration is called **diffusion** (see figure 1).

Diffusion will always occur when there are differences in concentration (called a **concentration gradient**). The larger the gradient, the faster diffusion. Your body has mechanisms by which it can usually maintain the right concentrations of substances in the blood and cytoplasm of cells to ensure diffusion will take place. The cells therefore get chemicals they need without having to supply any energy.

Diffusion is the main way by which substances enter and leave cells. As well as the concentration gradient, the rate of diffusion is also affected by the size of the particles, the distance the particles have to move and the temperature.

What is active transport and when is it used?

Sometimes diffusion is too slow for a cell or the cell needs to take up or get rid of a substance against a concentration gradient. In this case, cells will use a process called **active transport** (see figure 2). Active transport requires a great deal of energy which the cell must supply. This energy is provided by the mitochondria. You can always tell if a cell carries out a lot of active transport, because it will contain a lot of mitochondria.

Osmosis – a special kind of diffusion

The *net* movement of water molecules across a membrane is a special kind of diffusion called **osmosis**. This still requires a concentration gradient, but this time the gradient is created by solutions.

When two solutions of different concentrations are separated by a partially permeable membrane, and the solute, e.g. sugar molecules, are unable to pass through this membrane, the water molecules will still diffuse across it. They will diffuse from the weak solution (where there are lots of water molecules) into the stronger solution (where there are less). This process, called osmosis, will continue until the solutions have the same number of water molecules, or until a pressure builds up which stops the process (see figure 3).

Osmosis is very important to living cells. If your body fluids (blood and tissue fluid) suddenly become diluted, water starts to enter your cells by osmosis. The cells start to swell and may eventually burst. If your body fluids get too concentrated, more so than the cell contents, water will leave the cells by osmosis. Fortunately, your body has mechanisms by which it can keep these concentrations the same, i.e. **isotonic** to one another. These are described in chapter 8.1.

How do cells take up larger particles?

Some of your body cells, for example white blood cells, can take in very large particles. They do this by a process called **phagocytosis**, which means 'cell eating'. Full details are shown in figure 5.

What do **you** know?

You should now be able to:

- Explain why the cell membrane is described as partially permeable.
- Describe the 3 different kinds of particle that form matter.
- Explain why particles are always moving.
- Describe the process of diffusion and say why it happens.
- Name the factors that affect the rate of diffusion.
- Describe the process by which cells can take up substances against a diffusion gradient.
- Define osmosis and state why it takes place.
- Explain the term isotonic and describe what will happen when cells are not in isotonic solution.
- Draw diagrams to outline the process of phagocytosis.

Figure 1 *Diffusion occurs across a concentration gradient.*

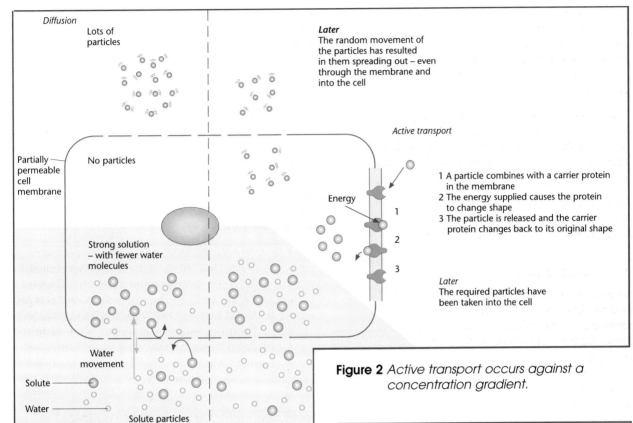

Figure 2 *Active transport occurs against a concentration gradient.*

Figure 3 *Osmosis occurs across a partially permeable membrane.*

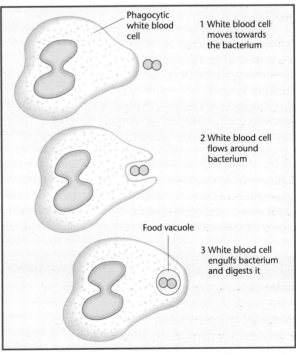

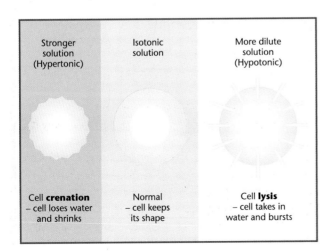

Figure 4 *Osmosis and living cells.*

Figure 5 *Some white blood cells can ingest (engulf) foreign particles such as bacteria. This is called phagocytosis.*

Chapter 1: Questions

1 The diagrams show four types of human cell.

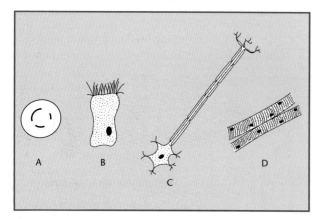

a Name each type of cell. *(4 marks)*

b For each of the cells A and B, give one function and describe one feature which helps the cell carry out its function. *(4 marks)*
(NEAB June 1997)

2 The diagram shows a cell from a plant.

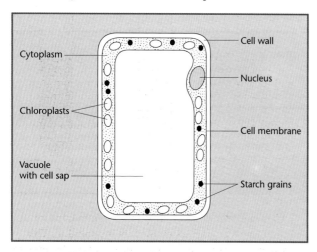

a List three structures present in this cell which you would also expect to find in a typical human cell. *(3 marks)*

b Give one way in which this plant cell is different from a human cell. *(4 marks)*
(SEG specimen 1995/96)

3 Powdered milk contains a protein called casein which forms a cloudy white suspension when mixed with water. Trypsin is a protein-digesting enzyme made in the digestive system of humans and other animals.

a i What chemical substance is formed when protein is digested? *(1 mark)*

ii If you mixed the protein-digesting enzyme with powdered milk suspension, what would you expect to see when digestion was completed? *(1 mark)*

b An experiment was carried out to find the effect of temperature on the activity of trypsin. The time taken for digestion of the protein at different temperatures was recorded. The results are shown in the table.

Temperature in °C	Time to complete the reaction in minutes
5	48
15	24
25	12
35	6
45	3
55	6
65	not completed

i What happens to the rate of reaction for each 10 °C rise in temperature between 5 °C and 45 °C? *(1 mark)*

ii Plot the data in the table as a line graph. Join the points with straight lines. *(5 marks)*

iii Suggest why the reaction was not completed at 65 °C. *(1 mark)*
(SEG June 1998)

4 The diagram below shows some of the major organs in the human body.

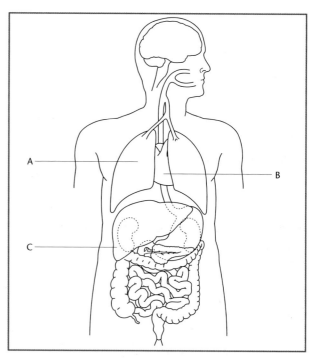

Use the information in the diagram to complete a table set out as the one at the top of next coloum.
(6 marks)

Letter	Name of organ	The main function of the organ
A		
B		
C		

(SEG specimen 1995/96)

5 a Equal quantities of red blood cells were placed in salt solutions of different strengths. Samples were withdrawn from each after ten minutes and examined under the microscope. Giving a reason in each case, briefly describe their appearance. Set out your answer in a table like the one shown.
(6 marks)

Strength of salt solution	Appearance	Reason
3.9%		
0.9%*		
0.09%		

* Blood plasma has the same osmotic concentration as a 0.9% salt solution.

b Why are isotonic solutions usually used when injecting substances into the circulatory system?
(2 marks)
(SEG June 1997)

6 a The diagram below shows a white blood cell.

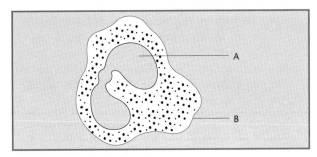

Name structures A and B. *(2 marks)*

b This diagram shows the first and last stages of the process by which a white blood cell engulfs a bacterium.
Draw in the white blood cell as it would appear at stage 2. *(1 mark)*

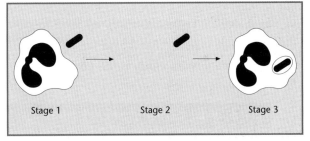

(SEG specimen 1998)

7 The diagram shows an experiment to investigate the enzyme amylase.

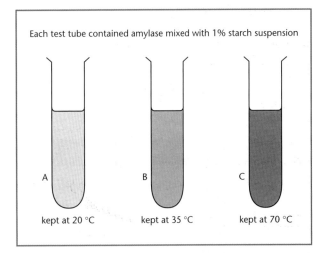

After one minute a few drops were removed from each test tube and tested with iodine solution. This test was repeated after 15 minutes and again after 25 minutes. The results obtained are shown in the table.

| Time (minutes) | Colour produced | | |
	Test tube A	Test tube B	Test tube C
1	Black	Black	Black
15	Black	Orange	Black
25	Orange	Orange	Black

a Suggest an explanation for these results. *(4 marks)*
b Suggest **one** precaution which should be taken when setting up an experiment like this to ensure that it is accurate. *(1 mark)*
c Suggest a suitable control for this experiment.
(2 marks)
(SEG June 1992)

2 Nutrition

You need a regular supply of food to stay alive and healthy. This chapter looks at the different types of food and why you need a balanced diet. It explains what happens to food inside your body once you have eaten it.

After you have worked through this chapter, you should be able to:

- Describe the components of food.
- Outline the reasons why you need food.
- Describe and explain the basic requirements of a healthy balanced diet.
- Discuss the variations in requirements of different population groups.
- Outline the principles of digestion.
- Describe the structure of the alimentary canal.

- Summarise the processes of digestion in the alimentary canal.
- Describe the structure and functioning of teeth.
- Explain the process of absorption.
- Describe the role of the small and large intestines in absorption.
- Explain how the products of digestion are used by your body.

Adverse reactions to food

Most people at some time in their life have had an unpleasant reaction to food, but recent studies suggest fewer than 10% will be true allergic reactions.

Adverse reactions to food

The causes of adverse reactions can be put into three groups:

- **Food poisoning** is a response to pathogenic micro-organisms in food (chapter 13.14).
- **Food intolerance** can be the result of:
  i) Not enough digestive enzymes to deal with a specific nutrient in food. For example, lactose is a sugar found in milk and its products. Adequate amounts of the enzyme **lactase** are required in the small intestine to digest this. If the enzyme levels are low, some undigested lactose reaches the large intestine where bacteria ferment it producing lactic acid. This lactic acid causes diarrhoea, pain and discomfort. This is the condition known as **lactose intolerance**.
  ii) The presence of toxic substances in food which irritate the lining of the intestine, e.g. caffeine.

Also some foods contain **histamine**, a chemical which causes inflammation in tissues, e.g. tuna and some mature cheeses.

- **Immune responses** are the true allergic responses. Proteins in foods can behave as antigens (chapter 13.8) and initiate an inflammation response and cause the production of antibodies.

What are the symptoms of food allergies?

Food allergies are thought to play a part in urticaria (skin rashes), eczema, nasal problems (e.g. runny nose) and asthma. They probably also cause abdominal pain, vomiting and diarrhoea. One particularly severe reaction, caused by foods such as peanuts and shellfish, is **anaphylatic shock** (see page 188). This can affect all parts of the body at the same time, resulting in swelling in the throat, nausea, vomiting and a rapid drop in blood pressure. If not treated, it can result in death.

Unusual behaviour such as hyperactivity has also been linked to foods, but this condition is extremely rare.

Psychological reactions to food

Anorexia nervosa and **bulimia nervosa** are very serious psychological reactions to food. Anorexia is a morbid fear of fatness which results in a sufferer refusing to eat. They can become so thin that normal body functions are affected. Symptoms include: extreme weight loss, cold extremities, distorted body image, loss of menstrual periods, disruption of heart functions, and in 10% of cases the heart stops, causing death.

A bulimic person will eat vast amounts of food (called binge eating) and then get rid of it by vomiting or using laxatives. Symptoms of this include weight fluctuations, damage to teeth, swollen salivary glands and bouts of depression. Both conditions need urgent medical treatment.

Which foods cause adverse reactions?

The most common foods causing adverse reactions are milk, eggs, fish, shellfish, nuts and peanuts, pork, soya, coffee and chocolate. Additives in foods can also cause problems, but this is rare. Generally, small children are more likely to experience reactions to foods, but they usually grow out of it. Adverse reactions to foods, such as milk, seem to run in families suggesting a genetic link.

How is food intolerance detected?

When a condition is thought to be caused by food, the first step in detection is to remove the suspected food from the diet and see if the symptoms disappear. The symptoms should re-appear when the food is re-introduced. The detection process also involves testing the blood for antibodies to the food.

If a psychological factor is suspected, a food challenge test is used. This is called a **double blind food challenge** because neither the subject or the observer knows when the food is being given.

There are various other tests which are sometimes used. One is the skin test which is often used for foods that contain metals such as nickel. This involves placing a small amount of the food on the skin and scratching the surface so that the food enters the outer skin layer. If redness and swelling appear it indicates a reaction to something in the food. It should be said that this test is not always reliable.

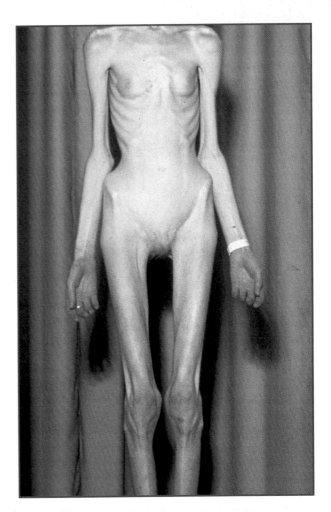

Figure 1 *An anorexic girl.*

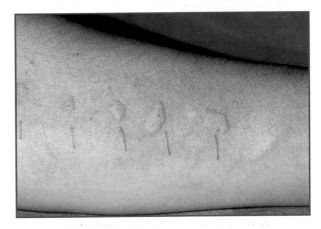

Figure 2 *Skin tests are used to identify substances which cause adverse reactions.*

2.1 Food

Why do you need food?

Food is necessary for life. All living things need a regular supply of it. The type of food, and the way they get it may differ but the way it is used is the same:

- Food provides cells with the **energy** to keep living and to carry out their work, e.g. the energy for muscle cells to contract and help you to move.
- Food provides the **raw materials for cells to grow** bigger, multiply and repair themselves when damaged.
- Food provides many of the **materials needed for metabolism** inside cells, and this keeps the body in a healthy state.

What is food?

Figure 1 shows the label of a typical fruit yogurt. The substances listed are called **nutrients**. Nutrients are molecules, the same molecules that are found in the protoplasm of cells. All foods are made up of different combinations of these molecules.

Carbohydrates

Carbohydrates are the **sugars**, **starches** and **cellulose** found in food. They are all compounds of the elements carbon, hydrogen and oxygen.

The simplest form of a carbohydrate is a single sugar, such as **glucose** or **fructose**. These are examples of **monosaccharides**. The more complex carbohydrates are formed by these single sugars joining together. For example, the sugar **maltose** is a made from two glucose molecules chemically linked together, and **sucrose** (table sugar) is made from one glucose and one fructose molecule linking together. These double sugars are called **disaccharides**.

Polysaccharides are the most complex carbohydrates because they are made from many monosaccharides linked together. The starch found in plants (**amylose**), is made from about 300 glucose molecules, and **glycogen** (animal starch) is made from about 1500 glucose molecules.

Cellulose is a complex carbohydrate found in plant cell walls. When we eat plants this contributes to our **dietary fibre** as it cannot be digested.

In your body, carbohydrates are mainly used to supply energy but they have to be converted to glucose first before they can take part in respiration (chapter 4.1) in animals. Glycogen is the main source of stored glucose and plants store glucose as amylose.

Foods that supply a lot of sugars include biscuits, cakes and fruit. Foods rich in starch include bread, potatoes, rice and pasta (see table 1).

Lipids

Lipids include the **fats**, **waxes** and **steroids**. These are all compounds of carbon, hydrogen and oxygen.

Most of the fats in your body are in the form of **triglycerides**. These are made from three **fatty acid** molecules chemically linked to one **glycerol** molecule. There are lots of different fatty acids but they are grouped into two main types; **saturated** or **unsaturated**. Fats in food contain both types, but animal fats often have a higher proportion of saturated fatty acids than plants. Fats containing a lot of saturated fatty acids are generally solid at room temperature, and those with mainly unsaturated fatty acids are liquid, and called oils.

The main use of fat in your body is as a source of stored energy. Gram for gram, it contains twice as much energy as carbohydrate or protein and, therefore, needs only half the space. Fat is stored around some of the vital organs in your body, where it provides protection from mechanical damage, as well as under your skin, where it also forms an insulating layer.

Cell membranes are made from a type of lipid called **phospholipid** and a steroid lipid called **cholesterol**. Many of the hormones in your body are also steroids, e.g. **oestrogen** and **testosterone**.

Foods rich in fat are butter, most other dairy products, nuts, fatty meat and oily fish (see table 1).

Proteins

Proteins are very large molecules made from simple 'building blocks' called **amino acids**. Amino acids are compounds of the elements carbon, hydrogen, oxygen and nitrogen. Some may also contain sulphur. There are only about 20 different amino acids, but these can chemically link together to form thousands of different proteins. The difference between one protein and another is in the numbers of each type of amino acid present and the sequence in which they are joined together. Proteins also vary in their shape. They can be straight fibrous molecules such as **keratin** in the hair and **collagen** in the skin, or folded into a globular shape such as **enzymes** and **haemoglobin** (the oxygen carrying pigment in blood).

Your body contains many thousands of different proteins. Many form structural components of cells, e.g. as part of the cell membrane, and so are needed for growth and repair, while others form enzymes and hormones, which are essential for the proper functioning of your body. Amino acids can also be used as a source of energy.

Good sources of protein include meat, fish, nuts and cheese (see table 1).

Food	Energy kJ	Carbohydrate g	Protein g	Lipid g	Fibre g	Average portion size g
Milk (whole)	279	4.8	3.4	3.9	0	200 (one glass)
Chicken	662	0	25	6	0	100
Eggs (Size 3)	619	0.4	12.3	10.9	0	60 (one)
Potatoes (boiled)	335	20	1.5	0	1	120
Bread (white)	1010	50	8	2	3	25 (one slice)
Whitefish (haddock)	428	0	17.1	0.9	0	100
Butter	3006	0	0.4	81	0	10 (per slice)
Cheese (Cheddar)	1700	0	26	34	0	50
Cabbage (cooked)	88	4.2	1.2	0	2.5	100
Baked beans	392	18	5	0.5	7.3	200
Apples	201	12	0.5	0	2	120
Bananas	337	19	1.1	0.3	3.4	100
Biscuit (digestive)	1969	66	8	21	1.2	30
Chocolate	2070	62	9	25	0	50
Peanuts (salted)	2497	8	24	53	8	50
Rice (boiled)	439	24.4	2.2	0.3	0.6	60
Pasta (spaghetti)	563	28.5	5.4	0.4	1.5	60
Cornflakes	1517	84	8	1	11	30

Table 1 *The average amounts of carbohydrates, proteins and lipids per 100 g of some common foods.*

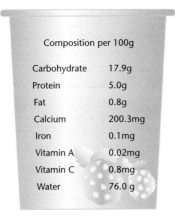

Composition per 100g

Carbohydrate	17.9g
Protein	5.0g
Fat	0.8g
Calcium	200.3mg
Iron	0.1mg
Vitamin A	0.02mg
Vitamin C	0.8mg
Water	76.0 g

Figure 1 *The nutrients in a typical fruit yogurt.*

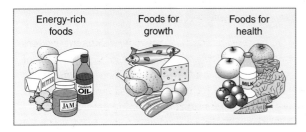

Figure 2 *Food provides us with energy, materials for growth and metabolism.*

What do **you** know?

You should now be able to:

- List the nutrients found in food.
- State the 3 main reasons why we need food.
- Name 2 monosaccharide sugars.
- Name the monosaccharides which make maltose and sucrose.
- State what the polysaccharides amylose and glycogen are made from.
- State the main uses of sugars and starches in your body.
- Explain what cellulose is and its use to us.
- Name 2 foods that are good sources of sugars and 2 that are good sources of starch.
- Name the 3 kinds of lipid.
- Describe the structure of a triglyceride.
- Name the 2 main kinds of fatty acid.
- Describe the main uses of the 3 different types of lipid in your body.
- Name 2 foods which have a high lipid content.
- Name the 'building block' of proteins.
- Name the elements found in protein but not in lipids or carbohydrates.
- Name 2 fibrous proteins and two globular proteins.
- Name 2 good dietary sources of protein.

Minerals and vitamins

Minerals

Minerals are elements such as **calcium**, **iron** and **iodine**. These all have very specific functions in your body. For example, calcium forms part of bone, making it hard. If the body does not get a regular supply of calcium the bones grow soft and a **deficiency disease**, such as **rickets** may result (see table 2 and figure 1).

Vitamins

Most vitamins are complex compounds. They all have names, but are usually just referred to by a letter. Like minerals, they are only needed in small amounts but deficiency leads to disease (see table 2).

Vitamins are usually classified into two groups; those which your body can store and those which it cannot. Vitamins your body can store are all found in the fat of fatty foods and are, therefore, called **fat soluble vitamins**. These include **A** and **D**. Vitamins your body cannot store include **B** and **C**. These are found in the water in foods and are, therefore, called **water soluble vitamins**. To prevent disease you must have a daily supply of these vitamins.

Is water an important nutrient?

Water forms about 70% of cell contents and is additionally found throughout the body in blood, tissue fluid (the fluid between cells), tears and digestive juices. Clearly, it is essential to life. Some of the uses of water in your body are:

● to **transport food materials**, such as glucose around your body

● to **transport waste materials**, like urea and carbon dioxide to the excretory organs

● to **remove soluble waste substances**, such as urea

● as a **solution in which metabolism** can take place

● for **the diffusion** of oxygen

● to **carry digestive enzymes**

● to **cool your body**, e.g. sweat

● to **protect the developing baby** (amniotic fluid in the womb)

● to act as a **lubricant**, e.g. mucus and synovial fluid.

Water is so important to the normal functioning of a body that even a small amount of **dehydration** can cause death. Table 1 shows how daily water losses are replaced.

Daily losses (cm³)		Daily gains (cm³)	
lungs (by evaporation)	400	food	850
urine	1500	drinks	1300
faeces	100	cell respiration	350
sweat	500		

Table 1 *Daily losses/gains of water in the body.*

What are food additives?

Additives are chemicals that are added to many processed or canned foods. Additives have no nutritional value, but are put in food to:

● colour it, E100–E180, e.g. E160 carotene

● as a preservative to protect it from spoilage by micro-organisms, E200–E290, e.g. E220 sulphur dioxide

● prevent **oxidation** of fats resulting in rancidity and vitamin losses, E300–E322, e.g. E300 ascorbic acid

● stabilise it so it keeps its consistency, E400–E495, e.g. E415 xanthan gum

● enhance or alter its flavour, e.g. E621 monosodium glutamate

● bulk it out, e.g. E460 cellulose.

Food manufacturers should list on the label all additives contained in their food. Additives prefixed by the letter E are allowed in the European Union. Those which do not have an E are only allowed in the UK.

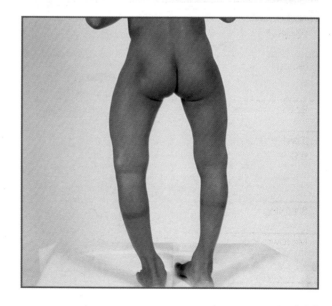

Figure 1 *Lack of vitamin D or calcium can cause rickets.*

Vitamin/Mineral	Body needs	Deficiency signs	RDA*	Sources
A	To produce the pigment in rod cells so that you can see clearly at night	Night blindness, increased infection	800 µg	Liver, dairy products, yellow/orange fruits and vegetables, e.g. carrots
B group	To help in the production of energy	Nerves, muscles and skin are all affected	varies with vitamin	Meat, fish, dairy products, cereals
C	To help keep your skin and gums healthy, wounds to heal, absorption of iron	Scurvy – bleeding, swollen gums, poor wound healing, increased infection	60 mg	Fresh citrus fruits, vegetables, e.g. potatoes
D	To help you absorb and make use of calcium in bones and teeth	Rickets – soft and weak bones, dental caries	5 µg	Action of sunlight on skin, liver, dairy products
Calcium	To help the building and maintenance of bones and teeth, in blood clotting, muscle contraction	Rickets, dental caries, poor blood clotting, muscle spasms	800 mg	Cheese, milk, yoghurt, sardines
Iron	To form part of the haemoglobin molecule	Anaemia – leading to tiredness, breathlessness	14 mg	Liver, red meat, brocolli
Iodine	To form part of the hormone thyroxine	Stunted growth and mental retardation in children (cretinism) Swollen thyroid gland in adults (goitre)	150 µg	Seafood, sea salt
Fluoride	To produce strong enamel on teeth	Dental caries	No RDA	Seafood, tea, water, some toothpastes

Table 2 *Some of the minerals and vitamins required by your body.*

* **RDA** Recommended Daily Amount to prevent deficiency symptoms (EC 1993)

Preparation/cooking	Effect on nutrients
Peeling	Removes vitamin C contained in skin
Slicing	Exposes vitamin C to oxygen resulting in its destruction
Boiling in water	Removes water soluble vitamins and minerals
Cooking in an oven e.g. roasting	High temperatures destroy some B group vitamins. Fat soluble vitamins can be lost in fat drippings
Stir frying	Seals the food preventing losses
Microwaving	Minimal losses compared with other methods

Table 3 *How food is prepared can effect its mineral and vitamin content.*

What do **you** know?

You should now be able to:

- State why you need calcium, iron and iodine in your diet and the symptoms associated with a lack of these.
- Name 2 good food sources of these minerals.
- State what may happen to your body if you did not get enough of the vitamins A, C, and D.
- Name 2 good food sources of each of these vitamins.
- Explain why if you cut fat out of your diet, you would suffer from vitamin A and D deficiency.
- Explain why deficiency of vitamin C is unusual.
- List some of the reasons why you should drink a lot of water.
- Explain why additives are sometimes put into foods.

2.3 A healthy diet

What should you eat?

You, like most people, probably have favourite foods. It would be nice if you could eat these all the time. But would these give you the full range of nutrients your body needs? Most probably not. A healthy person needs to have a healthy diet which is balanced to supply all the nutrients in the right proportions. This means a whole range of foods should be eaten every day to obtain:

- **Enough energy** for a healthy life. The energy taken in should equal the energy used. Your body's main source of energy is carbohydrates. In fact your brain cells can only use glucose but muscle cells can also use fatty acids, so it is best to include some of these in your diet. But remember, to stay healthy no more than 35% of your daily energy should come from fats and no more than 11% of this from saturated fats. Some fat is also required to supply the **essential fatty acids** (EFAs). These EFAs cannot be made in the body yet are required for the healthy formation of tissues.

- **Sufficient protein** to supply the amino acids for growth and repair of cells, and to produce your body's vital enzymes. Your body will need a selection of amino acids every day. It can only make some of these from the food you eat, those it cannot make are called **essential amino acids**. All of the essential amino acids are contained in most animal proteins, but not in plant proteins. So, to make sure you get all the essential amino acids, about 60% of your protein intake should come from animal products. Vegetarians get all the essential amino acids they need by eating a wide variety of plant material including foods like soya, pulses and nuts. Your body is unable to store surplus amino acids, so they are broken down in the liver producing urea and energy. To stay healthy, it is recommended that no more than 15% of your energy should come from proteins.

- **A selection of minerals and vitamins** to allow your body to function properly and therefore remain healthy. Mineral deficiency is rare in the UK as even tap water contains important minerals. Hard water contains calcium and magnesium, and soft water contains sodium and iron. Some water authorities also add **fluoride** to the water to help combat tooth decay (chapter 12.3).

Vitamin deficiency is more common, but usually only in a mild form. The general symptoms of this are tiredness and poor skin condition. Some foods have vitamins added to them. Margarine for example, has vitamin A and D added. Do not forget that some vitamins are found in the fatty parts of food, another reason for including some fat in your diet.

When working out how much food is needed to supply your daily vitamins, you must take into account vitamin losses during cooking and storing (see chapter 2.2). This can be substantial

- **Enough water** to replace that which is lost each day. This will usually be around 2.5 to 3 litres. Most people can go without fats, carbohydrates and proteins for weeks, but without water they would die within a few days. It is better to have too much water in the diet rather than too little, as the excess is easily excreted.

- **Some fibre** to add bulk to the food in the intestine. Cellulose from plant material such as fruit, vegetables and nuts is the main form of fibre in our diet (see figure 2). You cannot digest fibre, but you cannot do without it. We all need to eat about 18 g of fibre every day. Fibre absorbs water, swells and makes the contents of your intestines bulkier, making it easier for the muscles to move the food along and expel the waste. Lack of fibre can result in constipation and because wastes are not regulary removed you are more likely to suffer other digestive problems, such as bowel cancer, diverticulosis and irritable bowel syndrome.

Do we all need the same amounts of food?

You will get the best from your body if you eat the full range of nutrients. The amounts of these will depend upon your exact body requirements, which can change at different times of your life. For example, a growing child will need a higher proportion of protein and calcium to build muscle and bone. Menstruating females will need more iron to compensate for the iron lost with blood loss, and a pregnant woman will need more energy foods, extra protein and vitamins A and D for her growing baby. Even ill health can change your requirements. Usually more energy and extra vitamins are needed.

These changes to dietary requirements are described in more detail in the relevant chapters. Table 1 shows the maximum recommended amounts (except for energy) of nutrients different types of people require each day.

How can I achieve a healthy diet?

A healthy diet can be achieved by a combination and variety of different foods. Figure 1 shows the food groups. By selecting something from each group for every meal, in the right amounts, you will achieve a healthy balanced diet.

More information on diet can be found in chapter 12.4.

Age range	Energy* kJ	Protein g	Calcium mg	Iron mg	Vitamin A μg	Vitamin C μg
Children						
1 year-old	3850	14.9	525	7.8	350	25
4–6 years	7160	19.7	450	6.1	500	30
Males						
11–14 years	9270	42.1	1000	11.3	600	35
15–18 years	11510	55.2	1000	11.3	600	40
19–50 years	10600	55.5	700	8.7	700	40
50+ years	10600 max.	53.5	700	8.7	700	40
Females						
11–14 years	7920	41.2	800	14.8	600	35
15–18 years	8830	45	800	14.8	600	40
19–50 years	8100	45	700	14.8	600	40
50+ years	8000 max.	46.5	700	8.7	600	40
pregnant (last 3 months)	+0.8	+6	no increase	no increase	+100	+10
breastfeeding (3rd month)	+2.4	+11	+550	no increase	+350	+30

Table 1 *Recommended daily intake of nutrients (Department of Health, 1991).*

* Estimated average requirement (EAR) – will meet the needs of 50% of the population
The rest of the figures are Reference Nutrient Intakes (RNI) – sufficient intake for almost all people

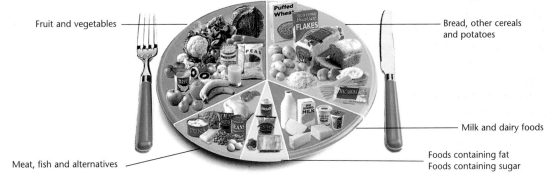

Fruit and vegetables — Bread, other cereals and potatoes — Milk and dairy foods — Foods containing fat / Foods containing sugar — Meat, fish and alternatives

Figure 1 *The segmented plate gives an indication of how much of each food group should be included in a balanced diet.*

What do **you** know?

You should now be able to:
- List the components of a healthy diet.
- Explain why should not exclude fat altogether from your diet.
- Explain why 60% of the protein should come from animal origin or foods like soya, pulses and nuts.
- Explain why your diet should include fibre and name 3 high fibre foods.
- Suggest how a healthy varied, yet balanced, diet might be achieved.
- Outline how dietary requirements can change at different times of your life.
- Suggest how your diet differs from the recommended daily intake of nutrients.

2.4 The digestive system

What is digestion?

All cells need a regular supply of nutrients so they can carry out their daily activities. They get these nutrients from the blood and tissue fluid. The blood gets them from the food we eat. It is the role of the digestive system to make these nutrients available to the blood in the right form. The digestive system breaks down the large lumps of food you eat into pieces that are small enough to pass through the gut wall and dissolve in the blood. Foods are broken down in the following ways:

- all **carbohydrates** are broken down into **simple sugars** like glucose

- **proteins** are broken down into **amino acids**

- **fats** are broken down into **fatty acids** and **glycerol**

- **minerals**, **vitamins** and **water** are released.

This breaking down process is called **digestion**. Digestion is just one part of processing food. The full sequence is shown in figure 1.

Where is your food digested?

Digestion takes place in the **digestive system** (see figure 2). The digestive system consists of:

- The **alimentary canal**. This is the muscular tube, about eight metres long, running from your mouth to your anus and has several distinct parts, each one fulfilling an important role in digestion.

- The **salivary glands**, **liver** and **pancreas**. These produce enzymes and other chemicals which help with digestion in the alimentary canal.

- The **teeth** and **tongue**. These are responsible for the physical breakdown of food in the mouth.

How does digestion take place?

Digestion is brought about in two ways:

- **Physically**, by your teeth and tongue, and by the muscles in the wall of the alimentary canal. There are two sets of muscle fibres in the gut wall. One set is arranged in rings (**circular muscle**), and the other set is arranged lengthwise (**longitudinal muscle**). These muscles work in opposition to one another. When the circular muscle contracts, the diameter of the gut is reduced and the food in it is squashed. When the longitudinal muscle contracts, this increases the diameter of the gut so the food can move into this area. By careful co-ordination of these muscles the food can be kept moving through the alimentary canal and at the same time be broken up into smaller pieces. It helps if your food has been bulked by fibre (chapter 2.3).

The co-ordinated actions of these muscles is called **peristalsis** (see figure 3).

- **Chemically**, by the enzymes and other chemicals made by glandular cells in the gut wall: the salivary glands, liver and pancreas. The enzymes are produced in a **digestive juice**. These juices also contain other chemicals to aid digestion, e.g. **mucus** to moisten the food.

The physical and chemical processes go on at the same time. The mechanical breakdown of food actually helps the enzymes to do their work by:

- mixing the food with the enzymes and

- increasing the surface area of the food for the enzymes to work on. It also helps move the food through the gut.

How long does it take to digest a meal?

This depends on the contents of the meal. A typical meal will take about 24 hours to digest. For the first 5 hours the food is in your stomach. This is followed by 5 hours in the small intestine, 7 hours in the colon and 7 hours in the rectum.

What do **YOU** know?

You should now be able to:

- Summarise what happens to the nutrients during digestion.
- Label a diagram of the digestive system.
- Annotate your diagram to show where the various stages of food processing take place.
- Explain the difference between physical and chemical digestion.
- Describe the process of peristalsis.
- Mark on your diagram where the main digestive juices are produced.

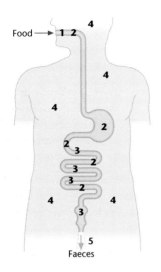

Food →

1 **Ingestion** – food is taken into the mouth where digestion starts

2 **Digestion** – the large lumps of food are physically broken down into small pieces. Enzymes break the large complex molecules into smaller soluble molecules which can be absorbed

3 **Absorption** – digested food passes through the gut wall and enters the blood and lymph

4 **Assimilation** – food is removed from the blood and used by the cells

5 **Egestion** – undigested waste is removed

Figure 1 *Food processing in the body.*

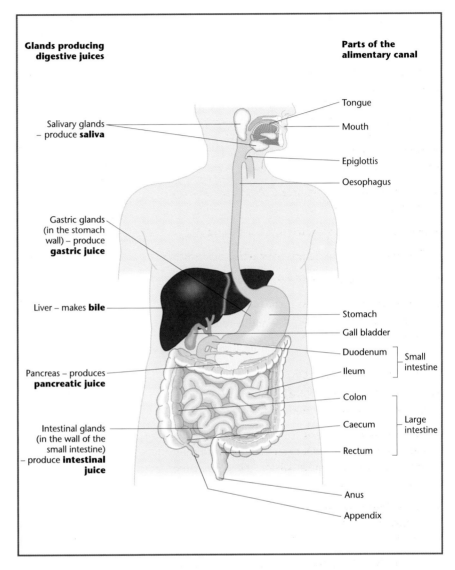

Glands producing digestive juices

Salivary glands – produce **saliva**

Gastric glands (in the stomach wall) – produce **gastric juice**

Liver – makes **bile**

Pancreas – produces **pancreatic juice**

Intestinal glands (in the wall of the small intestine) – produce **intestinal juice**

Parts of the alimentary canal

Tongue
Mouth
Epiglottis
Oesophagus
Stomach
Gall bladder
Duodenum — Small intestine
Ileum
Colon — Large intestine
Caecum
Rectum
Anus
Appendix

Figure 2 *The digestive system.*

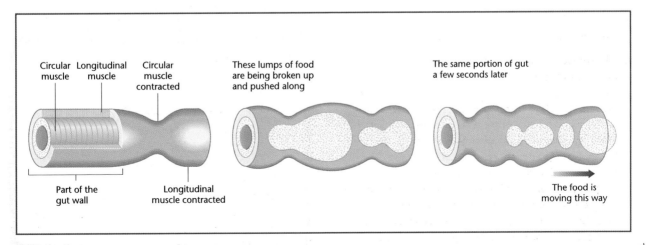

Circular muscle Longitudinal muscle Circular muscle contracted

These lumps of food are being broken up and pushed along

The same portion of gut a few seconds later

Part of the gut wall   Longitudinal muscle contracted

The food is moving this way

Figure 3 *Peristalsis helps to break up pieces of food and moves it through your gut.*

The structure of teeth

Why do you have teeth?

Your teeth are very important and are worth looking after. They are necessary for the first stage in breaking down food. For example, when you eat an apple you use your teeth to bite pieces out of it and then to crush these pieces before swallowing them. This makes digestion easier.

Teeth that are well cared for help you to speak clearly and avoid bad breath, and give a healthy smile (see figure 1).

What is a tooth made from?

A tooth has two distinct parts. The part above the gum is called the **crown** and the part which is set in the jawbone is called the **root**. A section through a tooth shows several different layers (see figure 2):

- The **enamel** covering the crown of the tooth. This is made mainly of calcium and phosphorus. It is very hard but once damaged, it will not be replaced.

- The bulk of the tooth is formed from **dentine**. This is very similar to bone in structure, but considerably harder. Dentine has very small canals running through it, containing fluid and extensions of the cells in the pulp cavity.

- The centre of the tooth is called the **pulp cavity**. This is the soft part of a tooth and contains living cells, blood vessels and a nerve ending.

- The root of the tooth is covered by bone-like **cement**. Tough fibres (**periodontal fibres**) are embedded in this and together they hold the tooth in place.

Are all teeth the same?

We have four types of teeth (see figure 1), each adapted to a different job and quite different in shape.

- **Incisors** are chisel-shaped, with sharp edges which can be used for cutting and biting food.

- **Canines** are pointed teeth, the top of the point being called a cusp. They are used to tear food.

- **Premolars** have two cusps and are used to tear and grind food.

- **Molars** can have up to five cusps and large roots. These are used to chew, crush and grind food.

When do we get our teeth?

You have two sets of teeth during your lifetime. A baby starts to get its first set, called the **milk**, or **deciduous teeth**, when it is about six months old. We say the baby

is **teething**. It may take up to three years for the complete set of 20 teeth to appear (see figure 3).

The milk teeth start to be replaced by the **permanent teeth** from about six years old. The milk teeth simply come loose and fall out and new teeth grow. By age 13 or 14 years, all the milk teeth have gone and have been replaced by 28 of the 32 permanent teeth: eight incisors, four canines, eight premolars and eight molars. The four remaining molars may, if your jaw is long enough, appear in your late teens or early twenties. Because they are late to appear, they are sometimes called **wisdom teeth**.

Why take care of milk teeth?

If you do not have a full, well-positioned set of milk teeth, you will never have a good set of permanent teeth. This is because the roots of the milk teeth guide the permanent teeth into position. Parents therefore, should make sure that young children take as much care of their milk teeth as they would their permanent teeth. (See chapter 12.3.)

Why are teeth sensitive?

Dentine is sensitive to touch and temperature. If enamel is damaged or the root exposed as your gums recede, the dentine becomes exposed. This can also happen from over-zealous brushing. Any sudden change in temperature or sugar concentration will affect the fluid in the canals running through the dentine causing it to move. The movement, sucking or pulling stimulates the nerve in the pulp cavity and causes pain. Some toothpastes claim to produce a protective barrier over the pores in the dentine, thereby stopping the fluid movement and any pain.

What do **you** know?

You should now be able to:

- Draw a diagram of a section through a typical tooth.
- Fully label your diagram and annotate each label with the function of that part.
- Draw a map of the teeth in your own mouth, clearly indicating which are incisors, canines, premolars and molars.
- Explain how you would use each type of tooth when eating an apple.
- State two differences between a set of permanent and a set of milk teeth.
- Explain why teeth are sometimes sensitive to heat and cold.

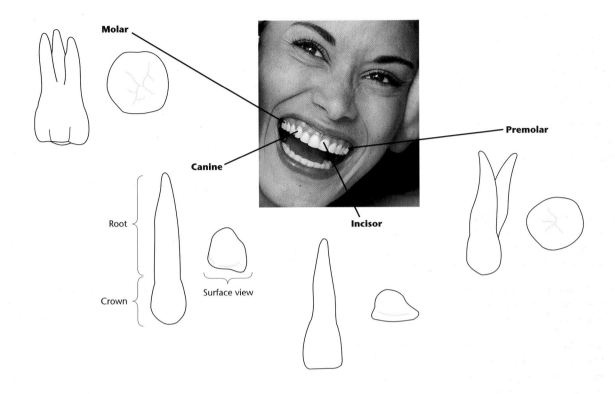

Figure 1 *We have four types of teeth.*

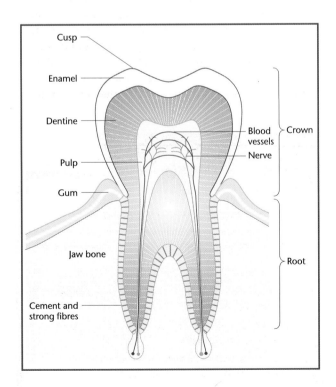

Figure 2 *A typical tooth has three main layers: the enamel, dentine and pulp.*

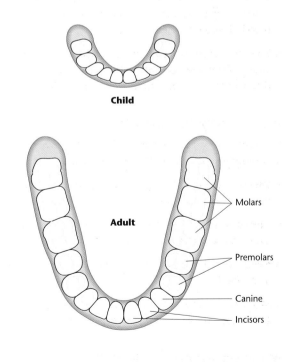

Figure 3 *A four-year-old child has 20 milk teeth. These are replaced in the adult by 32 permanent teeth.*

2.6 Digestion

What happens to food in your mouth?

Most people chew their food before swallowing it. This chewing action breaks the food down into smaller pieces and mixes it with the digestive juice **saliva**, produced by the salivary glands. Saliva contains two main substances:

- the enzyme **amylase** which starts the digestion of starch
- **mucus** which wets the food and makes it easier to swallow.

After chewing, the tongue moulds the food into a **bolus** and pushes it to the back of your mouth. Swallowing makes it slip into the oesophagus and move by peristalsis to the stomach. The **epiglottis** prevents it entering the trachea.

What happens in your stomach?

Once food is in your stomach, the stomach is sealed by two strong circular muscles, one at either end. These are the **sphincter muscles**. For the next hour or so **peristaltic waves** pass along the wall of the stomach. These continue to physically break down the food and also mix it with the **gastric juice** made and secreted by cells in the stomach wall. Gastric juice contains:

- the enzyme **pepsin** which starts the breakdown of proteins
- **acid** to provide the acidic conditions (pH 2) that pepsin needs and which kill any germs present in the food
- **mucus** to moisten the food. This mucus also lines the wall of the stomach, preventing damage by the pepsin and acid.

The gastric juice of infants also contains the enzyme **rennin** to clot milk.

A meal may spend up to 5 hours in the stomach. The mixture leaves your stomach as creamy white pulp called **chyme**, and enters the small intestine.

What happens in your small intestine?

Your small intestine is about 6 m long and has two regions. The first 25 cm is called the **duodenum** and the rest is the **ileum**. Muscles in its wall continue to physically break down the food. Chemical digestion is brought about by three new juices:

- **bile** is produced by the liver and stored in the **gall bladder** before entering the duodenum via the bile duct (see figure 1). Bile contains **bile salts** to

emulsify any lipids present, i.e. change them from large droplets into smaller droplets. This increases the surface area available for enzymes to work on and thereby speeds up digestion of the lipids. Bile is alkaline and helps raise the pH in the duodenum to pH 8. This creates suitable conditions inside the intestines for the enzymes to work.

- **pancreatic juice** is produced by the **pancreas** and secreted into the duodenum. It is alkaline juice that contains the enzymes **trypsin**, **amylase** and **lipase**. Trypsin starts to breakdown the polypeptides produced by pepsin in the stomach. The amylase breaks down any remaining starch, and the lipase breaks down the lipids.
- **intestinal juice** is produced by special cells in the intestine wall. It contains **protease** enzymes to complete the digestion of proteins and **carbohydrase** enzymes to complete the digestion of starch.

Chemical digestion is completed in the small intestine. The result is a mixture of soluble sugars, amino acids, fatty acids, glycerol, minerals, vitamins and water. These can now pass through the intestine wall and enter the blood and lymph (chapter 3.3). Any waste passes through the large intestine.

What happens in your large intestine?

The first part of the large intestine is the **colon**. By the time the food reaches this, many of the useful substances have been removed. What is left is a watery waste containing a few minerals, vitamins and undigested materials such as fibre. Bacteria that live in the colon ferment any remaining carbohydrates, lipids or proteins producing gases like methane. They also produce some vitamin B and K. As the mixture slowly travels through your colon, a lot of the water and most of the remaining minerals and vitamins pass into your blood. By the time it reaches the rectum the remains are quite dry and can be moulded into **faeces**. These faeces can be stored for a day or so, but must eventually be passed out through the **anus** (a double sphincter muscle).

If the movement through your colon is too fast a lot of the water remains in the waste resulting in **diarrhoea**. If the movement is too slow, too much water is removed leaving hard, dry faeces which are difficult to pass through the anus resulting in **constipation**.

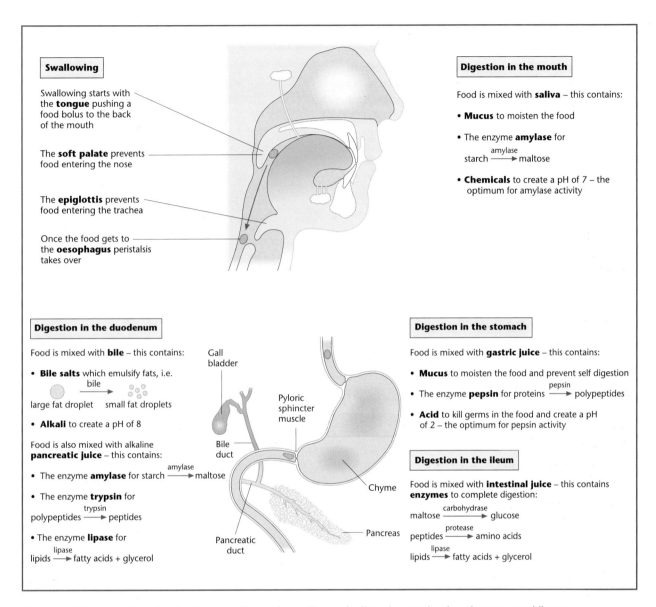

Swallowing

Swallowing starts with the **tongue** pushing a food bolus to the back of the mouth

The **soft palate** prevents food entering the nose

The **epiglottis** prevents food entering the trachea

Once the food gets to the **oesophagus** peristalsis takes over

Digestion in the mouth

Food is mixed with **saliva** – this contains:

• **Mucus** to moisten the food

• The enzyme **amylase** for

starch $\xrightarrow{\text{amylase}}$ maltose

• **Chemicals** to create a pH of 7 – the optimum for amylase activity

Digestion in the duodenum

Food is mixed with **bile** – this contains:

• **Bile salts** which emulsify fats, i.e.

large fat droplet $\xrightarrow{\text{bile}}$ small fat droplets

• **Alkali** to create a pH of 8

Food is also mixed with alkaline **pancreatic juice** – this contains:

• The enzyme **amylase** for starch $\xrightarrow{\text{amylase}}$ maltose

• The enzyme **trypsin** for polypeptides $\xrightarrow{\text{trypsin}}$ peptides

• The enzyme **lipase** for lipids $\xrightarrow{\text{lipase}}$ fatty acids + glycerol

Gall bladder

Bile duct

Pancreatic duct

Pyloric sphincter muscle

Chyme

Pancreas

Digestion in the stomach

Food is mixed with **gastric juice** – this contains:

• **Mucus** to moisten the food and prevent self digestion

• The enzyme **pepsin** for proteins $\xrightarrow{\text{pepsin}}$ polypeptides

• **Acid** to kill germs in the food and create a pH of 2 – the optimum for pepsin activity

Digestion in the ileum

Food is mixed with **intestinal juice** – this contains **enzymes** to complete digestion:

maltose $\xrightarrow{\text{carbohydrase}}$ glucose

peptides $\xrightarrow{\text{protease}}$ amino acids

lipids $\xrightarrow{\text{lipase}}$ fatty acids + glycerol

Figure 1 *Digestion begins in the mouth and continues in the stomach, duodenum and ileum.*

What do **you** know?

You should now be able to:

● Describe what happens to food in your mouth.
● Describe the process of swallowing a piece of food.
● Describe what happens to food in your stomach.
● Outline the role of the acid in the stomach.
● Explain why the acid does not damage your stomach wall.

● Name the 2 juices food is mixed with in the duodenum.
● Outline the chemical digestion in the duodenum.
● Explain the importance of bile in the digestion of fats.
● State precisely where starch, protein and lipid digestion takes place in the alimentary canal and name the enzymes involved.

Absorption and assimilation

What happens after digestion?

The products of digestion pass through the gut wall and dissolve in the blood. This process is called **absorption**. Carbohydrate digestion produces simple sugars like **glucose**. Protein digestion produces **amino acids**, and lipid digestion produces **fatty acids** and **glycerol**. It is these substances, together with the **water**, **vitamins** and **minerals** that are absorbed into the blood and **assimilated** (used up) by the cells.

Where does absorption take place?

Most absorption takes place from the intestines. Sugars, amino acids, fatty acids, glycerol, most of the vitamins and minerals, and 90% of the water are absorbed into the blood from the **small intestine**. This is where the majority of the absorption takes place. The remaining water, minerals and vitamins are absorbed from the **large intestine**. A few substances, such as alcohol and some drugs may be absorbed from the **stomach**.

The small intestine has a structure which greatly increases the speed and efficiency of absorption (see figure 1). The internal surface is very folded and small projections, called **villi**, stick out from it. The cells lining these villi also have folded membranes called **microvilli**. These folds and projections provide a greatly increased surface area for the rapid absorption of the nutrients.

Each **villus** has an extensive supply of blood capillaries for the nutrients to enter so they can be transported away quickly. This maintains a concentration gradient for diffusion. Each villus also contains a lymph vessel (called a **lacteal**) into which fatty acids and glycerol pass.

Most absorption is by **diffusion**, but **active transport** is also used. The cells lining the villi have lots of mitochondria to provide the energy for this. Water is absorbed by **osmosis**.

What happens to the absorbed nutrients?

All the nutrients that enter the blood from the intestines are taken in the **hepatic portal vein** straight to the **liver** (see figure 2).

- The **blood glucose level** (chapter 8.2), is adjusted and any remaining glucose is converted into **glycogen** which can be stored in the liver and muscle cells. When both these storage areas are full, surplus glucose is converted into fat and stored in adipose tissue.

- Some of the amino acids are removed by the liver cells and used to make **plasma proteins**. Some are left in the blood for the body cells to use to make their own proteins. Surplus amino acids cannot be stored and are therefore **deaminated** by the liver cells. Deamination

is the splitting of an amino acid into the part which contains the nitrogen, that is the **amino group**, and a part which can be converted into glucose. The amino group is then combined with carbon dioxide to form **urea**. This urea travels in the blood to the kidneys, where it is filtered out and becomes part of **urine**.

- Surplus iron, and vitamins A and D are removed and stored in the liver cells.

- Most of the fatty acids and glycerol are absorbed into the lacteals and by-pass the liver. They are carried by the lymph to a vein near the neck (see figure 3), where they rejoin the blood to be carried to all parts of the body.

- Absorbed water stays in the blood. Any excess is removed by the kidneys and excreted.

- The concentrations of other minerals such as calcium and sodium are adjusted by hormones. Excesses are either stored or excreted.

Vitamin D is needed for the absorption of calcium and vitamin C can affect the absorption of iron. Many of the fat soluble vitamins (A, D, E and K) have to be absorbed along with the fat.

How do the cells assimilate the nutrients?

Glucose is used to provide energy for the cell to do work. Amino acids are used for the formation of new proteins in the cytoplasm, the repair of damaged parts and the formation of enzymes, plasma proteins and hormones. Some of the fats are used to build cell membranes, and the rest are used to provide energy.

What do **you** know?

You should now be able to:

- List the products of digestion and state which part of the gut they are absorbed from.
- List the processes involved in absorption.
- Describe why the small intestine is very efficient area for absorption.
- Name the blood vessel which takes absorbed products to the liver.
- Describe how the liver deals with the absorbed products.
- Explain what happens to fatty acids and glycerol which enter the lacteal.
- Describe how body cells make use of the products of digestion.
- Name a substance which is needed for the absorption of calcium.

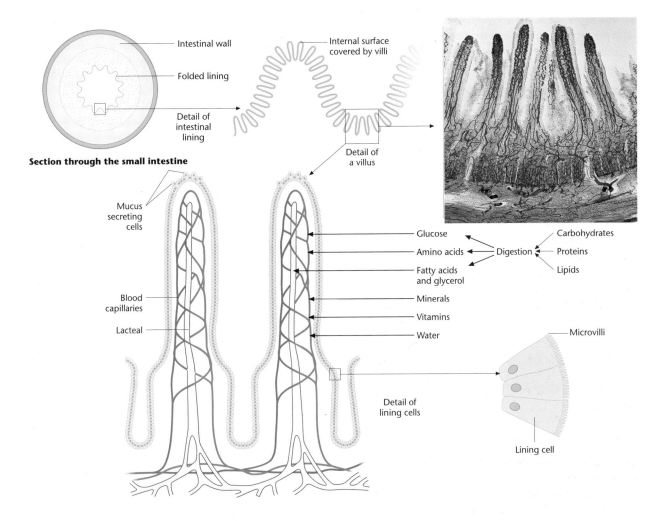

Section through the small intestine

Intestinal wall

Folded lining

Detail of intestinal lining

Internal surface covered by villi

Detail of a villus

Mucus secreting cells

Blood capillaries

Lacteal

Glucose ← Digestion ← Carbohydrates

Amino acids ← Digestion ← Proteins

Fatty acids and glycerol ← Lipids

Minerals

Vitamins

Water

Microvilli

Detail of lining cells

Lining cell

Figure 1 *The structure of the small intestine makes it very efficient for absorbing food.*

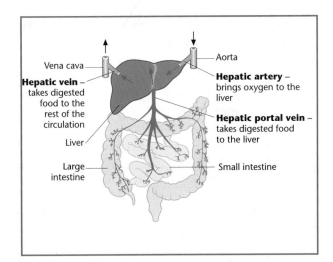

Vena cava

Aorta

Hepatic vein – takes digested food to the rest of the circulation

Hepatic artery – brings oxygen to the liver

Hepatic portal vein – takes digested food to the liver

Liver

Large intestine

Small intestine

Figure 2 *All the nutrients that pass into the blood from the small intestine are first taken to the liver before assimilation into the body cells.*

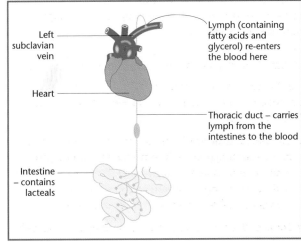

Left subclavian vein

Lymph (containing fatty acids and glycerol) re-enters the blood here

Heart

Thoracic duct – carries lymph from the intestines to the blood

Intestine – contains lacteals

Figure 3 *Absorbed fat bypasses the liver by entering the lymphatic system.*

Chapter 2: Questions

1 The table shows the seven types of food needed in a healthy human diet and their uses in the body. The names of three types of food are missing. Write out the missing names in order. *(3 marks)*

Type of food	Use in the Body
Carbohydrates	Energy supply
Fats/Lipids	Energy storage and insulation
	Body building, making enzymes and antibodies
Vitamins	Help in chemical reactions, maintain health
	Healthy gut functioning, aids peristalsis and prevents constipation
Mineral salts	Healthy body functioning, help in chemical reactions and form body structures
	Solvent, medium for chemical reactions and for transport

(SEG specimen 1998)

2 The table shows some enzymes used in digestion, where they are made in the alimentary canal, the substances they act upon (substrates) and the products of digestion.

Enzyme	Where enzyme is made	Substrate	Product
	Mouth	Starch	Maltose sugar
Pepsin		Protein	Amino acids
Lipase	Pancreas		Fatty acids and glycerol

a Copy and complete the table. *(3 marks)*

b Give two reasons why it is necessary to digest food. *(2 marks)*

(SEG June 1995)

3 a The table gives information about a meal bought in a hamburger bar.

Nutrients	Hamburger	Regular fries	Milk shake
Energy in kJ	1090	1220	945
Carbohydrate in g	30.0	46.0	16.5
Protein in g	14.0	4.7	11.5
Fat in g	9.8	6.0	6.5
Sodium in g	0.4	0.3	0.2

This meal is very rich in energy.

   i Give two uses of energy in the human body. *(2 marks)*

   ii What is the total amount of energy provided by this meal? *(1 mark)*

  iii Which nutrient will contain the most energy per gram? *(1 mark)*

  iv Which nutrient will supply materials for body building? *(1 mark)*

   v The main carbohydrate in this meal is starch. The types of food present in the meal are listed in the table below. Draw your own table and tick two boxes to show which foods have a high starch content. *(2 marks)*

Type of food	High starch content
Bread	
Beef	
Milk	
Onions	
Potato	

  vi How would you test some food for starch? Describe what you would see if starch were present. *(2 marks)*

b The diagram shows the human alimentary canal.

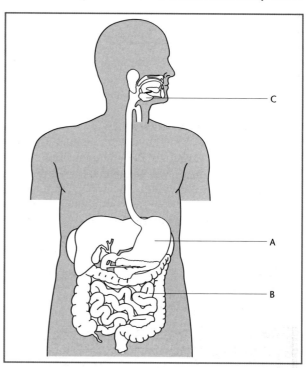

   i Look at the diagram, name structures A and B. *(2 marks)*

  ii Name the enzyme produced in structure C which helps in the digestion of starch. *(1 mark)*

  iii What substance is formed when starch is digested? *(1 mark)*

iv Name the main site of absorption of the products of digestion. *(1 mark)*

v Name one process by which absorption of the products of digestion occurs from the gut into the blood. *(1 mark)*
(SEG June 1998)

4 The sugars produced in digestion are absorbed from the alimentary canal through the villi. The diagram shows a single villus.

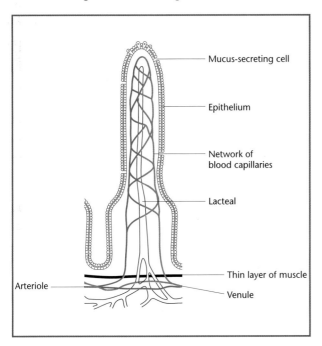

a Where in the alimentary canal would villi be present? *(1 mark)*

b State three features of the villus, which you can see in the diagram, which help it to absorb sugars quickly. *(3 marks)*

c Name one process by which sugars pass from the inside of the alimentary canal into the blood. *(1 mark)*
(SEG June 1999)

5 An experiment was carried out to investigate the effect of bile salts on the digestion of fat (lipid). Two flasks were set up as shown in the table.

Contents of flask	Flask 1 volume in cm³	Flask 2 volume in cm³
Milk (contains fat)	10	10
Sodium carbonate solution	14	14
Lipase solution	2	2
Bile salts solution	2	—
Water	—	2

The pH of each solution was recorded over several minutes using a pH meter connected to a microcomputer. The computer printout is shown below.

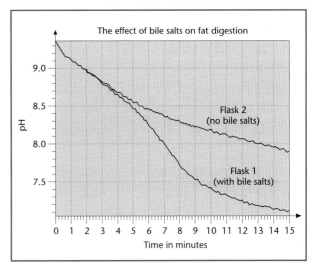

a i What caused the drop in pH during the experiment? *(2 marks)*

ii What evidence is there in the graph to suggest that bile salts help in fat digestion? *(1 mark)*

iii Suggest two reasons why the rate of fall in pH in flask 1 slowed down after about 14 minutes. *(2 marks)*

b Name the organ in the human body which makes bile salts. *(1 mark)*
(SEG June 1997)

6 a Explain why food needs to be digested. *(2 marks)*

b Smelling food causes a reflex response.
Nerve impulses pass to the brain.
The brain then passes impulses to the salivary glands in the mouth.
The salivary glands then release saliva containing mucus, water and an enzyme.
Using this information and your own knowledge:
i Name the stimulus in this reflex. *(1 mark)*
ii Describe how the stimulus is detected. *(3 marks)*
iii Describe the response to this stimulus. *(1 mark)*

c i Name the enzyme present in saliva. *(1 mark)*
ii Describe how this enzyme is used in digestion. *(2 marks)*

d When food enters the stomach another reflex causes it to release gastric juice. Stress may cause gastric juice to be released all of the time. The gastric juice irritates the stomach lining and may cause ulcers.
Suggest why the secretion of gastric juice all of the time may cause ulcers. *(2 marks)*
(OCR June 1999)

3 Transport

If you cut yourself it soon becomes clear that you have blood circulating your body. But do you know what the components of blood are and why you need it? This chapter describes blood and why you cannot live without it. It also describes how it travels around your body and why your heart is so important.

After you have worked through this chapter, you should be able to:

- List the general functions of blood.

- Describe the composition, structure and functions of the blood components.

- Detail the differences between arteries, veins and capillaries.

- Name the major blood vessels in the circulation.

- Outline the changes in blood composition as it passes through the major organs of your body.

- Outline the structure and role of the lymphatic system.

- Identify the main internal and external structures of the heart.

- Outline the cardiac cycle and its co-ordination.

- Explain why the heart is described as a double pump.

- Explain the reason for the heart rate increasing during exercise.

- Explain the causes of high blood pressure.

- List and explain the causes of coronary heart disease.

- Explain the significance of blood groups.

Heart disease

The various forms of heart disease account for more deaths in the UK than any other disease. By far the biggest killer is **coronary heart disease** (CHD).

In CHD the coronary arteries which supply blood to the heart muscle become narrower reducing the blood flow (chapter 3.5). The first sign of this is a pain in the chest when exercising. This is called **angina pectoris**. If left untreated, the disease will progress to a full **heart attack**. There are several ways to prevent this, but first the problem must be confirmed:

- an **angiogram** can be taken. A contrast substance which will show up on an X-ray is injected into the blood vessels and an X-ray of the vessels is taken. This will help identify any narrowed regions.

- an **electrocardiogram** (ECG) can be taken. An ECG machine is used to montior heart rhythmns by

picking up the tiny electrical signals which co-ordinate the contractions of the heart muscle (see figure 1). When the blood supply to an area of the heart is reduced, its electrical activity alters and this shows on an ECG. It can even detect which area is affected.

If diseased arteries are confrmed, there are several treatments which can be used to prevent further development:

- **Angioplasty** can be used to reduce the constriction in an artery, thereby restoring full blood flow. The procedure involves inserting a thin tube, with a balloon attched to the end, into the narrow part of the coronary artery. As the balloon is inflated, it widens the artery. Sometimes a small stent is left inside the artery to keep it open (see figure 2).

- **Heart bypass surgery** can be used if the disease is severe enough. Surgeons remove part of a vein in a leg and join it to the blocked artery and aorta, bypassing the diseased part (see figure 3). The patient may need a single, double or triple bypass depending on how many coronary arteries are affected.

- **Drugs** can be used to reduce stress on the heart. Many drugs act directly on the heart muscle to alter the rate and rhythm of the heartbeat. **Beta blockers**, for example, stop the HR increasing too much during periods of excitement, by preventing it responding to the hormone adrenaline. Drugs based on **digitalis** increase the force of each contraction so each heartbeat is more efficient.

Other drugs alter blood pressure. **Vasodilators** and **vasoconstrictors** do this by altering the diameter of the blood vessels. **Diuretics** reduce the blood volume by increasing the excretion of water.

There are several drugs which lower the blood cholesterol level. These must be taken as part of a reduced fat diet.

Anti-coagulants are used to reduce the chances of blood clots forming inside blood vessels. One which has been the subject of much research is **aspirin**. It is said that half an aspirin a day is sufficient to protect you.

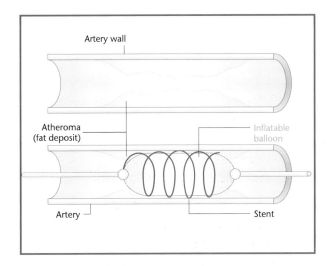

Figure 2 *Balloon angioplasty restores blood flow by inflating a balloon in the affected artery.*

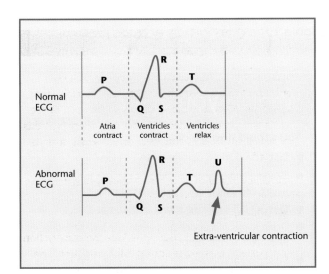

Figure 1 *An ECG machine monitors heart rhythms. The letters P, Q, R, S and T show equivalent contractions and U shows the extra-ventricular contraction in the abnormal heart.*

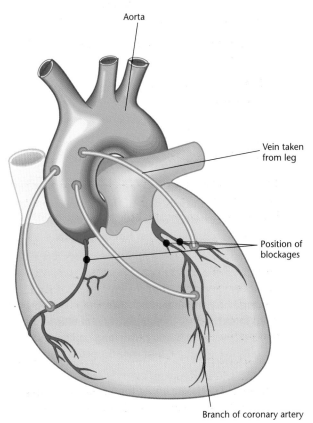

Figure 3 *This shows a triple heart bypass where the blocked arteries are bypassed.*

3.1 The composition of blood

Your own transport system

If you live near a big town you will know that it needs a good transport system so that people and materials can get around. In the same way your body depends on a good transport system to distribute substances to its cells. The transport system of the human body is the **blood circulatory system**. This is made up of a fluid tissue called **blood** that circulates around the body in a series of tubes called **blood vessels**. The **heart** acts as a central pump that keeps the blood moving round.

The human body has another part to its transport system, called the **lymphatic system** (see chapter 3.3). This works with the blood circulatory system in delivering food materials to cells and removing wastes.

What is blood?

You may think blood is only a red liquid, but about 45% of blood is made up of cells. It can be described as a fluid tissue because the cells float in a liquid and can flow around your body (see figure 1).

Blood is made in the **red bone marrow** of many of your bones. The average adult weighing 70 kg will have about 5–6 litres of blood. The various components of blood are shown in figure 2 and described below.

- **Plasma**, the liquid part of the blood, is a pale straw colour. About 90% of plasma is water. The rest consists of various dissolved food and waste substances, some mineral ions (e.g. sodium, potassium, chloride), hormones, blood clotting proteins and antibodies. Some of these, for example carbon dioxide and the hormones, are being transported from one part of the body to another; whereas some, like the blood clotting proteins, are always present in the blood.

- **Red blood cells** are the only cells in your body that do not contain a nucleus. The nucleus disintegrates very early on in the red cell's formation and is replaced by a substance called **haemoglobin**. Haemoglobin is an oxygen-carrying protein. It gives your blood its red colour.

  Red cells are shaped like a biconcave disc (a doughnut without the hole in the middle). This shape presents the maximum surface area for oxygen to diffuse into the cells as they pass through the lung capillaries. Red blood cells live for about four months before being destroyed by the liver.

- **White blood cells** are larger than the red cells and there are fewer of them. There are several kinds but the two main types are:

1 **phagocytes** which are irregular in shape with an unusual shaped nucleus and cytoplasm containing granules. The granules contain digestive enzymes. Phagocytes engulf foreign substances such as bacteria, and use the enzymes to digest them. This process, called **phagocytosis**, is described in chapter 1.5.

2 **lymphocytes** which are spherical in shape, with a very large nucleus and a small amount of non-granular cytoplasm. There are two kinds of lymphocyte. **B lymphocytes** which produce **antibodies** to deal with micro-organisms; and **T lymphocytes** which destroy cells that have become infected with viruses or become cancerous.

- **Platelets** are produced by cells which break up into small fragments. These fragments do not contain a nucleus, but are capable of producing enzymes involved in blood clotting.

Is everybody's blood the same?

There are four different kinds of blood called type **A**, type **B**, type **AB** and type **O**. These form the **blood groups**. It is important to know your blood group because not all are compatible. Possible blood transfusions are shown below.

Blood group	Can donate to	Can receive from
A	A and AB	A and O
B	B and AB	B and O
AB	AB	A, B, AB and O
O	A, B, AB and O	O

Table 1 *The compatibility of blood groups.*

What do **you** know?

You should now be able to:

- List the 4 main components of blood.
- State precisely where blood cells are made and where red blood cells are destroyed.
- List 10 substances found in plasma.
- Draw a red blood cell and describe how the shape is suited to its function.
- Describe and draw the structure of a phagocyte and lymphocyte.
- Briefly describe the functions of the white blood cells.
- List the 4 kinds of blood group.

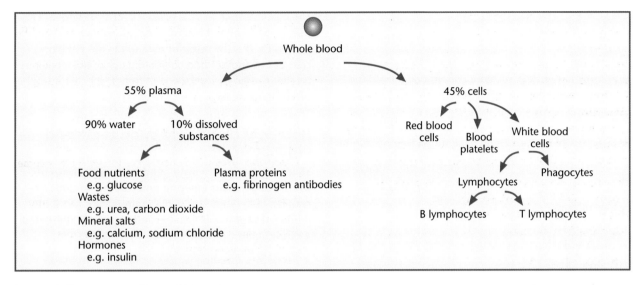

Figure 1 *The composition of blood.*

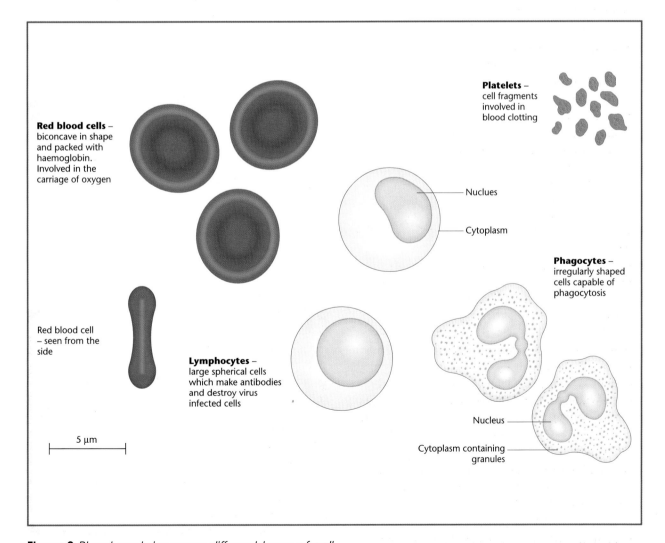

Figure 2 *Blood contains many different types of cell.*

3.2 The functions of blood

Why do you need blood?

Blood has many important functions in your body. Some of these are:

- to transport various substances from one part of the body to another
- to act as a source of materials for cells to draw on
- to distribute heat and help regulate body temperature
- to defend your body against disease causing organisms.

If your blood was to stop circulating, you would die within minutes.

Which substances does blood transport?

The plasma, the fluid part of your blood, transports:

- **food substances**, such as glucose, amino acids, fatty acids, mineral salts and vitamins from your intestines to the cells of your body. Here they are used immediately or stored for future use. Some of these substances, glucose for example, is always present in the blood so that cells can use it when they need energy (see chapter 8.2).

- **waste substances** produced by cells during their normal metabolism. The main ones are carbon dioxide, water and urea (see chapter 8.2). These are transported from your cells to your excretory organs. If these were allowed to build up, they would soon kill you.

- **heat**, produced in the liver and muscles, to all areas of your body. This is your central heating system, which helps to keep your body temperature at 37 °C (see chapter 8.5).

- **hormones** from your endocrine glands to their target cells. These hormones control and influence many important processes that take place in your body. More details can be found in chapter 7.4.

The red blood cells transport **oxygen** from your lungs to your other body cells. As the red blood cells pass through the blood vessels in your lungs, oxygen diffuses into them and immediately combines with the **haemoglobin**, forming **oxyhaemoglobin**.

$$\text{Haemoglobin} + \text{oxygen} \underset{\text{tissues}}{\overset{\text{lungs}}{\rightleftharpoons}} \text{oxyhaemoglobin}$$

Oxyhaemoglobin releases this oxygen as the red blood cells pass through an active tissue, such as muscle. The oxygen can now diffuse into the tissue cells.

Some people may have a disease called **anaemia**. This affects their ability to supply enough oxygen to their body cells. It is the result of having too few red blood cells or not enough haemoglobin. Lack of haemoglobin is often caused by a shortage of iron in the diet and can be easily corrected.

How does blood fight disease-causing organisms?

Your body has many ways of preventing **pathogenic micro-organisms** entering and causing damage (see chapter 13.8). Your skin is the main barrier, but if this is damaged your blood then becomes involved. The blood defends against disease in five ways:

- **Bleeding**. Bleeding carries germs away from the wound, but it is dangerous for it to go on too long. To prevent serious loss of blood and the entry of more germs, the wound is naturally plugged by a blood clot.

- **Blood clotting**. The production of a blood clot is outlined in figure 2. A few people have an inherited condition in which their blood will not clot. This is called **haemophilia** (chapter 11.5).

- The **inflammation response**. This is a rapid response to tissue damage, initiated by the release of chemicals (one being **histamine**), by damaged cells and white blood cells. It is characterised by redness and warmth, due to an increased blood flow in the area; swelling caused by the formation of extra tissue fluid; and pain as a result of the pressure on the nerve endings in the area. Inflammation speeds up the healing process by increasing the supply of nutrients and increasing the concentration of **phagocytic** white blood cells in the area, which prevents the spread of infection.

- **Phagocytosis**. Phagocytic white blood cells engulf any germs in or around the damaged area and digest them (see chapter 1.5). They also start to clean up the area by destroying damaged cells. **Pus**, the yellow substance that collects at wounds, is a mixture of these phagocytes, tissue fluid and the germs. Germs which penetrate deeper than the immediate wound area are filtered out of the tissue fluid as it passes through the **lymph nodes** and are then engulfed by more phagocytes.

- **Immune response**. If any micro-organisms avoid the phagocytes, they will be tackled by the lymphocytes. This is described in chapter 13.9.

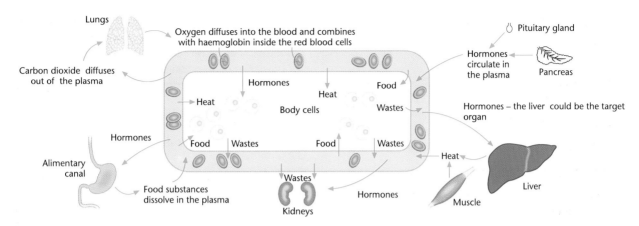

Figure 1 *The blood transports substances around your body.*

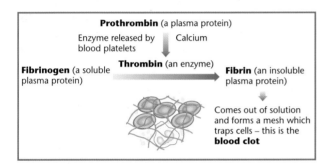

Figure 2 *Blood clots are formed by a series of complex reactions requiring the presence of 13 clotting factors, including calcium.*

What do **you** know?

You should now be able to:

- Describe 4 important functions of your blood.
- List 5 food substances transported in your blood plasma. State where to and from.
- List 3 waste substances transported by your blood and again state where to and from.
- List 2 more substances transported in your blood.
- Describe the role of haemoglobin in the carriage of oxygen.
- Explain what anaemia is and its causes.
- Describe how the composition of blood changes as it passes through the intestines and the lungs.
- Describe the sequence of events that take place when your skin is damaged.
- Explain the roles of bleeding, blood clotting and inflammation.
- Outline the process of blood clotting.

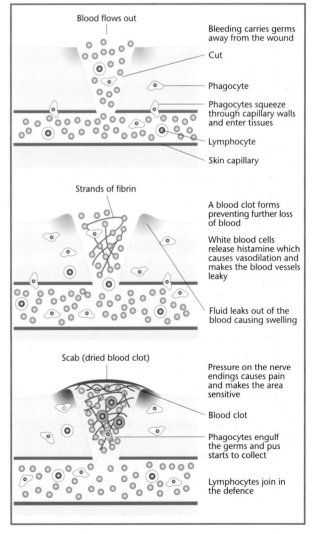

Figure 3 *When your skin is cut a whole series of events take place to prevent germs entering and causing disease.*

3.3 The circulation of blood

Blood delivers food and oxygen to every cell of your body. It does this in a series of tubes called **blood vessels**, through which it also returns to the heart and lungs.

The circulation of blood is sometimes called a **double circulation** because the circulation to and from the lungs is separate from the one to and from the other parts of the body (see figure 1).

The blood vessels

There are three main kinds of blood vessel; **arteries**, **capillaries** and **veins** (see figure 2). Together these form a network of tubes in your body through which your blood can flow.

- **Arteries** (except the pulmonary artery) take oxygenated blood away from the heart towards the tissues. They have thick muscular and elastic walls to withstand the very high pressure generated by the heart pumping blood through them. When the heart forces blood into an artery, it expands slightly as the muscle and elastic fibres are stretched. These fibres then contract pushing the blood towards the capillaries. When you press an artery against something solid like a bone, you can feel this slight expansion and contraction. It happens once every heartbeat and is known as the **pulse**. As arteries get nearer to the tissues, they get narrower and narrower. The narrowest arteries are called **arterioles**.

- **Capillaries** are found at the ends of arterioles and take the blood through a tissue. Every tissue contains a large network of capillaries so that every cell is served by the blood. The wall of a capillary is only one cell thick and very 'leaky'. As the blood enters the capillaries, the blood pressure forces some of the plasma through the capillary walls, and into the spaces between the tissue cells. Here it is known as **tissue fluid**. The cells remove food and oxygen from this tissue fluid and excrete their wastes into it. Most of the tissue fluid returns back into the capillaries before they leave the tissue. The rest goes into **lymph capillaries** and is transported back to the blood via the **lymphatic system**.

- **Veins.** Before leaving a tissue, the blood from the capillaries flows into slightly larger vessels called **venules**. These join up to form the veins. Veins (except the pulmonary vein) take the deoxygenated blood back to the heart. Their walls contain muscle and elastic fibres but are much thinner than the walls of arteries, because they do not have to withstand quite so much pressure. Most of the pressure that keeps blood moving has been lost in the capillaries as some

of the plasma leaks out and becomes tissue fluid. The pressure in the veins is often so low it cannot keep the blood moving. However, most major veins are sandwiched between skeletal muscles and when these contract, the veins are squashed, forcing the blood in them to move (see figure 3). To ensure movement in one direction, the veins contain one way valves called **pocket valves**.

The names of some of the main arteries and veins are shown in figure 1.

What is the lymphatic system?

The lymphatic system consists of a series of vessels which eventually join up with the blood system in the shoulders. All tissues contain lymph vessels and these form an alternative route for tissue fluid to leave the tissues. Tissue fluid which passes into the lymph vessels becomes known as **lymph**. Lymph eventually rejoins the blood, but first is filtered several times to remove dead cells and any foreign substances, such as bacteria. The filters are called **lymph nodes**. The main lymph nodes in your body are in your neck, armpits, abdomen and groin (see figure 5). These filter the lymph formed in these areas of your body.

Lymph nodes contain phagocytes that devour dead cells and infection particles. If the lymph contains a lot of infection particles, such as bacteria, the lymph nodes become very active and swell. This is often one of the first signs of an infection. Lymphocytes also accumulate here and are important in the immune response (chapter 13.8).

The lymph is kept moving in the lymph vessels in much the same way as the blood is kept moving in the veins (see figure 3).

What do **you** know?

You should now be able to:

- Construct a table, including diagrams, to compare the structure and functions of the 3 kinds of blood vessel.
- Describe how blood moves in the different vessels.
- Explain what cause the pulse.
- Explain how tissue fluid is formed from blood.
- Outline what happens to this tissue fluid.
- Outline the role of the lymphatic system.
- Name the organs associated with the pulmonary, hepatic and renal blood vessels.
- Explain the term double circulatory system.

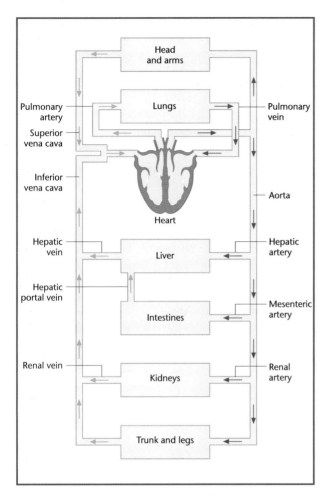

Figure 1 *Some of the main blood vessels in the blood circulatory system.*

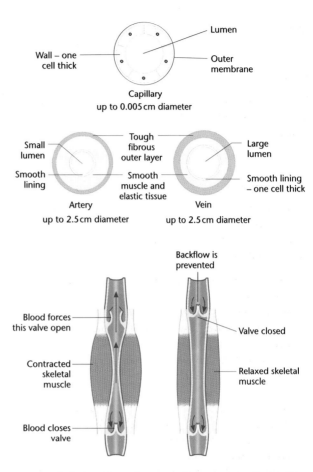

Figures 2/3 *Sections through the vessels. The veins contain valves to make sure the blood flows in the right direction.*

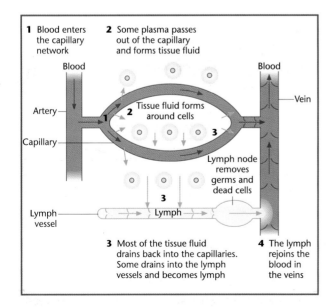

1 Blood enters the capillary network
2 Some plasma passes out of the capillary and forms tissue fluid
3 Most of the tissue fluid drains back into the capillaries. Some drains into the lymph vessels and becomes lymph
4 The lymph rejoins the blood in the veins

Figure 4 *How tissue fluid and lymph are formed.*

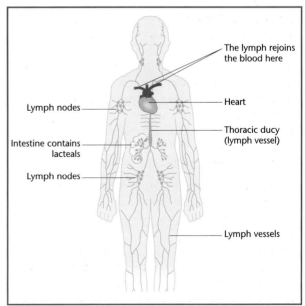

Figure 5 *The lymphatic system.*

3.4 The heart

Your heart is a double pump

Blood is kept moving in your circulatory system by the pumping action of the heart. It is two pumps joined together. The right side pumps blood to the lungs and the left side pumps blood to the rest of the body.

What does your heart look like?

The heart is a hollow structure about the same size as an adult's clenched fist. The walls are made from **cardiac muscle**. This is a specialized muscle: it has to contract, on average, 70 times a minute for 70 years or more without tiring! This amount of activity requires a lot of energy and food and oxygen to produce this. The cardiac muscle gets these from its own blood supply, the **coronary vessels** (chapter 3.5).

The inside of the heart is divided into four chambers. The left and right side each have an upper chamber called an **atrium** (plural atria) and a lower chamber called a **ventricle**. Blood can flow from an atrium into a ventricle through a valve called a **cuspid valve.**

Veins bring blood to the atria and arteries take blood away from the ventricles. There are also valves in the beginning of the arteries leaving the ventricles. These are called **semi-lunar valves** and, together with the cuspid valves, they make sure that the blood only flows through the heart in one direction.

More details of heart structure are shown in figure 1.

How does the heart pump blood?

As each chamber of the heart fills with blood it then contracts to force this blood out. This happens in a organised sequence which is illustrated in figure 2.

One complete filling and emptying of the heart is called the **cardiac cycle**. During this cycle, each chamber of the heart goes through two phases:

1 **Diastole**, a period when the muscular wall relaxes and the chamber enlarges and fills with blood.

2 **Systole**, a period of contraction resulting in the chamber getting smaller and forcing the blood out.

The timing of these phases is controlled by the **pacemaker**, a small patch of tissue on the wall of the right atrium. This makes sure your heart beats about 70 times a minute when you are resting. During periods of exercise, your brain will stimulate the pacemaker to increase your heart rate. This will ensure that your muscles are supplied with the food and oxygen they require to produce the extra energy they need. Your heart rate may also increase when you are excited or frightened, or even if you are unwell.

The heart sounds, often described as a '**lubb dup**' noise, are created by the closure of the cuspid and semi-lunar valves.

How is heart rate controlled?

The changes to your heart rate during exercise are controlled by a reflex action involving the **carbon dioxide concentration** of your blood and the **medulla** of your brain. The carbon dioxide concentration in blood is monitored in the aorta and carotid arteries. During exercise it increases and the medulla is informed. The medulla in turn sends out a message (nerve impulse) to the heart pacemaker to increase the heart rate. A similar message goes to the lungs to increase breathing rate. This is an example of a **negative feedback system** (chapter 8.1) because a rise in the carbon dioxide level will initiate changes to reduce it. A similar reflex action will reduce the heart and breathing rates if the blood carbon dioxide levels fall.

What do **you** know?

You should now be able to:

- Label a diagram of the heart.
- Identify the structures on a photograph of the heart.
- Describe the route taken by a red blood cell as it moves from the vena cava to the aorta.
- Explain why the heart is a double pump.
- Outline the events of the cardiac cycle.
- Name and describe the roles of the valves in the cardiac cycle.
- Suggest why one side of the heart is more muscular than the other.
- Draw the pacemaker on your heart diagram and describe its function.

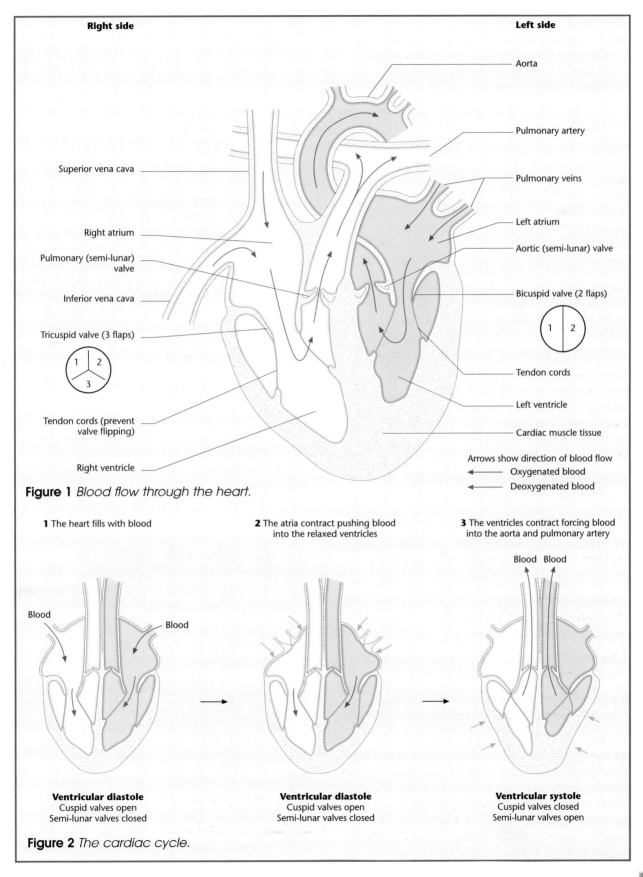

Right side   **Left side**

Aorta

Pulmonary artery

Superior vena cava

Pulmonary veins

Right atrium

Left atrium

Pulmonary (semi-lunar) valve

Aortic (semi-lunar) valve

Inferior vena cava

Bicuspid valve (2 flaps)

Tricuspid valve (3 flaps)

Tendon cords

Left ventricle

Tendon cords (prevent valve flipping)

Cardiac muscle tissue

Right ventricle

Arrows show direction of blood flow

Oxygenated blood

Deoxygenated blood

Figure 1 *Blood flow through the heart.*

1 The heart fills with blood

2 The atria contract pushing blood into the relaxed ventricles

3 The ventricles contract forcing blood into the aorta and pulmonary artery

Blood   Blood

Blood

Blood

Ventricular diastole
Cuspid valves open
Semi-lunar valves closed

Ventricular diastole
Cuspid valves open
Semi-lunar valves closed

Ventricular systole
Cuspid valves closed
Semi-lunar valves open

Figure 2 *The cardiac cycle.*

3.5 Heart disease

What is blood pressure?

When the heart pumps blood into your arteries, it creates a pressure called **blood pressure** (BP). This pressure is at its greatest when the heart muscle is contracting and lower when relaxing. The two pressures, called the **systolic** and **diastolic** pressures, can be measured using a **shygmomanometer**. The readings are usually taken on the brachial artery in the arm. Normal blood pressure is different for different age groups (see figure 1).

What affects blood pressure?

Blood is like water travelling through a hosepipe: turn the tap on more so more water enters, or squeeze the pipe to make it narrower and the pressure goes up; the longer the hosepipe, the greater the loss in pressure as the water travels through it. Blood pressure goes up if the volume of blood being pumped into the blood vessels increases or the diameter of the vessels is reduced. The further you get away from the heart, the lower the blood pressure. This drop in blood pressure helps the blood to flow round the circulatory system.

The amount of blood being pumped into the vessels will increase during exercise, so your blood pressure will increase. Your body has mechanisms to limit this increase, but if your resting BP is already too high, this could be dangerous.

What about high blood pressure?

Permanent high blood pressure is called **hypertension**. In diagnosing hypertension, the diastolic pressure is more important. A permanent resting diastolic pressure of over 90 mmHg is considered high. This can be very damaging to health. Some of the main problems it causes are:

- small blood vessels may rupture. If blood capillaries supplying the brain rupture, it is called a stroke.

- kidney function may be impaired and the kidneys damaged.

- artery walls may thicken, narrowing the lumen and further increasing BP.

- the lining of the blood vessels may be damaged resulting in an inflammation response and the build up of fatty deposits or a blood clot.

- the heart will have to work harder, which may result in a heart attack.

What is coronary heart disease?

Coronary heart disease (CHD) accounts for 30% of premature deaths in males and 14% in females in the UK. It is by far the largest cause of premature death in the UK.

CHD is really a disorder of the **coronary arteries** that supply blood to the heart muscle (see figure 2). If these are damaged or blocked, the oxygen supply to the heart muscle is reduced, the heart stops contracting, and a **heart attack** ensues. If a large part of the heart is affected this can cause instant death, or if it is less serious recovery is possible.

CHD usually starts with the build up of fatty deposits on the inside of the coronary vessels. This reduces the diameter of the vessels, and therefore the flow of blood to the heart muscle. The first symptom is a chest pain when exercising. This is called **angina**. The fatty deposits, or **atheroma**, may eventually completely block the coronary vessel, or more usually cause blood clots to form and lodge in the narrowed areas. This can cut off the blood supply to the heart muscle altogether and the heart muscle, without sufficient food and oxygen, stops contracting. Figure 2 gives a fuller explanation.

What sort of people get CHD?

CHD can be triggered by many factors:

- High blood pressure (see figure 1). The higher the BP, the more work the heart has to do.

- Smoking. The nicotine in cigarette smoke constricts the blood vessels raising BP. Nicotine also increases the blood cholesterol level and raises the heart rate. Carbon monoxide in the smoke reduces the oxygen carrying capacity of the blood. It is estimated that 18% of deaths from CHD can be attributed to smoking.

- Diet. A high fat diet, especially saturated fat will raise blood cholesterol levels and result in obesity. A high blood cholesterol level is a trigger factor for the formation of an atheroma. Obese people are less likely to exercise and put great stress on their heart. A high salt intake, excessive caffeine or alcohol will also raise BP.

- Stress. Stress raises BP because hormones released cause constriction of the blood vessels.

- Lack of exercise. Exercise strengthens the heart and maintains a healthy blood flow in the coronary arteries. It also reduces stress.

- Genetic factors. CHD seems to run in families Blood cholesterol level is in part genetically determined.

- Diseases such as diabetes.

Detecting CHD and current methods of treatment are described in chapter 3.1.

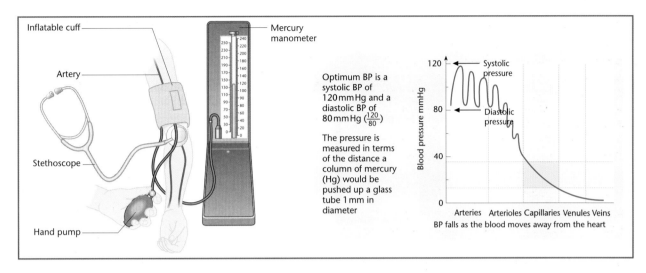

Figure 1 *Blood pressure (BP) is usually measured in the arm using a sphygmomanometer.*

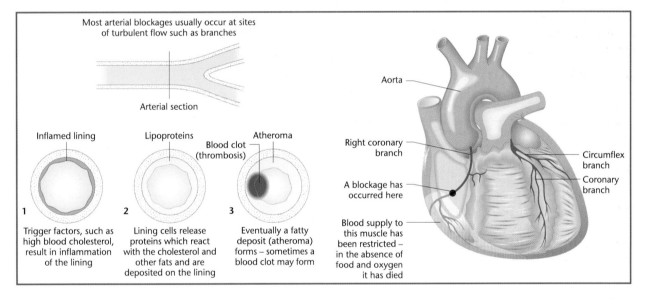

Figure 2 *The events leading to a heart attack.*

What do **you** know?

You should now be able to:

- Explain what blood pressure is and how it is measured.
- Explain the difference between systolic and diastolic pressures.
- Name 2 factors which can affect blood pressure.
- Describe the problems hypertension can cause.

- Describe two ways the diameter of a blood vessel can be altered.
- Explain what CHD is.
- Describe a heart attack and angina.
- Draw diagrams to show how an atheroma can build up.
- List and explain the risk factors for CHD.

Chapter 3: Questions

1 Copy and complete the table below to show differences between red blood cells and white blood cells. Drawings of these cells are shown to help you.

(4 marks)

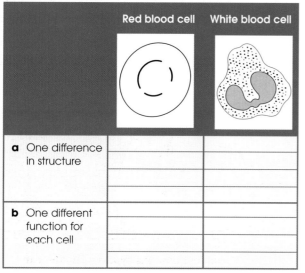

	Red blood cell	White blood cell
a One difference in structure		
b One different function for each cell		

(SEG June 1989)

2 The diagram shows a wound in the skin as seen in sectional view.

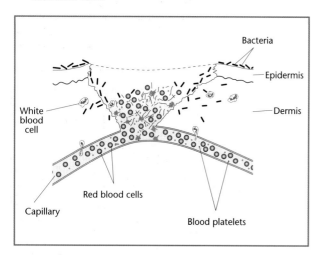

Briefly describe what this diagram shows about the way the body defends itself against the entry of bacteria. Only use information visible in the diagram.

(5 marks)
(SEG June 1991)

3 The diagram shows the pathway of blood between the heart, lungs and other body organs.

   a Name the types of blood vessel labelled A and D.

(2 marks)

   b One of the valves of the heart is labelled on the diagram. What is the function of the valves of the heart?

(1 mark)

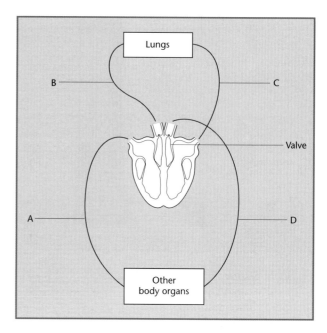

   c Draw a simplified diagram and add arrows to show the direction of blood flow in the blood vessels labelled B and C.

(2 marks)

   d The table shows how the output of blood from the heart changes as the heart rate changes.

Heart rate (beats per minute)	Output of blood (litres per minute)	Output per beat (litres)
65	4.8	0.073
70	4.6	0.066
75	4.9	0.065
80	5.1	0.063
85	5.3	0.062
90	5.5	0.061
95	5.7	0.060
100	5.9	0.059
105	5.9	0.056
110	5.8	0.052
115	5.6	0.048
120	5.2	0.043
125	4.8	0.038

   i As the heart rate increases the output of blood changes. Describe these changes. *(3 marks)*

   ii How does an increase in heart rate affect the output per beat from the heart? *(1 mark)*

   e Describe the exchange of gases between blood and the air in the lungs.

(5 marks)
(NEAB June 1998)

4 **a** This diagram shows the outside of the human heart seen from the front.

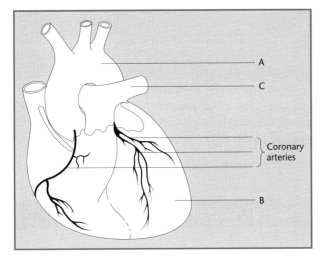

i Name structures A and B. *(2 marks)*

ii Name a part of the body which receives blood from vessel C. *(1 mark)*

b Sometimes damage may occur to the coronary arteries, causing coronary heart disease. This is more likely to occur in people who smoke cigarettes and who eat large amounts of fatty foods. Some materials in cigarette smoke can cause the blood cells to become more sticky and can also cause the release of blood clotting factors.

The graph shows the relationship between cigarette smoking and deaths from coronary heart disease for British men aged between 45 and 54 years.

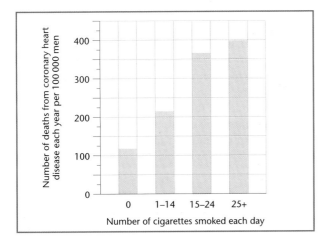

i How many more men who smoked 25 or more cigarettes each day died of coronary heart disease compared with non-smokers?

(1 mark)

ii Explain how eating too much fatty food and smoking cigarettes can lead to coronary heart disease. *(5 marks)*

iii A coronary bypass operation can be performed to help overcome coronary heart disease. The diagram shows a triple coronary bypass graft.

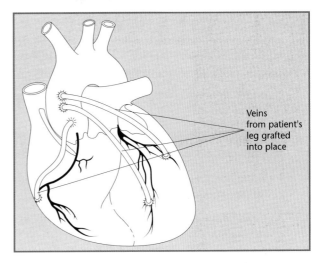

1 Explain how this bypass operation can help to overcome the effects of coronary heart disease. *(2 marks)*

2 Give a biological reason why it is better to transplant veins from the patient's leg rather than from the leg of another person.

(1 mark)
(SEG specimen 1998)

5 The diagram shows part of the circulation of the blood.

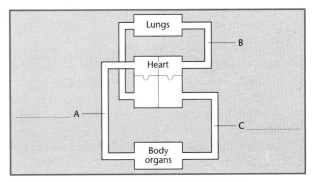

a What is the function of the heart? *(1 mark)*

b Look at the diagram, name the types of blood vessel labelled A and C. *(2 marks)*

c In blood vessel B does the blood flow to the heart or to the lungs? *(1 mark)*

d Blood is made up of the following:
plasma, red blood cells, white blood cells, platelets
Which of these:

i carries oxygen? *(1 mark)*

ii destroys microbes? *(1 mark)*

iii carries dissolved food? *(1 mark)*
(OCR June 1999)

4 Respiration

Everything you do requires energy. To produce this energy you need a constant supply of oxygen. In this chapter you will find out how you get this oxygen and what happens if you cannot get enough. You will also see how people damage their breathing apparatus by smoking.

After you have worked through this chapter, you should be able to:

- Explain what energy is, why we need it and where it comes from.

- Describe the processes of aerobic and anaerobic respiration.

- Describe the structure and functioning of the respiratory system.

- List the features of a respiratory surface to maximise gas exchange

- Describe the breathing mechanism.

- Explain the reasons for the variations in breathing rate due to exercise.

- Explain how breathing rate is controlled.

- Discuss the effects on health of smoking.

- Describe an occupational disease caused by dusts.

Energy and sport

As soon as a race starts, the energy requirements of an athlete can increase by up to twenty times. So, where does this extra energy come from?

Energy supply systems

Muscle cells (and all other cells) get their energy from a high energy compound called **adenosine triphosphate** (ATP). When the body is at rest, small stocks of this are built up in the cells. When the stocks are used up, which takes less than 3 seconds during strenuous exercise, they have to be replenished. This can be achieved in several ways:

- The muscle cells contain another high energy compound called **creatine phosphate** (CP). This can be used to rapidly re-energise some ATP, but stores of it are limited and will only last for about another 7 seconds. ATP and CP together will enable maximum exertion for about 10 seconds, then the ATP has to come from elsewhere.

- Some ATP can be produced from **anaerobic** processes utilising **glycogen** stored in the muscle cells. However, it also produces **lactic acid**, which can (in sufficient quantities) stop muscles contracting altogether.

Glucose (from glycogen) $\longrightarrow$ lactic acid + ATP

Anaerobic respiration on its own can, at maximum, supply ATP for approximately two minutes before cramp sets in.

- Most ATP is generated by **aerobic respiration**, but this requires oxygen. It takes about three minutes to reach the maximum oxygen supply, but once achieved, it can take over energy supply for the duration of the exercise. At first, it mostly uses glucose from the blood, but as exercise progresses more and more fatty acids are used.

the first 10 seconds (the start)	energy from stored ATP and CP system
the next 2 minutes	anaerobic respiration
from 1 minute onwards	aerobic respiration by 3 minutes, it is almost entirely aerobic
the final sprint	aerobic supplemented by anaerobic respiration

Table 1 *The energy supply during a 10 000 metre race lasting about 29 minutes.*

As you can see all three energy systems are used. The one which supplies most of the energy is determined by the intensity and duration of exercise. Table 2 below gives an indication of the relative importance of the three energy systems in different running events.

The anaerobic threshold

The more energy that is obtained from anaerobic respiration, the faster the lactic acid builds up. If an athlete runs too quickly, the lactic acid will build up to an intolerable level before the end of the race. The intensity of effort at which lactic acid starts to build up is called the **anaerobic threshold**. For a fully trained athlete, this is usually at around 85% of his maximum heart rate.

An athlete has to judge his speed so that the energy supplied by anaerobic respiration is not so high as to cause the build up of damaging lactic acid, otherwise he will get cramp before he crosses the line. He must also make sure his muscles do not contain too much lactic acid to make his final sprint impossible.

Explosive events like the 100 metre sprint depend more on the power of the muscles rather than the ability to get oxygen. The energy for these events comes from the stored ATP and CP system.

Recovery after exercise

After the exercise has finished, each energy system must be restored to the normal resting situation (see figure 1).

The first thing to be restored is the CP. This is re-energised from ATP in the cell within the first two minutes. In theory 100 metre sprinters should be able to run again after this.

Next, the lactic acid has to be removed. It has to be oxidised to carbon dioxide and water, a process which requires oxygen. The amount of oxygen required for this is called the oxygen debt. The maximum **oxygen debt** a person can have is about 17 dm^3. It can take up to one hour to clear this.

Finally the glycogen reserves in the muscles need to be replenisehed. This can take up to two days. Incidentally, the 'hitting the wall' effect during long distance running is the feeling of complete exhaustion due to the liver and muscle glycogen reserves running out.

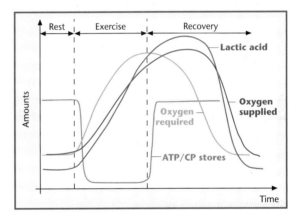

Figure 1 *After exercise there must be a recovery period.*

Event	Duration	% Anaerobic	% Aerobic	Main energy system
100 metre sprint	10s	100	0	ATP/CP
400 metre	45s	90	10	Anaerobic races less than 3 minutes
		80	20	
800 metre	1m 45s	70	30	
		60	40	
1500 metre	3m 45s	50	50	Aerobic races longer than 3 minutes
		40	60	
		30	70	
5000 metre	14m	20	80	
10000 metre	29m	10	90	
Marathon	135m	0	100	

Table 2 *The main energy source depends on the intensity and duration of exercise.*

4.1 Energy

What is energy?

Energy makes things happen and is described as the power to do work. Your body cells are working all the time and, therefore, must have a continual supply of energy: without this energy, they would soon die.

Energy comes in several forms, as **chemical**, **light**, **sound**, **heat** and **mechanical** energy. It is possible to change one form into another. For example, when coal is burnt, the chemical energy contained within it is turned into heat energy and light energy.

In what form does your body get energy?

Our energy comes from the food we eat. This food contains chemical energy that our cells are able to release and use to perform work. The process that releases energy from food is called **respiration**.

Respiration is a series of chemical reactions that take place in the cytoplasm and mitochondria of cells. The main food substance used is glucose, but other sugars, fatty acids and even amino acids can also be used. To get all the available energy from a food requires a supply of oxygen. Energy production with oxygen is called **aerobic respiration** (see figure 1). Some of the energy is released as heat. This enters the blood and is used to keep your body warm. The rest is stored in a substance called **ATP** (adenosine triphosphate), until the cell needs to use it.

Different types of food release different amounts of energy when they are used in respiration. Energy is measured in **joules**. This is a very small amount, so we usually measure energy in **kilojoules**. A kilojoule is 1000 joules. Carbohydrates supply 16 kilojoules per gram, proteins supply 17 kilojoules per gram and lipids supply 37 kilojoules per gram. The amount of energy a food can supply will therefore depend on how much of these nutrients it contains (see figure 2).

How much energy do you need?

You need energy all the time, even when you are sleeping. Your cells need this energy to keep their metabolism going. The amount of energy your cells consume over a period of time, e.g. per day, is determined by your **metabolic rate** (chapter 1.3). When your cells are doing just enough to keep you alive, the energy they are consuming is used to express the **basal metabolic rate** (BMR). The BMR is different for different people, and at different periods of their lives (see figure 3). It is influenced by age, size (surface area), gender, and state of health. Your overall metabolic rate will include the additional energy your cells need to do the extra work for the day's activities.

Why do people get cramp?

When muscles are working hard, they need lots of energy, the release of which requires a lot of oxygen. If this oxygen does not get to the muscles fast enough, they will start producing energy without it. Energy production without using oxygen is called **anaerobic respiration**.

We only use anaerobic respiration in an emergency because, although the extra energy is useful, **lactic acid** is produced which builds up in the muscles and stops them working. This is what causes the painful condition we know as **cramp**.

Anaerobic respiration is summarised in figure 1. The glucose is not completely broken down to release all its energy. In fact, only about one tenth of it is released so it is not very efficient for humans and the muscles will only return to normal working when all the lactic acid has been removed. Lactic acid requires oxygen to convert it to harmless substances. The deep and rapid breathing after exercising is to supply this oxygen. The extra oxygen required to remove the lactic acid is called the **oxygen debt**.

Fermentation sometimes called **alcoholic fermentation** is a kind of anaerobic respiration carried out by plants, bacteria and fungi, such as yeast. Alcohol and carbon dioxide are formed instead of lactic acid. We make use of these substances in brewing and baking (see chapter 14.5).

What do **you** know?

You should now be able to:

- Describe what energy is, which forms it comes in and the form we get it from.
- Comment on the different energy needs of different people.
- Define the term respiration.
- Write a word equation to summarise aerobic respiration and draw a diagram to show where it takes place within a cell.
- Describe what happens to the energy released during respiration.
- Outline the differences between aerobic and anaerobic respiration.
- Explain why anaerobic respiration releases less energy than aerobic respiration.
- Explain why some people get cramp and build up an oxygen debt.

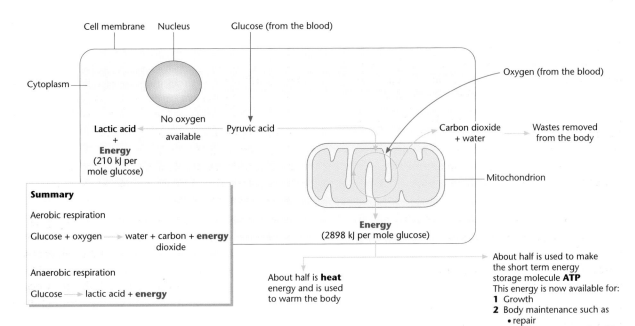

Figure 1 *Both aerobic and anaerobic respiration occur in animal cells.*

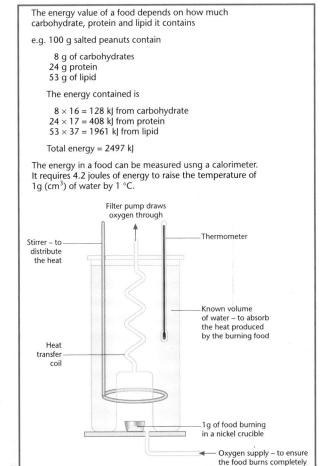

The energy value of a food depends on how much carbohydrate, protein and lipid it contains

e.g. 100 g salted peanuts contain

8 g of carbohydrates
24 g protein
53 g of lipid

The energy contained is

$8 \times 16 = 128$ kJ from carbohydrate
$24 \times 17 = 408$ kJ from protein
$53 \times 37 = 1961$ kJ from lipid

Total energy = 2497 kJ

The energy in a food can be measured usng a calorimeter. It requires 4.2 joules of energy to raise the temperature of 1g (cm^3) of water by 1 °C.

Filter pump draws oxygen through

Stirrer – to distribute the heat

Thermometer

Known volume of water – to absorb the heat produced by the burning food

Heat transfer coil

1g of food burning in a nickel crucible

Oxygen supply – to ensure the food burns completely

Figure 2 *The measurement of energy in food.*

	Weight/ kg	BMR MJ/day	BMR MJ/kg/day
Infant (1 yr old)	10	2.3	0.23
Boy (17 yrs old)	70	7.9	0.11
Girl (17 yrs old)	60	6.3	0.10
Man (35 yrs old)	76	7.3	0.10
Woman (35 yrs old)	62	5.7	0.09

Table 1 *Your BMR is different at different times of your life.*

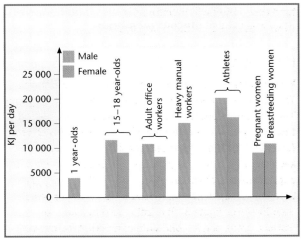

Figure 3 *Different people require different amounts of energy.*

4.2 Supplying oxygen

How do cells get oxygen for respiration?

Your cells get all the oxygen they need from your blood. The blood obtains oxygen from the air. This happens in your lungs. Your lungs are part of your **respiratory system**. This system makes oxygen available to the blood which picks it up and transports it to the cells in your body. The respiratory system also transports the carbon dioxide made in the cells to the lungs.

The respiratory system

The respiratory system (see figure 1) consists of:

- A **gas exchange surface** across which oxygen can pass from the air into the blood, and carbon dioxide can pass from the blood into the air. This surface is formed from about 300 million tiny pockets, or sacs, called **alveoli** (see figure 4). Together these provide a very **large surface area** in excess of 160 m^2 over which the diffusion of gases can take place. The linings of the alveoli are kept moist because the gases need to be in solution to diffuse across the membrane, and are thin to allow efficient diffusion. Each alveolus is also surrounded by an extensive **network of blood capillaries** containing lots of blood. This blood carries the incoming oxygen away quickly, thereby maintaining a **diffusion gradient**.

- A **series of air passages** to take the air into and out of the alveoli. These passages are formed by the **nose** and **nasal cavity**, the **throat** and **mouth**, the **trachea**, the two **bronchi** (singular **bronchus**) and many tiny **bronchioles**. Most of these passages are lined by a membrane that contains some special cells. **Goblet cells** produce **mucus** which keeps the lining moist and traps the dirt and dust in the air. **Ciliated cells** move the mucus and debris towards the throat where it can be swallowed. This kind of lining is often called a ciliated **mucous membrane**.

- The **ventilating structures** which move air in and out of the alveoli and air passages, and also support the lungs. These structures are the **diaphragm**, the ribcage with its **ribs** and **intercostal muscles** and the **pleural membranes**.

What happens in the lungs?

Table 1 shows the content of the air we breathe in (inspired air) and the air we breathe out (expired air). There are several differences:

- There is less oxygen in expired air. Some of the oxygen has diffused into the red blood cells and combined with haemoglobin ready to be transported away to the body cells for use in respiration.

$$\text{Oxygen} + \text{haemoglobin} \underset{\text{active tissues}}{\overset{\text{lungs}}{\rightleftharpoons}} \text{oxyhaemoglobin}$$

- There is about 100 times more carbon dioxide in expired air. This extra carbon dioxide is a waste product from respiration. It has diffused out of the blood plasma into the alveoli, from where it is expired.

- Expired air is warmer, cleaner and saturated with water vapour. The water vapour comes from the mucous membranes lining the air passages and the heat from the blood. To function properly, the alveoli must be kept moist, free of dust and not exposed to extremes of temperature. Air we breathe in is usually fairly dry, very dusty and often very cold. Before it gets to the alveoli it must therefore be moistened, filtered and warmed. This is done as it passes through the trachea and other air passages.

Gas	Inspired air	Expired air
Nitrogen	79%	79%
Oxygen	21%	16%
Carbon dioxide	0.04%	4%
Water vapour	a little	saturated

Table 1 *Content of gases in inspired/expired air.*

What do **you** know?

You should now be able to:

- Label a diagram of the respiratory system.
- State which part forms the respiratory surface and describe 4 features which increase its efficiency.
- Explain the features of a mucous membrane.
- Outline the importance of the air passages.
- Account for the differences between inspired and expired air.
- Write an equation to show how oxygen is transported.
- State where carbon dioxide is transported.
- Annotate a diagram of an alveolus to explain gas exchange.

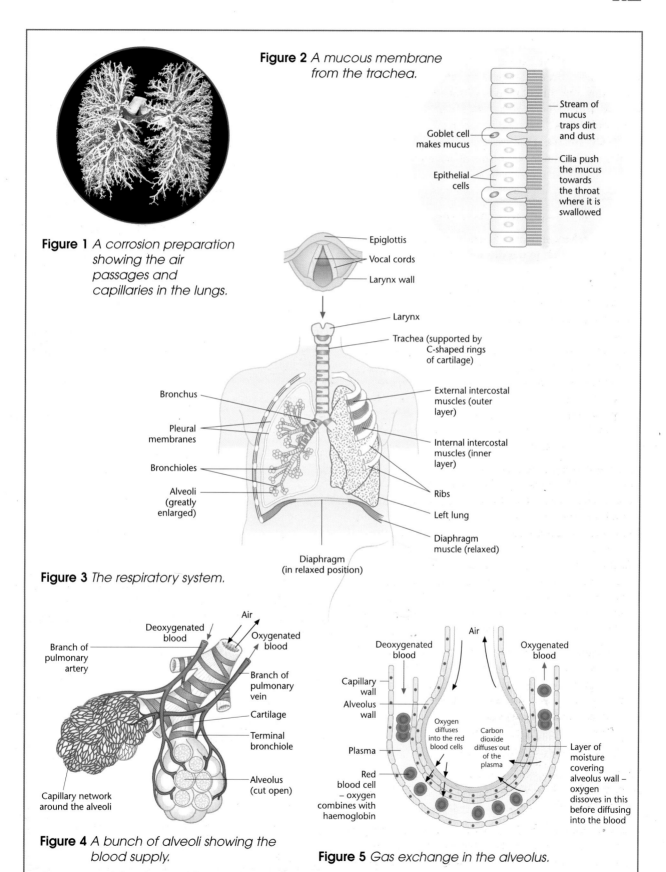

Figure 2 *A mucous membrane from the trachea.*

Goblet cell makes mucus

Epithelial cells

Stream of mucus traps dirt and dust

Cilia push the mucus towards the throat where it is swallowed

Figure 1 *A corrosion preparation showing the air passages and capillaries in the lungs.*

Epiglottis

Vocal cords

Larynx wall

Larynx

Trachea (supported by C-shaped rings of cartilage)

Bronchus

External intercostal muscles (outer layer)

Pleural membranes

Internal intercostal muscles (inner layer)

Bronchioles

Alveoli (greatly enlarged)

Ribs

Left lung

Diaphragm muscle (relaxed)

Diaphragm (in relaxed position)

Figure 3 *The respiratory system.*

Air

Deoxygenated blood

Oxygenated blood

Branch of pulmonary artery

Branch of pulmonary vein

Cartilage

Terminal bronchiole

Alveolus (cut open)

Capillary network around the alveoli

Figure 4 *A bunch of alveoli showing the blood supply.*

Air

Deoxygenated blood

Oxygenated blood

Capillary wall

Alveolus wall

Oxygen diffuses into the red blood cells

Carbon dioxide diffuses out of the plasma

Plasma

Red blood cell – oxygen combines with haemoglobin

Layer of moisture covering alveolus wall – oxygen dissoves in this before diffusing into the blood

Figure 5 *Gas exchange in the alveolus.*

4.3 Breathing

How is air moved in and out of the alveoli?

The alveoli are ventilated by the action of the **diaphragm** and **intercostal muscles**. These can alter the volume of the thorax creating pressure differences between the air in the lungs and the air outside. Air will move in or out to equalise these pressures.

The diaphragm is a sheet of tendon surrounded by muscles. It separates your thorax from your abdomen. When relaxed, it is forced into a dome shape by the organs in your abdomen. When the diaphragm muscles contract, it becomes flatter (see figure 1). If you are resting, the up and down movements of the diaphragm are often all that is needed to move sufficient air in and out of your lungs. It is only when you start to exercise and more oxygen is needed that the intercostal muscles are used to move the ribcage. This is why you can only feel and see the ribcage moving during and immediately after exercising.

You have two sets of intercostal muscles between the ribs, an outer set (external) and an inner set (internal). When the external set contract, your ribcage pivots on the backbone upwards and outwards. When the internal set contract your ribcage pivots downwards and inwards.

Figure 1 shows how the intercostal muscles and diaphragm work together during breathing.

How much air do your lungs hold?

The size of your lungs depends upon your age, sex and physique. If the average man filled his lungs, they would contain about 5 litres of air. If this same man then tried to empty his lungs, he would only be able to breathe out about 4 litres of this air. The maximum amount of air, which a person can breathe out from full lungs, is known as the **vital capacity**.

The 1 litre of air which has remained in the lungs, can never be expelled and is called the **residual air**. This occupies the area inside the trachea, bronchi and bronchioles, often called the dead space. These will always contain some air because they never completely collapse.

The air which a person normally breathes in and out is called the **tidal air**. For the average man at rest, this is approximately 0.5 litre, but during exercise, his depth of breathing gradually increases until his vital capacity is reached.

How does exercise affect your breathing?

When you exercise, your muscle cells need more energy and therefore more food and oxygen to produce it. This extra oxygen must be made available to your blood by your respiratory system and so you need to increase your breathing rate and depth of breathing to achieve this.

At rest, the average adult person breathes 16 times per minute. The air exchanged will be 8 litres (16 × 0.5 litre), containing 1.68 litres of oxygen (21%). During exercise, the breathing rate can more than double and the tidal air volume can increase by up to 8 times. This is equivalent to 128 litres (32 × 0.5 litre) of air, or 26.88 litres of oxygen. The blood circulation also speeds up so that more blood goes through the lung capillaries, thereby picking up more oxygen to transport to the cells.

How is your breathing rate controlled?

Breathing is automatic and under the control of your brain. The rate of breathing is set to meet the oxygen demand of your cells. One of the factors it uses to set the rate is the amount of carbon dioxide in the blood. This is monitored as the blood flows through the brain. An increase in blood carbon dioxide will result in an increase in both your breathing rate and depth of breathing, to remove the extra carbon dioxide. As the level falls, breathing rate is adjusted accordingly.

Mouth to mouth resuscitation

The fact that increased carbon dioxide can stimulate breathing is used by first aiders. By breathing expired air into a persons lungs, you are, (i) supplying oxygen because this air will still contain 16% oxygen, and (ii) increasing blood carbon dioxide because the air contains 100 times more carbon dioxide than normal air. This should help stimulate breathing.

What do **you** know?

You should now be able to:

- Name the structures involved in breathing.
- Explain how these structures create the pressure changes needed to take air in.
- Explain the processes involved in breathing air out.
- Explain the terms tidal air, vital capacity, residual air and dead space.
- Interpret a graph produced by a spirometer showing breathing rate, tidal volume and oxygen used.
- Explain the role of carbon dioxide concentration in the control of breathing rate.
- Explain why mouth to mouth resuscitation works.

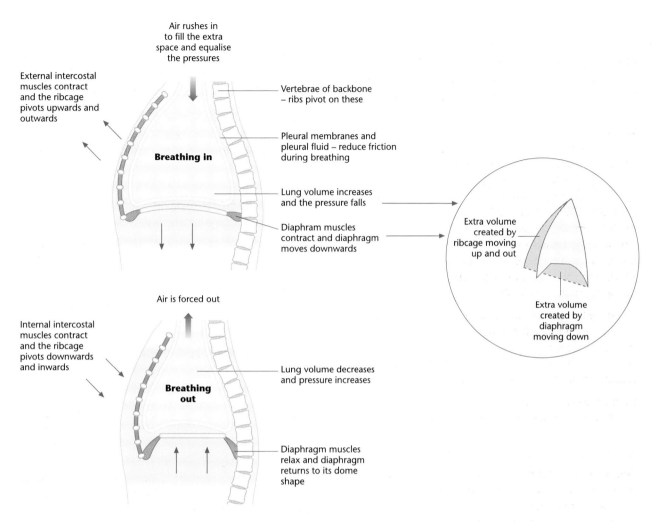

Figure 1 *Breathing involves your diaphragm, intercostal muscles and ribcage creating pressure changes.*

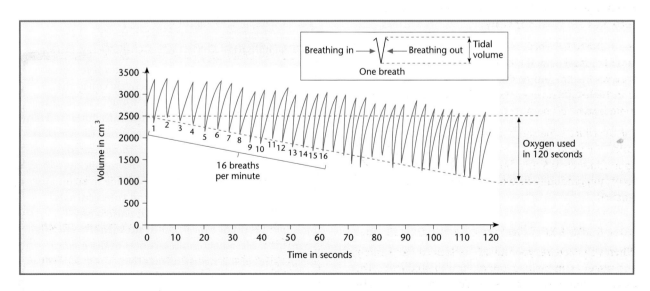

Figure 2 *Breathing rate, tidal volume and oxygen used can be measured using a special machine called a spirometer. This graph was produced from this.*

Smoking damages your health – it's official!

There is evidence from documented research to show that smoking can increase your risk of developing coronary heart disease (CHD), lung cancer, bronchitis, emphysema and many more life-threatening diseases. Yet one in four UK adults still smoke and in 1999, 21% of boys and 25% of girls aged 15 claimed to smoke regularly. It has been estimated that 17% of all deaths in the UK, 18% of deaths from CHD, 66% of deaths from bronchitis and emphysema and a staggering 81% of deaths from lung cancer are related to smoking.

Why is smoking so harmful?

Cigarette smoke contains over 1000 different substances, many of which can damage your body. Some of the main ones are:

- **Nicotine**. Nicotine is a **drug** which in small doses stimulates your brain cells (chapter 12.7). It also causes narrowing of your blood vessels which increases blood pressure (BP). This has two effects in your body:
  (i) it makes your heart work harder, so your heart muscle requires more oxygen, but another substance in cigarette smoke, carbon monoxide, prevents oxygen reaching your heart;
  (ii) the high BP damages the blood vessel lining making the build up of an **atheroma** or **blood clot** more likely (chapter 3.5). Nicotine also increases the levels of fatty acids in the blood, which lead to blood clotting.

- **Carbon monoxide**. Carbon monoxide is a poisonous gas which irreversibly combines with the haemoglobin in your red blood cells leaving you **breathless**. The haemoglobin would normally carry oxygen.

- **Tar.** Tobacco tar is a brown sticky substance made up of many different chemicals, many of which are **carcinogens** (cancer producing). Others are **irritants**. Because it is sticky, tar tends to accumulate and 'clog up the works'. It stops the **cilia** on the **mucous membranes** from moving allowing the build up of **mucus**. A cough often develops to clear this mucus. Persistent coughing can damage the delicate alveoli resulting in **emphysema**, a serious and chronic condition. Tar can also build up in the alveoli preventing gas exchange.

- **Irritants**. Some of the irritants in smoke are dusts such as **soot**, others are chemicals like **ammonia** and **hydrogen cyanide**. All have the same effect in that they irritate the delicate mucous membranes lining your air passages, resulting in **bronchitis**

(inflammation of the tube lining). The extra mucus, produced by the goblet cells, traps dust and germs hastening infections such as **pneumonia**.

Some of the irritant chemicals are known to be carcinogenic and result in **lung cancer**.

- **Heat**. Even the heat from a burning cigarette can cause damage. Every time you draw on a cigarette, the heat burns away some of the cilia lining your trachea.

Why is it so difficult to give up smoking?

Nicotine creates both **physical** and **psychological dependence** (chapter 12.6). It provides a relaxing effect but unfortunately, your body also builds up a **tolerance** to it so, with time, you need to increase the dose. Eventually, you may smoke 40 cigarettes a day, but the dosage will still seem too small. You are left feeling irritable and bad tempered all the time. It is difficult to give up smoking so it's best to avoid starting.

What are the effects of passive smoking?

A recent survey showed that 39% of women and 23% of men are exposed to 'sidestream' smoke at work. Also people who visit pubs have up to a 30% higher risk of developing lung cancer, due to exposure to smoke. They will also suffer more minor problems, such as headaches, eye irritation, sore throats and breathing difficulties, than people who are not subjected to cigarette smoke.

Smoking when pregnant

It is unwise to smoke during pregnancy as you are not only affecting your own health, but also the health and future of your unborn baby (see chapter 9.7).

Occupational diseases caused by dusts

The inhalation of harmful dusts or fibres is responsible for a large group of diseases collectively called the **pneumoconiosises**. **Asbestosis** is one of these. It is caused by the inhalation of blue asbestos fibres and may develop after only a few weeks exposure. The symptoms of pneumoconiosises are similar to those caused by heavy smoking, only they develop more quickly. Sufferers of pneumoconiosis may die due to secondary infections such as **pneumonia** and **tuberculosis**. Those who survive often develop a particularly malignant form of cancer, called **mesothelioma**, many years later. Mesothelioma is a cancer of the pleural membranes and is nearly always fatal.

Fortunately the dangers of inhaling these dusts are now recognised and workers are protected by laws which lay down strict regulations for working practice.

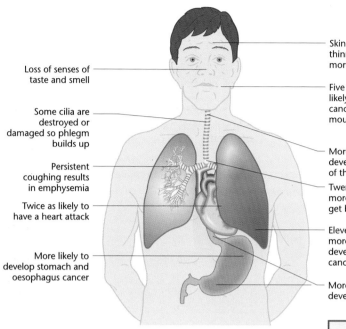

Skin up to 40% thinner and more wrinkles

Loss of senses of taste and smell

Five times more likely to develop cancer of the mouth and larynx

Some cilia are destroyed or damaged so phlegm builds up

More likely to develop cancer of the trachea

Persistent coughing results in emphysema

Twenty times more likely to get bronchitis

Twice as likely to have a heart attack

Eleven times more likely to develop lung cancer

More likely to develop stomach and oesophagus cancer

More likely to develop ulcers

Figure 1 *Some of the problems which can result from smoking 20 cigarettes a day.*

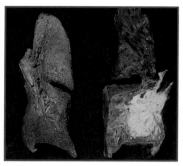

Section through a healthy lung and a lung of a smoker.

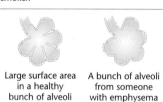

Large surface area in a healthy bunch of alveoli

A bunch of alveoli from someone with emphysema

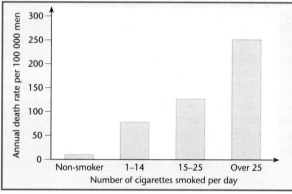

Figure 2 *The increased risk of developing lung cancer.*

Time since quitting	Beneficial health changes that take place
20 minutes	Blood pressure and pulse rate return to normal.
8 hours	Nicotine and carbon monoxide levels in blood reduce by half, oxygen levels return to normal.
24 hours	Carbon monoxide will be eliminated from the body. Lungs start to clear out mucus and other smoking debris.
48 hours	There is no nicotine left in the body. Ability to taste and smell is greatly improved.
72 hours	Breathing becomes easier. Bronchial tubes begin to relax and energy levels increase.
2–12 weeks	Circulation improves.
3–9 months	Coughs, wheezing and breathing problems improve as lung function is increased by up to 10%.
5 years	Risk of a heart attack falls to about half that of a smoker.
10 years	Risk of lung cancer falls to half that of a smoker. Risk of heart attack falls to the same as someone who has never smoked.

Table 1 *The benefits of giving up smoking.*

What do **you** know?

You should now be able to:

- Describe 2 harmful effects of nicotine.
- Explain why carbon monoxide leaves you breathless.
- Explain how tar and other irritants can result in bronchitis, pneumonia and emphysema.
- Explain what bronchitis and emphysema are.
- Review the evidence suggesting smoking causes lung cancer.
- Explain why it is inadvisable to smoke when pregnant.
- List the effects of passive smoking.
- Explain why it is so difficult to give up smoking.
- Describe one occupational disease caused by inhaling a dust.

Chapter 4: Questions

1 a The diagram shows the human breathing system.

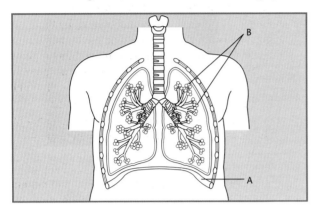

i Name structures A and B.

ii Copy and complete the following passage by writing the correct word or words in the spaces provided. Choose your answers from the list in the box.

bronchioles	carbon dioxide	decrease
downwards	increase	oxygen
rib cage	upwards	

To breathe in, the muscle in structure A must contract. The centre of A will move _____ . At the same time, the intercostal muscles will also contract, moving the _____ upwards and outwards. These two actions increase the volume of the chest cavity and so _____ the pressure inside the lungs. Air is therefore sucked into the lungs. Gaseous exchange occurs at the structures labelled B. This involves the movement of _____ gas into the blood from the inhaled air and the movement of _____ gas from the blood into the air. *(5 marks)*

b A person breathed air into and out of a special machine. The graph shows changes in the volume of air inside the machine. Each time the person breathed in, the line on the graph drops. Each time the person breathed out, the line rises.

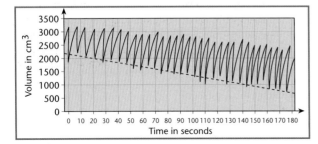

i How many times did the person breathe in during the first minute? *(1 mark)*

ii The dotted line shows the uptake of oxygen. What was the rate of oxygen uptake per minute? (*Show your working.*) *(2 marks)*

iii Breathing into and out of the machine involved a certain amount of work. Give two pieces of evidence from the graph which indicate that the person did work during the experiment. *(2 marks)*

c The table shows a comparison for two athletes who ran in races of different distances.

Athlete	Distance of race (m)	Oxygen needed in the race (dm³)	Oxygen entering blood in the race (dm³)
A	100	10	0.5
B	10 000	150	134.0

i The difference between the oxygen needed and the oxygen actually entering the blood during the race is known as the oxygen debt. What is the oxygen debt for each of the athletes? *(1 mark)*

ii When a race is over both athletes continue to breathe more rapidly and more deeply than normal for some time as they rest. Suggest the reason for this. *(2 marks)*

iii Both of the athletes obtained some of their energy from anaerobic respiration. What is meant by the term **anaerobic respiration?**
(1 mark)
(SEG various)

2 The diagram shows some cells from the lining of the trachea (windpipe).

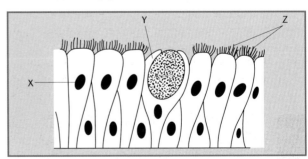

a Name structure X. *(1 mark)*

b Cells of type Y secrete mucus onto the inside surface of the trachea. Give two functions of mucus in the trachea. *(2 marks)*

c How do structures Z help to keep the lungs healthy?
(2 marks)
(SEG June 1999)

3 **a** The bar graph shows the number of deaths from chronic bronchitis and emphysema in women who smoked different numbers of cigarettes.

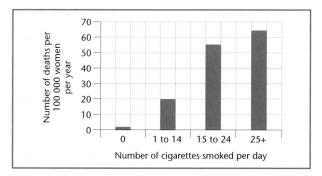

Describe the relationship between the number of cigarettes smoked each day and the number of deaths from chronic bronchitis and emphysema.
(2 marks)

b The diagrams show lung tissue from a healthy person and from a person suffering from emphysema. Both diagrams are drawn to the same scale.

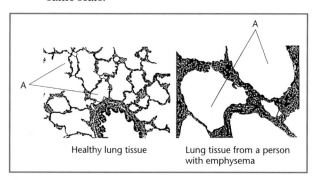

Healthy lung tissue   Lung tissue from a person with emphysema

i Name structure A. *(1 mark)*

ii Emphysema causes changes in the lung tissue. Several of these can be seen in the diagram. Copy and complete the table to describe how each of the two listed features is changed due to emphysema. Also state how each of these changes would affect how quickly oxygen is taken up by the blood passing through the lung. *(4 marks)*

Feature	Change due to emphysema	Effect on how quickly oxygen is taken up
1 Surface area available for diffusion of gases		
2 Thickness of the surface used for diffusion of gases		

c The disease bronchitis is caused by infection of the lungs with bacteria. This causes the production of large amounts of mucus by the cells lining the air passages. The person has to cough to remove the mucus from the lungs.

i What is the normal function of mucus in the lungs? *(1 mark)*

ii Apart from coughing, how is this mucus normally removed from the lungs? *(1 mark)*

iii Explain how cigarette smoking can cause bronchitis.
(You will be awarded up to **one** mark if you write your ideas clearly.) *(5 marks)*

d Name **one** other disease caused by cigarette smoking. *(1 mark)*
(SEG June 1997)

4 **a** Cigarette smoke contains the following substances:
Tar which stops the lining of the breathing passages working.
Nicotine which narrows arteries.
Carbon monoxide which reduces the ability of the blood to carry oxygen.
Dust particles which irritate the lining of the breathing passages.
Using this information explain why a person who smokes may show the following effects:

i 'Smokers cough'

ii high blood pressure

iii breathless after exercise *(3 marks)*

b **i** What is the function of the lining of the breathing passages? *(1 mark)*

ii Explain how smoking stops the lining of the breathing passages working properly. *(1 mark)*

c A man who has smoked 20–30 cigarettes per day for 20 years is worried about the effects of smoking on his health and has decided to give up smoking.

i Name one example of a lung disease that may develop as a result of his smoking habit. *(1 mark)*

ii Suggest which component of smoke is most likely to be responsible for the disease you have named in **i**. *(1 mark)*

iii Suggest two ways in which his family may help him to give up smoking. *(2 marks)*

iv Suggest one reason why this person may find it difficult to give up smoking. *(1 mark)*
(OCR/MEG June 1998)

5 Support and locomotion

Your body contains over 600 muscles and 200 bones. This chapter explains how these work together to produce movement, provide support and maintain posture. It also looks at some of the things that can go wrong and the modern solutions to these problems.

After you have worked through this chapter, you should be able to:

- Name the main bones in the human skeleton.
- List the functions of the skeletal system and describe in detail the specific functions of the skull, backbone, ribcage, girdles and limbs.
- Describe the structure of a long bone.
- Compare the structure and functions of cartilage and bone tissue.
- Explain why bones are strong.
- Discuss osteoporosis.
- Describe the structure of an elbow and hip joint.

- Discuss the problems which stop joints working properly.
- Outline the process of joint replacement.
- Outline the structure and properties of skeletal, smooth and cardiac muscle tissue.
- Describe how muscles can be used to move bones and create movement.
- Define good posture and describe how your muscles help maintain it.
- Discuss some of the problems created by a poor posture.

Orthopaedic solutions

No matter how well we look after our joints, sometimes things can go wrong. Most people will develop some **osteoarthritis** as they get older, probably due to wear and tear. Some will develop **rheumatoid arthritis** for no apparent reason. We are all prone to problems caused by trauma and athletes, in particular, suffer from **torn cartilages** and **damaged joint ligaments**.

Can joints be repaired or replaced?

In cases of severe and irreversible damage to a joint, part of, or even the whole joint can now be replaced. Forty-five thousand complete hip replacement operations are carried out every year in the UK. During the operation the head of the femur is replaced by an alloy and the socket in the pelvis is refashioned and replaced with a high density plastic (see figure 1). The materials are chosen carefully to resist corrosion and withstand the stresses on the joint. But even so, artificial joints only have an expected life span of 10 years.

Repairing joints

Replacing a joint is only ever considered if the pain and disability is so bad that it affects daily activities. Attempts to repair the joint and alleviate the pain are the first course of action. There are several options available:

- **Medical options**. Anti-inflammatory and steriod drugs can be used to reduce pain and inflammation.

- **Surgical options** other than joint replacement include:
  i **Arthroscopy**. Occasionally a piece of cartilage or bone can break free within a joint and cause problems, such as causing the joint to lock. This happens with knee joints especially, because they contain two extra pieces of cartilage which act as shock absorbers. These often tear when subjected to trauma such as a sudden twisting. A procedure called **debridement** is carried out, usually by **keyhole surgery** using an **arthroscope** to remove the damaged tissue. Rather than opening

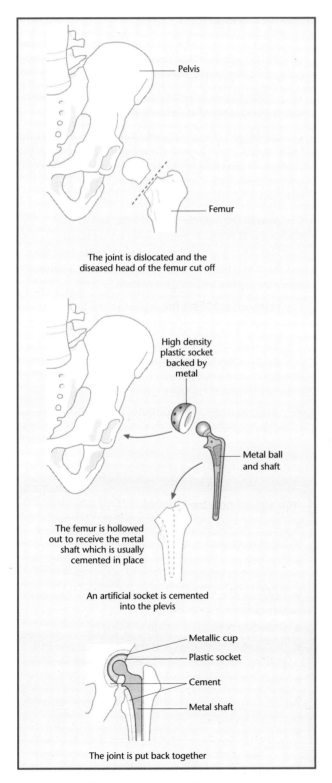

The joint is dislocated and the diseased head of the femur cut off

High density plastic socket backed by metal

Metal ball and shaft

The femur is hollowed out to receive the metal shaft which is usually cemented in place

An artificial socket is cemented into the plevis

Metallic cup

Plastic socket

Cement

Metal shaft

The joint is put back together

Figure 1 *Arthroplasty – the replacement of a joint.*

the knee up, the surgeon makes two small incisions at either side of the joint. Through one incision he slides a small rod-shaped telescope and fibre optic cable. The interior of the knee can now be displayed on a closed circuit TV screen. Small surgical instruments are inserted through the other incision enabling the surgeon to remove or repair damaged structures within the joint (see figure 2).

Sometimes washing the joint out (called **lavage**) to remove debris is sufficient to alleviate the problem.

ii **Osteotomy**. This is carried out on younger people with less severe osteoarthritis. The bone near the problem joint is reshaped so the ends of the bone forming the joint meet at a slightly different angle. This can relieve the pain caused by damaged surfaces rubbing together. It is an operation that is often carried out on the big toe.

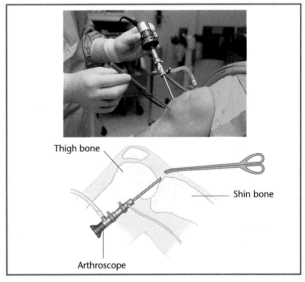

Thigh bone

Shin bone

Arthroscope

Figure 2 *Keyhole surgery using an arthroscope.*

iii **Arthrodesis**. Sometimes arthritic joints are fused together to alleviate pain. For example, collapsed vertebrae can be fused together to stop them pressing against the nerves leaving the spinal canal. One cause of back pain is the result of the fifth lumbar vertebra sliding forward over the sacral vertebra below it. This can be successfully treated by arthrodesis. Arthrodesis is particularly useful for small joints such as fingers and toes.

5.1 The skeleton

Why do you have a skeleton?

The skeleton provides a basic framework inside your body. It supports your body and gives it a shape. Without it, you would collapse.

The bones of the skeleton also:

- help to bring about movement or locomotion by working with the many muscles which are attached to it
- protect some of your vital body organs, such as your brain, heart and lungs
- produce new blood cells in a tissue called **red bone marrow**, which is found in some bones.
- help blood clotting and muscle contraction by providing calcium, a vital mineral to these processes.

What is your skeleton made of?

The human skeleton is made of 206 separate bones. Each bone can be considered an organ (chapter 5.2) but together they form two functional parts:

1 The **axial skeleton** which consists of the skull, ribcage and backbone. All these parts provide protection for vital organs:

The **skull** protects the brain, eyes and ears. It is made from 22 bones most of which are fused together. You can see many of these joins on the cranium (see figure 1). They are known as **sutures**. The bones forming the cranium of a newly born baby are not fully fused together. There are soft membranous spots between them called **fontanelles**. These allow the skull to compress a little during birth. After birth, the soft spots are rapidly replaced by bone.

The **backbone** protects the spinal cord, gives support for the upper body and provides attachment for the back muscles and ribs. It is made from 33 small bones called vertebrae (see figure 2). With the exception of the top two, these all have the same general structure. Each **vertebra** has areas for the attachment of the back muscles and a central canal through which the spinal cord can pass. There are slight differences between vertebrae, depending on where they are located in the backbone. For example, those in the chest region (thoracic vertebrae), have areas that form joints with the ribs, and those in the pelvic region (sacral vertebrae), need to be able to join with the pelvis. The two vertebrae at the top of the neck are called the **atlas** and **axis** vertebrae. These are very different from all the others in that they are modified to support the skull and allow all the different movements the head can make.

The 33 vertebrae are held together by **ligaments**, but in between each one is a small pad of cartilage called an **intervertebral disc**. These discs allow the backbone to bend.

The **ribcage** protects the heart and lungs and is involved in breathing. It is made from 12 pairs of ribs and the **sternum** (breastbone).

2 The **appendicular skeleton** consists of the **pectoral** and **pelvic girdles**, the arms and the legs. These parts are mainly involved in movement:

The girdles connect the limbs with the backbone and are important areas for muscle attachment.

The **pectoral** (shoulder) girdle connects the arms to the backbone. It is made from the **scapula** (shoulder blade) and **clavicle** (collar bone). The scapula provides a large flat area for attachment of the many muscles involved in moving the arm at the shoulder joint.

The **pelvic** (hip) girdle connects the legs to the backbone. It is made from several bones fused together. This provides great strength to support the weight of the body and can also transmit the thrust produced by the legs to the backbone.

The pelvis also protects the organs in the lower part of the abdomen.

The limbs act as levers when creating movement. The pattern of bones in the arm and leg is very similar. The hand contains 19 bones and is one of the most complex structures in the human body. The way the bones and muscles are arranged allows for a wider range of movements than any other animal.

What do **you** know?

You should now be able to:

- List the main functions of the skeleton.
- Label a diagram of the skeleton.
- Colour the appendicular and axial parts in different colours and explain the basis of this split.
- Describe the functions of the skull, backbone and ribcage.
- Draw and annotate a typical vertebra.
- State where the atlas and axis vertebrae are located in the backbone and describe their function.
- Suggest why the lumbar vertebrae are the largest.
- Describe how the vertebrae are held together and explain the function of the intervertebral disc.
- State the functions of the pectoral and pelvic girdles.
- Explain why we have arms and legs.

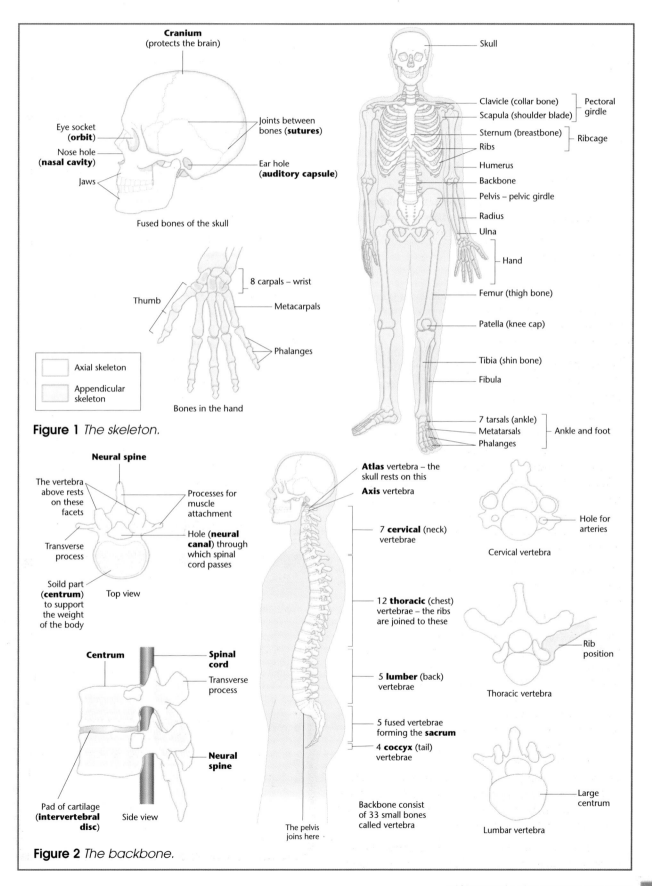

Cranium
(protects the brain)

Skull

Eye socket
(**orbit**)

Nose hole
(**nasal cavity**)

Jaws

Joints between
bones (**sutures**)

Ear hole
(**auditory capsule**)

Fused bones of the skull

Clavicle (collar bone)
Scapula (shoulder blade)

Pectoral
girdle

Sternum (breastbone)
Ribs

Ribcage

Humerus
Backbone
Pelvis – pelvic girdle
Radius
Ulna

Hand

Femur (thigh bone)

Patella (knee cap)

Tibia (shin bone)
Fibula

7 tarsals (ankle)
Metatarsals
Phalanges

Ankle and foot

8 carpals – wrist

Thumb

Metacarpals

Phalanges

Axial skeleton

Appendicular
skeleton

Bones in the hand

Figure 1 *The skeleton.*

Neural spine

The vertebra
above rests
on these
facets

Processes for
muscle
attachment

Hole (**neural
canal**) through
which spinal
cord passes

Transverse
process

Soild part
(**centrum**)
to support
the weight
of the body

Top view

Atlas vertebra – the
skull rests on this

Axis vertebra

7 **cervical** (neck)
vertebrae

Hole for
arteries

Cervical vertebra

12 **thoracic** (chest)
vertebrae – the ribs
are joined to these

Rib
position

Thoracic vertebra

Centrum

**Spinal
cord**

Transverse
process

**Neural
spine**

5 **lumber** (back)
vertebrae

5 fused vertebrae
forming the **sacrum**

4 **coccyx** (tail)
vertebrae

Pad of cartilage
(**intervertebral
disc**)

Side view

The pelvis
joins here

Backbone consist
of 33 small bones
called vertebra

Large
centrum

Lumbar vertebra

Figure 2 *The backbone.*

5.2 Bones

What are bones made of?

Bones come in many different shapes and sizes. Some, like the ribs and bones of the skull, are thin and flat. These mostly provide protection for vital organs. Others, like the bones in the limbs, are thick and long to provide support and transmit movement. Whatever their shape and function, they are all made of two kinds of living tissue:

● **Bone tissue**. This consists of special bone cells called **osteocytes**, embedded in a matrix which they produce. This matrix is partly flexible protein (**collagen**), and partly a hard mixture of calcium salts (mainly calcium phosphate). The properties of both these non-living substances contribute to the great strength and durability of bone.

There are two kinds of bone tissue:

1 **Compact bone tissue** on the outside of bone. This contains a higher proportion of calcium salts making it strong and hard.

2 **Spongy bone tissue** underneath the compact tissue. This contains fewer calcium salts, but is still strong. It is called spongy because it contains spaces, just like a sponge, which makes it lighter. In some bones, these spaces are filled with **red bone marrow**, a blood producing tissue.

● **Cartilage tissue**. Cartilage is a tough, yet flexible, material containing cartilage cells called **chondrocytes**. These secrete a matrix of **glycoproteins** (proteins with a carbohydrate molecule attached). Embedded in this are varying amounts of collagen and elastic protein fibres, producing three functional types of cartilage: **hyaline**, **fibrous** and **elastic**. The cartilage in the pinna of the ear is very flexible (elastic), but the cartilage covering the ends of bones is quite rigid and very smooth (hyaline).

Some of the larger bones in your body have a hollow centre to make them lighter. This cavity is filled with bone marrow, which in adults is mainly fat and therefore called **yellow bone marrow**.

All bones are enclosed in a protective membrane containing blood vessels and nerves. The tendons and the ligaments are attached to this.

Can bones grow?

All bones begin as cartilage. When a baby is born most, but not all, of this cartilage has already been turned into bone by a process called **ossification**. The remaining areas of cartilage can be identified on X-rays of a child's skeleton (see figure 2). They appear as gaps in the bones. These areas of cartilage are the growth areas of the bone (see figure 3). As the skeleton reaches full size, all the cartilage becomes ossified and the bone can no longer grow, although it can still repair itself when damaged.

Although long bones stop growing around the age of 18 years, they undergo changes as we continue to age. They are also continually being remodelled to accommodate changing stresses and blood calcium levels. These changes, to a large extent, are controlled by our hormones and are affected by our diet, health and exercise. In general, bones are usually strongest in early adulthood, but then start to lose minerals and weaken with age. This happens more quickly in women because of the hormonal changes during the menopause.

Why do children need to drink lots of milk?

Milk contains calcium and vitamin D. Calcium makes bones hard and rigid, without it bones become soft and bend easily. This condition is called **rickets**. Vitamin D is needed for the absorption of calcium from our food.

What is osteoporosis?

Osteoporosis is a condition that generally affects older people, especially older women. It occurs as a result of removal of more minerals from bone tissue than are deposited, leaving the bones weak and brittle. This happens to everyone over the age of 35 years, and by the age of 70 years, most people's bone density will have fallen by a third. Women are particularly vulnerable because of the hormonal changes that accompany the menopause.

There are no cures for osteoporosis, but it can be slowed down by maintaining a healthy diet containing adequate amounts of calcium and vitamin D.

What do **you** know?

You should now be able to:

● Label a diagram of a long bone and annotate it with the functions of the parts.
● Explain the difference between hard and spongy bone tissue.
● Explain the difference between red and yellow bone marrow.
● State the functions of the calcium salts and collagen in bone tissue.
● Use diagrams to explain how bones grow.
● Explain why X-rays of the bones of a child's hand show gaps between the bones.
● Explain why it is important for children to drink milk.
● Explain what osteoporosis is and suggest who is most at risk and why.

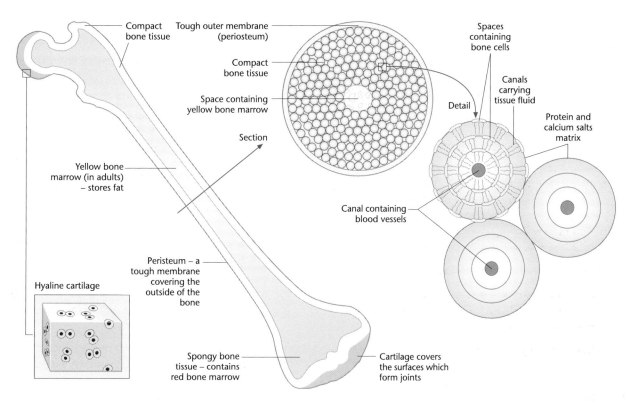

Figure 1 *Section through a long bone.*

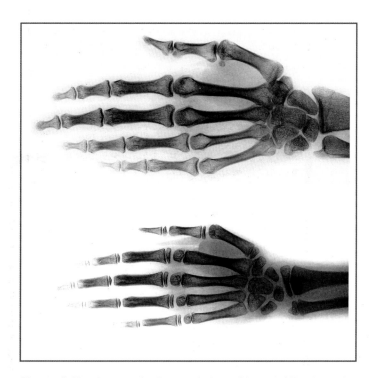

Figure 2 *The lower photograph is an X-ray of the hand of a child. It shows the areas of cartilage where the bone grows. Compare it with the adult's hand above.*

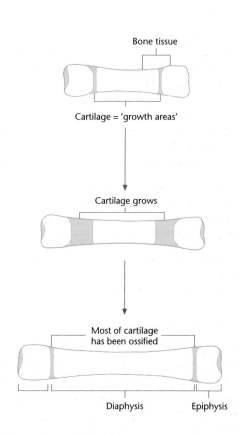

Figure 3 *How a bone gets bigger.*

5.3 Joints

What are joints?

Joints are formed where the end of one bone meets another. There are over 200 places in your skeleton where this happens. The obvious joints are in your shoulder, elbow, hip, knee, hands and feet. Your hand alone has over 20 joints. Joints that enable parts of your skeleton to move are referred to as **movable joints**.

Some joints, however, e.g. the **sutures** in the cranium, do not allow movement and are called **fixed joints.**

Are all movable joints the same?

Some movable joints only allow a small amount of movement. These are often called **slightly movable joints**. An example is the joint between the vertebrae of your backbone. There is a pad of fibrous cartilage in the junction between the vertebrae and this only permits a slight amount of movement between the bones.

Most joints in your body are **freely movable**. These are often called **synovial joints** because of their structure. They are adapted for friction-free movement. The ends of the bones are covered in slippery cartilage and a lubricating fluid is produced by the joint membrane.

Movable joints are often classified by the type and range of movement they allow. Details of the main types are shown in figure 1.

Why do bones stay together at joints?

Bones are held together at joints by pieces of strong fibrous connective tissue called **ligaments**. These ligaments often form a complete capsule around the joint, and control its movement and stability. Ligaments are elastic, but even so, they can be damaged. This happens when bones are pulled apart, **dislocating** the joint, or you **sprain** a joint by twisting it. Damaged ligaments will soon become weak and prone to further damage. Many athletes have to give up sport because of ligament damage.

What is a torn cartilage?

Footballers often get torn cartilages in the knee. The knee has two extra pieces of cartilage, called the **menisci**, to strengthen and protect the joint. If these tear and pieces lodge between the bones, the joint can lock. Usually, an operation is needed to remove the damaged cartilage tissue. This operation is carried out using an **arthroscope** in a technique called **keyhole surgery**. This avoids cutting open the joint (see page 60).

What is arthritis?

Arthritis is the term used to describe painful swollen joints. The inflammation can be caused by several things, but there are two main forms of arthritis:

- **Osteoarthritis**. This is a result of the cartilage at the ends of the bones wearing away more quickly than it can be repaired and replaced. This is often due to injury or old age, but can also result from over-exercising, especially as a child, while the bones are still growing. Eventually, the bone surfaces become exposed and rub together creating unpleasant grating. The joint becomes inflamed and painful (see figure 3). The hip and knee joints are the main ones affected by osteoarthritis.

- **Rheumatoid arthritis**. The causes of this are unclear, but it is probably, in part, due to an **autoimmune** response whereby the body attacks its own tissues. The inflammation begins in the synovial membrane which swells up and then starts to disintegrate. Cartilage on the ends of the bones becomes soft and wears away very quickly, leaving the joint stiff and very painful. Rheumatoid arthritis usually affects several joints at the same time and may disappear and reappear. Women are more prone to it than men.

Joints which are particularly badly damaged may often be replaced. Full details can be found on page 60.

What do **you** know?

You should now be able to:

- List the 3 main kinds of joint in your body and name 1 place each type is found.
- Label a diagram and annotate the functions of the main parts of a typical synovial joint.
- Label a diagram of an elbow joint and describe the kind of movement it is capable of.
- Label a diagram of a hip joint and describe the kinds of movement it is capable of.
- Describe the roles of ligaments at joints and describe how they can be damaged.
- Explain the differences between osteo- and rheumatiod arthritis.
- Describe how an arthroscope is used to look at knee cartilages.
- Describe how a hip joint can be replaced.

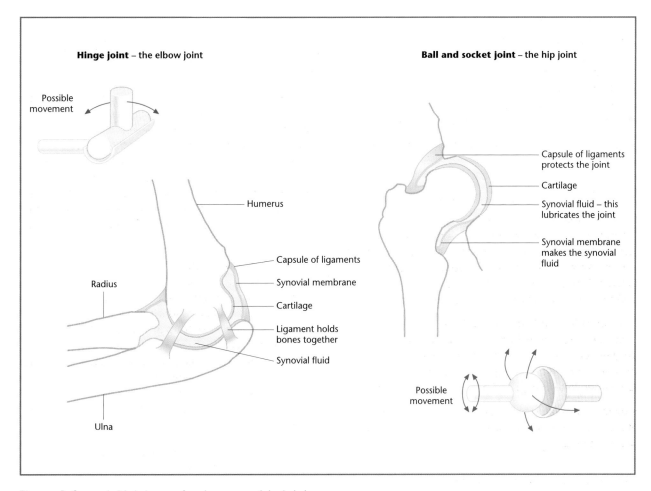

Hinge joint – the elbow joint

Possible movement

Humerus

Radius

Ulna

Capsule of ligaments

Synovial membrane

Cartilage

Ligament holds bones together

Synovial fluid

Ball and socket joint – the hip joint

Capsule of ligaments protects the joint

Cartilage

Synovial fluid – this lubricates the joint

Synovial membrane makes the synovial fluid

Possible movement

Figure 1 *Synovial joints are freely moveable joints.*

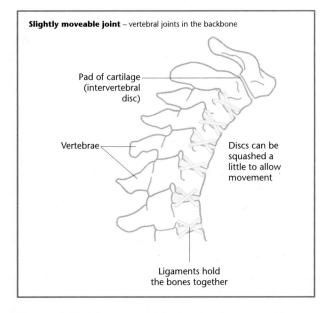

Slightly moveable joint – vertebral joints in the backbone

Pad of cartilage (intervertebral disc)

Vertebrae

Discs can be squashed a little to allow movement

Ligaments hold the bones together

Figure 2 *Slightly moveable joints allow a small amount of movement between bones.*

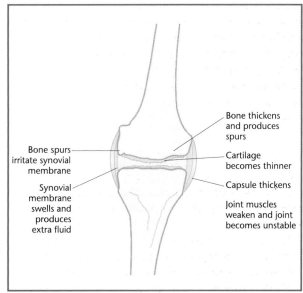

Bone thickens and produces spurs

Cartilage becomes thinner

Capsule thickens

Joint muscles weaken and joint becomes unstable

Bone spurs irritate synovial membrane

Synovial membrane swells and produces extra fluid

Figure 3 *Osteoarthritis mostly affects the hip and knee joints.*

5.4 Muscles and movement

What is muscle tissue?

Muscle tissue makes up about 50% of your body weight. There are three kinds of tissue, each having specific functions, but all are made from cells containing **contractile proteins**. Using available energy, these proteins contract, thereby shortening the cells in the muscle tissue (muscle contraction) and causing movement.

The types of muscle tissue

- **Skeletal muscle tissue**. The cells of skeletal muscle are joined together to form long fibres. These fibres are found bundled together and several of these bundles together form a 'muscle' (see figure 2a).

  Skeletal muscles are all attached to the skeleton. They are also sometimes called **striped muscle** because of their appearance when viewed through a microscope. Skeletal muscles pull on the bones to produce movement and maintain **posture**. They are generally large and powerful muscles, capable of very fast or very slow contractions. Unfortunately they also tire quickly (become **fatigued**).

  Because you choose when you want to use these muscles, they are sometimes called **voluntary muscles**.

- **Smooth muscle tissue**. Smooth muscle is made from long thin tapered cells held together by a fibrous connective tissue (see figure 2b). This type of muscle is found in the walls of hollow tubular organs such as the gut, ureters and blood vessels. The cells are arranged so that the protein fibres either run along or around the organ. These form the **circular** and **longitudinal** muscles respectively, which enable the passage of substances through the organs by **peristalsis** (chapter 2.4). Smooth muscle is ideal for this because it does not tire, can produce smooth and regular contractions and requires no conscious thought, i.e. the movements are involuntary. Peristalsis is happening inside your body all the time, but you would never know!

  These muscles are sometimes called **involuntary muscles**.

- **Cardiac muscle tissue.** Cardiac muscle is very similar in structure to skeletal muscle except that the parallel fibres are cross-linked together at intervals (see figure 2c). Its properties, however, are very different. Cardiac muscle is only found in the heart. It contracts on average 70 times a minute for 70 years, without ever tiring and without outside control. It initiates its own contractions which are described as **myogenic**,

that is they originate in muscle independent of nervous stimulation. The brain, however, can influence the heart's natural **pacemaker** (chapter 3.4), making it speed up or slow down the rate of contractions.

How do muscles move bones?

The skeletal muscles are attached to bones by pieces of non-stretching fibrous connective tissue called **tendons**. One end of a muscle (described as the **origin** end) is always attached to a bone which does not move and the other end (the **insertion** end) is attached to a bone near a joint which does move. When the muscle contracts, it pulls on the bones and the bone near the joint moves in the direction of the pull. Movement is therefore produced by a **lever system**, the joint acting as the fulcrum, the bone as the lever and the muscle providing the effort (the force) to overcome any resistance (the load).

How is the arm moved?

Figure 3 illustrates how the biceps muscle moves the bones in the lower part of your arm. To straighten your arm, another muscle is required to pull on the bones at the opposite side of the elbow joint. All muscles work in pairs like this. The muscle that bends the joint is called the **flexor** muscle and the muscle that straightens it is called the **extensor** muscle. The flexor and extensor muscles are known as an **antagonistic pair** of muscles. Remember, muscles must always work in pairs because muscles can only contract on their own. They have to be pulled back into a relaxed state.

What do **you** know?

You should now be able to:

- Outline the structure of the 3 kinds of muscle tissue.
- Explain why cardiac muscle is described as myogenic.
- Describe how muscles are attached to bones and explain the terms origin and insertion.
- Explain the different functions and properties of tendons and ligaments.
- Name the two antagonistic muscles in the upper arm. Describe which muscle is the flexor and which is the extensor.
- Describe, using diagrams, how these muscles bend and straighten the arm.

5.4

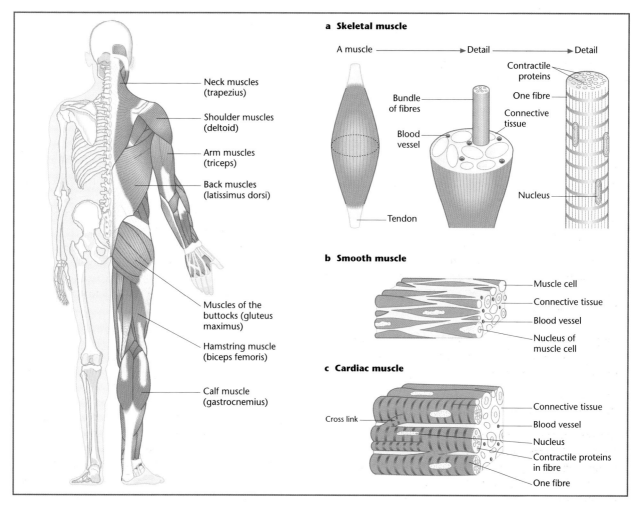

Figure 1 *There are over 600 skeletal muscles. These are some of the main ones.*

Figure 2 *There are 3 types of muscle, each with a different function.*

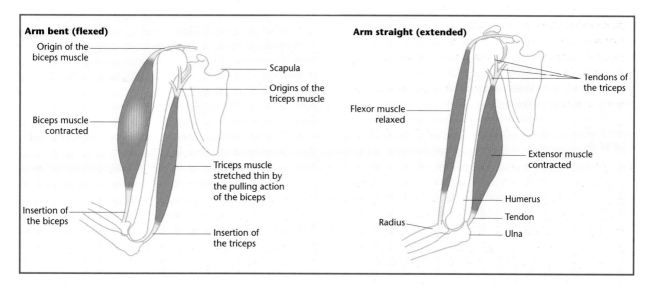

Figure 3 *The muscles of the arm work as an antagonistic pair.*

5.5 Posture

What is posture?

Your posture is the position in which your body is held by your muscles and ligaments. This will depend upon many factors, some of the more obvious ones being:

- muscle strength and muscle tone
- flexibility of your joints
- age and health, e.g. degree of stress, state of feet, and so on.
- diet, e.g. lack of calcium could cause rickets
- weight and body build

What is muscle tone?

Skeletal muscles never completely relax. Some fibres are always slightly contracted so they are in an active state and ready for further contraction. This slight contraction is called **muscle tone**.

Muscle tone is important in maintaining posture. A good posture is one where the antagonistic groups of muscles in your body (i.e. flexors and extensors) have the same degree of muscle tone so they exactly balance each other. In this condition the muscles of your body are using as little energy as possible. The muscles involved in maintaining posture are collectively called **anti-gravity muscles** (see figure 1). If the degree of muscle tone of even one of these muscles varies, your whole postural balance can be disturbed.

What is a good posture?

A good posture is one in which the bones of the body are held in such a way as to allow all the organs of the body to work and grow properly. The joints should be able to achieve the full range of movements, and the muscles should be using as little energy as possible in maintaining the posture.

Your **centre of gravity** is the point through which gravity acts on your body. In a good posture the centre of gravity will always be such that the loads on the skeleton will be distributed evenly on all sides. If your body is balanced in this way, there will be no strain on your muscles, ligaments or joints.

There are recognised good postures for standing, sitting and lifting. These are illustrated in figure 2.

Your backbone has four natural curves (chapter 5.1). A good posture will maintain and support these. Bad posture may exaggerate or flatten these leading to some quite serious problems. Three main problems are illustrated in figure 4.

How is posture maintained?

You maintain your posture in three ways:

- by visual clues
- by messages from the organs of balance in your ears
- by involuntary reflex actions involving receptors in your joints, muscles and tendons.

What are the effects of poor posture?

If your body is not held in a good position, many organs cannot work or grow properly. For example, if your shoulders sag forward, your chest will be cramped and your lungs will not be able to expand fully, preventing you getting enough oxygen. A bent backbone will cramp your digestive system, causing digestive problems. This will also put strain on the muscles and ligaments of your back, which could result in serious back problems.

Generally, a poor posture will result in muscle aches, weakened ligaments, stressed and therefore painful joints, cramped organs, poor blood and lymph flow and a feeling of tiredness.

Do badly fitting shoes affect posture?

A foot has two arches (see figure 3) which are crucial to locomotion, support and balance. Wearing badly fitting shoes or high heel shoes can damage these arches and, therefore, affect the way you move and your posture. High heels, for example, will accentuate the longitudinal arch and throw your body forwards. You automatically compensate by moving your chest backwards creating a hollow back and plenty of backache.

Badly fitting shoes can also cause a number of other problems, some of which are described in chapter 12.3.

What do **you** know?

You should now be able to:

- Explain what 'good posture' is and how it is maintained.
- Explain the importance of muscle tone in posture.
- List the factors that can affect your posture.
- Describe a good standing and sitting posture.
- Explain how to lift a weight safely.
- Explain how poor posture can result in a hump back, a hollow back and a lateral spine.
- Describe some of the other effects of bad posture.
- Explain why badly fitting or high heel shoes can affect your posture.

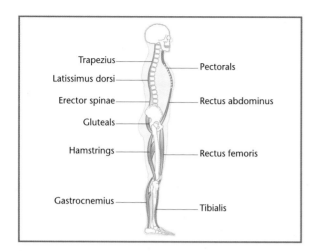

Figure 1 *Some of the anti-gravity muscles.*

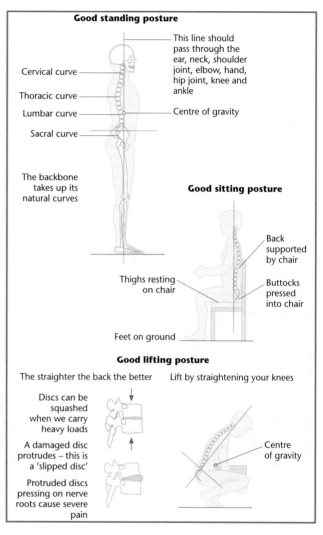

Figure 2 *Good sitting, standing and lifting posture.*

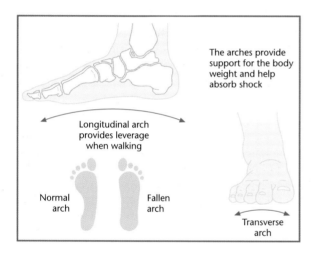

Figure 3 *The foot has two arches.*

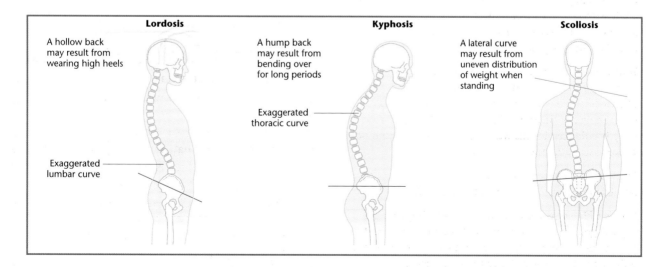

Figure 4 *Some common postural problems.*

Chapter 5: Questions

1 a The presence of calcium salts in bone make it hard and rigid. Briefly describe the method and results of an experiment you could do to show this. *(1 mark)*

b The diagram shows a femur cut open vertically along its length.

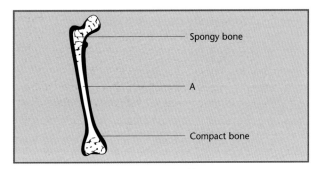

Spongy bone

A

Compact bone

i What tissue is present in region A? *(1 mark)*

ii What is the advantage of the spongy bone having the structure that is shown in the diagram? *(1 mark)*
(SEG June 1990)

2 a The diagram below shows a synovial joint in the skeleton.

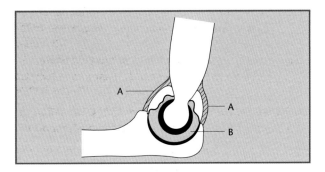

A

A

B

i Give one property of the tissue which protects the articulating surfaces. *(1 mark)*

ii What is the function of the material which fills the space labelled B? *(1 mark)*

iii Give two properties of the tissue labelled A. *(2 marks)*

b The diagram below shows two lumbar vertebrae as they would be joined in the vertebral column.

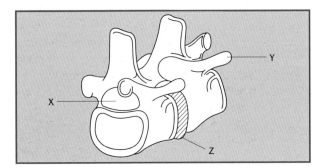

Y

X

Z

i What passes through the cavity labelled X in the living body? *(1 mark)*

ii What is the function of the projection labelled Y? *(1 mark)*

iii What is the function of the structure labelled Z? *(1 mark)*
(SEG June 1988)

3 The drawing shows the bones and muscles of the elbow joint.

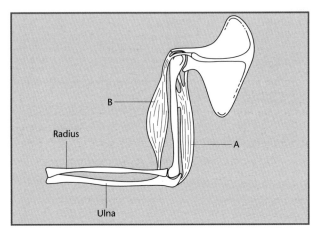

B

Radius

A

Ulna

a Name muscles A and B. *(2 marks)*

b Describe how the action of muscle A would straighten the arm at the elbow joint. *(2 marks)*
(SEG June 1999)

4 The diagrams below show a person with a poor standing posture and one with a good standing posture.

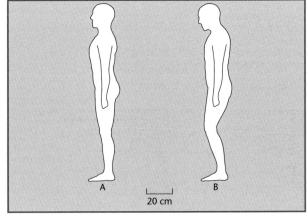

A

20 cm

B

a Give three ways in which posture shown in Diagram A is different from the posture shown in Diagram B.

b i Which diagram, A or B, shows the good posture? *(1 mark)*

ii Give one reason for your answer. *(1 mark)*
(SEG June 1988)

5 The diagram below shows a section through a hip joint.

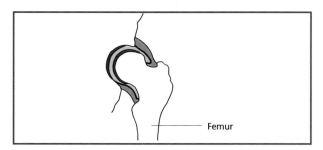

Femur

a Draw the diagram, label the following with a clear guideline and the name of the part:
  i synovial fluid;
  ii cartilage;
  iii ligament. *(3 marks)*
b Some elderly people need to have a hip replacement operation. In this operation, the top of the femur (the 'ball') is removed and replaced by a new 'ball', made of either metal or plastic, as shown in the diagrams below.

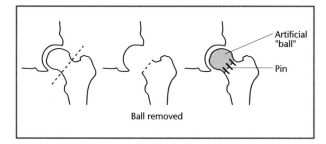

Artificial "ball"

Pin

Ball removed

The new 'ball' must have certain properties if it is to be used in a hip replacement operation. Suggest two of these properties. *(2 marks)*
(NEAB Sample assessment)

6 It is possible to replace a diseased or damaged hip joint with an artificial joint. One method of doing this is shown in the diagrams.

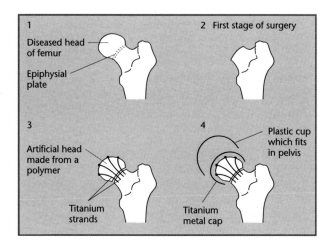

1
Diseased head of femur
Epiphysial plate

2 First stage of surgery

3
Artificial head made from a polymer
Titanium strands

4
Plastic cup which fits in pelvis
Titanium metal cap

a Use the diagrams to describe the stages in this method of joint replacement. *(4 marks)*
b The part of the joint which is fixed into the femur has a ball-shaped 'head' and is covered with Titanium (a metal). Suggest a reason why the 'head' is
  i ball-shaped, *(1 mark)*
  ii covered with metal. *(1 mark)*
(SEG June 1995)

7 The diagram shows the position of the human foot bones whilst wearing high-heeled shoes. Examine the picture carefully, then answer the questions that follow.

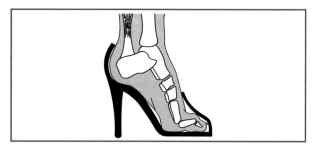

a Suggest two ways in which high-heeled shoes can damage the feet. *(2 marks)*
b What damage can wearing high-heeled shoes cause to the wearer's body other than to the feet? *(2 marks)*
c Give one reason why it is important for young children to wear shoes that fit correctly. *(2 marks)*
(SEG June 1995/6)

8 The diagram shows the back view of a person sitting on a bench. Some features of the skeleton are also shown.

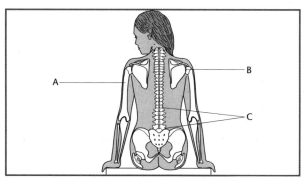

A
B
C

a Name the bone labelled A. *(1 mark)*
b Name a tissue, other than bone. that you would expect to find in the joint labelled B. *(1 mark)*
c i Name the region of the vertebral column labelled C. *(1 mark)*
  ii Suggest one way in which the posture of the person is a good one for sitting on a bench without a back rest *(1 mark)*
(SEG June 1994)

6 The senses

Prick yourself with a needle and it hurts. Walk past a fresh bread counter and the smell makes your mouth water. A sudden noise behind you and you turn round to look. These may all seem quite simple responses to every day situations, but they all involve a very complex system of communication within your body. In this chapter you will learn more about this communication system and how it helps you to respond and react to the constant changes which are taking place in your environment.

After you have worked through this chapter, you should be able to:

- Outline the sequence of events in responding to change.

- Describe the role of receptors in detecting change.

- Describe the location of your main sensory receptors.

- Describe the structure of the eye and the functions of its main parts.

- Explain how the eye focuses on an object.

- Describe how you are able to focus on both near and distant objects.

- Explain the causes and solutions to the eye defects: long and short sight; astigmatism; cataracts.

- Describe the structure of the ear.

- Explain the process of hearing.

- Explain how you keep your balance.

Pain sensations

What is pain?

Pain is a very complex phenomenon and many factors contribute to it. It is defined as 'the feeling of distress, suffering or agony caused by stimulation of specialised nerve endings.' We could add to this and say that it is always unpleasant and always an emotional experience. Each person learns, from their past experiences, the feeling of pain. No two people will experience or describe their pain in the same way.

What is the purpose of pain?

Pain is a requirement for normal life. It acts as a warning sign of actual or imminent tissue damage and enables us to take protective action. A healthy person can usually tolerate more pain than a person who is ill.

Types of pain

Pain is classified as **acute** or **chronic**, **somatic** (to do with the outer covering of the body) or **visceral** (to do with the internal organs). Acute pain is always somatic and is 'felt' very quickly after stimulation. It is usually described as sharp, such as being cut with a knife, or piercing, such as a prick with a needle.

Chronic pain can be both somatic and visceral and is not 'felt' as quickly as acute pain. It may even build up in intensity until it becomes excruciating. Chronic pain is often described as burning, aching or throbbing.

The pain pathway

Pain receptors are called **nociceptors**. They are located in almost all tissues: in skin, bones, muscles, connective tissues and the internal organs.

Nociceptors respond to any stimulus, for example heat, cold, pressure, touch, and so on, that is strong enough to cause tissue damage. For this it must be above a certain threshold. Overstimulation of some of the other sensory receptors is also registered as pain, for example overstimulation of sound receptors.

The nociceptors change the stimuli into nerve impulses, which are conducted along nerve fibres into the central nervous system (CNS). Recognition of the type of pain, that is gripping, sharp, cutting, etc takes place in the brain. The cerebral cortex in the brain interprets the message of pain (chapter 7.1). For somatic pain, the pain is usually felt in the area first stimulated. With visceral pain the pain is felt in the skin or connective tissue above the organ. This is because the nerves taking the pain messages into the CNS are bundled up with the sensory nerves from the skin. The nerve impulses somehow manage to cross into these so pain from the heart for example is felt in the skin over the heart and down the left side of the left arm. This is called **referred pain** and is a valuable clue for doctors when diagnosing internal problems (see figure 1).

The part of the nervous system which deals with visceral pain also controls the heart rate (HR), breathing rate (BR) and digestive processes so when stimulated by pain, you often also feel nauseous, dizzy and your HR and BR go up.

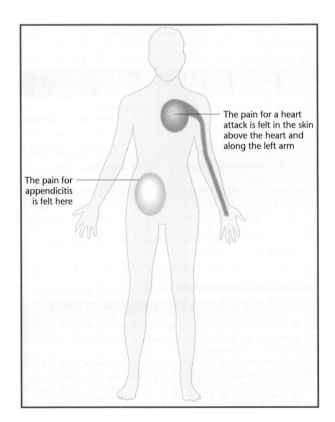

Figure 1 *Referred pain is the term used for pain 'felt' in the skin above the organ.*

The pain for a heart attack is felt in the skin above the heart and along the left arm

The pain for appendicitis is felt here

The management of pain

Pain is a symptom and the long term relief of it depends on treating the cause. Temporary pain relief can be achieved by using chemicals. Your body makes its own natural painkillers called **endorphins**. These block the cell-to-cell transmissions in the brain, stopping pain messages being passed on to the relevant parts of the brain.

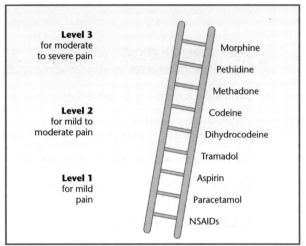

Level 3 for moderate to severe pain

Morphine
Pethidine
Methadone

Level 2 for mild to moderate pain

Codeine
Dihydrocodeine
Tramadol

Level 1 for mild pain

Aspirin
Paracetamol
NSAIDs

Figure 2 *The ladder of pain relief.*

Drugs which can be taken to control pain in the body are called **analgesics**. There are two main groups:

● **Non opioids** are drugs like **paracetamol**, aspirin and **NSAIDs** (non steroidal anti-inflammatory drugs). These are used against mild or moderate pain. With the exception of paracetamol, they block pain at the site of stimulation. They have what is called a ceiling effect, in that they have a maximum effective dose and going above this does not improve the pain relief.

● **Opioids** are drugs like **codeine**, **heroin** and **morphine**. These are very powerful pain killers which work (as does paracetamol) in a similar way to your own endorphins. It is because they replace endorphins, that you get withdrawal symptoms should you become dependent on them.

In managed pain relief, as for cancer pain, it is usual to start with the non-opioids and move onto the weak opioids, such as dihydrocodiene, before trying the strong potent opioids like morphine.

6.1 Sensory perception

Responding to change

Your surroundings change all the time. It gets dark as night falls; there are noises in the street; it is cold outside and warm inside; your new clothes feel rough on your skin. We detect all these changes with special sensory cells, called **receptors**. Each receptor is connected to a nerve which will take a message to the brain. The brain interprets this message. If a response is required, it will send a message along another nerve to an **effector**. The main effectors in your body are your muscles and glands. The receptors are grouped together forming **sense organs** (see figure 2).

What do we respond to?

Anything that produces a response is called a **stimulus**. The main changes in our environment, which act as stimuli are due to light, sound, heat, cold, touch, pressure and chemicals. We have separate receptors to detect each of these stimuli.

How do receptors work?

A receptor is a cell which can change the energy from a stimulus into a nerve impulse, i.e. can **transduce** energy. For example, the light energy which enters your eye can be changed into a nerve impulse by **light receptors** (called **rod** and **cone cells**) at the back of your eye. The nerve impulse travels along a nerve to the brain, which uses the message to form a picture and may also send a message to an effector to produce a response.

Responding to chemicals

The receptors which are stimulated by chemicals are located in your **tongue** and an area of your nasal cavity called the **olfactory area** (see figure 2). These areas are permanently covered by a layer of moisture in which the chemicals must first dissolve if they are to be detected.

There are four kinds of receptor in your tongue, each sensitive to a different chemical. These chemical stimuli are **salt**, **sweet**, **bitter** and **sour** (see figure 2). The flavour of a food is determined by how many of each of these receptors are stimulated, together with the smell. Your tongue also contains receptors which can sense the texture and temperature of food.

The sensation of smell is created when the chemical receptors in your olfactory area are stimulated.

The skin as a sense organ

Your skin is the largest of your sense organs. It contains a number of different receptors (see figure 2). Each type of receptor can respond to several stimuli, but is more sensitive to a one particular kind. Some are more sensitive to light pressure (**touch**), some to heavier **pressure**, some to **heat** and some to **cold**. There are even receptors which specialise in creating the sensation of **pain**. However, overstimulation of any of the receptors is also registered as pain.

Are parts of my skin more or less sensitive?

The skin receptors are distributed over your body surface in such a way that some parts are more sensitive than others. The sensitivity is determined by the number of receptors per square millimetre of skin surface. For example, the lips, finger tips, soles of your feet and external sex organs have more touch receptors per square millimetre than other areas. This makes them more sensitive.

Stimulus	Receptor	Sense organ
Chemicals	Taste buds and olfactory cells	Tongue Nose
Touch	Touch receptors	Skin
Pressure	Pressure receptors	Skin
Warmth and cold	Temperature receptors	Skin
Pain	Pain receptors	Skin
Light	Rods and cone cells	Eye
Sound	Sensory hair cells	Ear
Movement and gravity	Sensory hair cells	Ear

Table 1 *The main stimuli and corresponding receptors in the body.*

What do **you** know?

You should now be able to:

- Outline the sequence of events in responding to change.
- List the main stimuli we respond to.
- Describe, with an example, how a receptor works.
- Name the 5 main sense organs and the kind of receptors they contain.
- Draw a diagram to show the position of the main sensory receptors in the skin.
- Explain why some areas of skin are more sensitive than others.
- Describe why you can taste, smell, detect the texture and the temperature of your food.

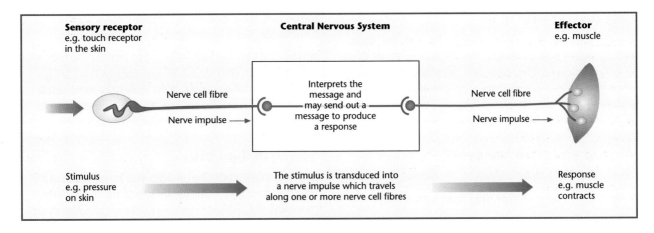

Figure 1 *Responding to change involves many different structures.*

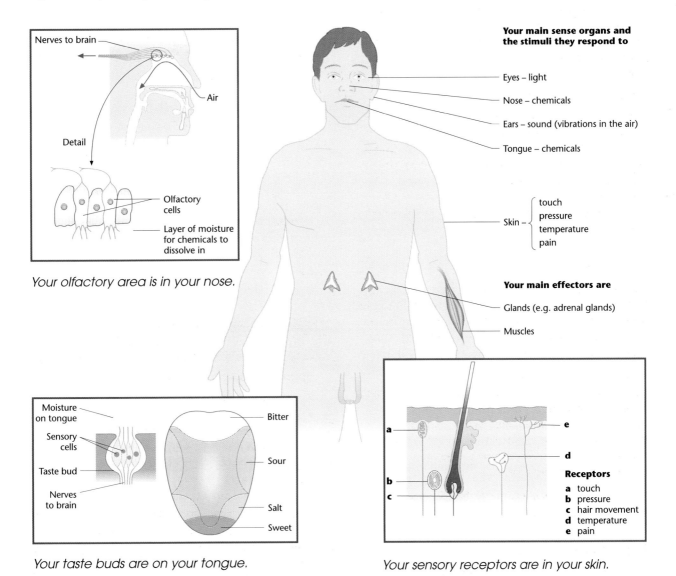

Your main sense organs and the stimuli they respond to

Eyes – light

Nose – chemicals

Ears – sound (vibrations in the air)

Tongue – chemicals

Skin – touch
pressure
temperature
pain

Your main effectors are

Glands (e.g. adrenal glands)

Muscles

Your olfactory area is in your nose.

Your taste buds are on your tongue.

Your sensory receptors are in your skin.

Figure 2 *Your main senses.*

6.2 The eyes and vision

How do you see?

The eye is the sense organ responsible for detecting light. Your brain receives messages from the eyes and uses them to 'form a picture'. The response is instantaneous so that, when your eyes are open, they are constantly stimulated and your brain constantly 'forming a picture'. This is the sensation we call **vision**.

Why do you have two eyes?

There are at least three advantages to having two eyes:

- you can see over a larger area than with one eye

- you can judge short distances

- can you see an object in three dimensions (3D), that is, you see the depth of objects as well as their height and width. With 3D vision (sometimes called **binocular vision**), you can judge the size and shape of objects and the speed of a moving object much more accurately.

The structure of the eye

The eye (see figure 1) contains:

- light sensitive cells (receptors). These form the **retina** at the back of the eye. The nerve fibres which take the messages from these cells to the brain form the **optic nerve**.

- structures to focus the light onto the retina, i.e. the **cornea** and **lens**.

- structures to protect and support the eye, i.e. the **sclera**, **choroid layer**, **iris** and the **aqueous** and **vitreous humours**.

Each eye is housed in a bony socket (**orbit**) at the front of the skull. It is held in position by six muscles which can move it up, down or sideways (see figure 2). This enables you to move your eyes around to look at things in different places.

The surface of the eye is constantly cleaned and kept moist by tears produced by the **tear glands**. Tears contain an enzyme called **lysozyme** which kills bacteria. Blinking spreads the tears over the exposed surface of the eye.

The light sensitive receptor cells are found in the retina of the eye (see figure 4). There are two kinds, **rod cells** and **cone cells**. Rod cells can be stimulated by all wavelengths of light except red light, but your brain only registers these as shades of black and white. They can however, respond in low light intensities (dim light).

There are three kinds of cone cell, each sensitive to one of the primary colours (red, green and blue). Your brain registers these colours, and when required, mixes them to produce other colours. Cones are only stimulated in bright light, such as daylight or a well-lit room.

A typical retina contains about 150 million rod cells and 7 million cone cells. The rods are more or less evenly spread out, whereas most of the cones occupy a small region of the retina called the **fovea**. Light striking this area produces the clearest images in the brain.

Seeing in the dark

You may have noticed that after you have switched a bright light off, you cannot see anything at all. Only gradually do you begin to see things, but only in shades of grey. This is because your cone cells are no longer being stimulated by the dim light and your rod cells cannot initially respond. They have been overstimulated by the very bright light and need time to recover and start working again. Getting use to the darkness is called **dark adaptation**. The size of the pupil also alters in bright and dim light.

How does your eye work?

You are able to see objects because every object reflects rays of light and some of these rays enter your eyes. To see an object clearly (described as **in focus**), these light rays must be bent (**refracted**) inwards so they meet exactly on the retina at the back of your eye and stimulate the same receptor cell. If they are bent too little, or too much, your image of the object will be blurred (**out of focus**). This rarely happens as the focusing of light rays is done automatically by the eye. The light rays are refracted by the cornea and the lens so that they are always in focus (see figure 3).

What do **YOU** know?

You should now be able to:

- Label a diagram of the eye.
- Annotate your diagram with the functions of the cornea, iris, lens, ciliary muscles, suspensory ligaments, retina, and optic nerve.
- Describe the positions of, and compare the roles of the rods and cones.
- Outline how the eye perceives colour.
- Explain dark adaptation.
- Draw a diagram to show how the eye focuses on an object.
- Name the parts of the eye which refract light.
- Explain the advantages of having two eyes.

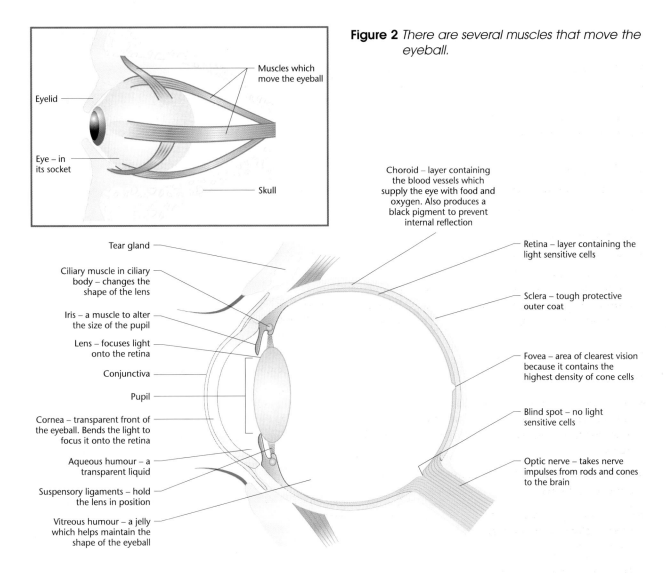

Figure 2 *There are several muscles that move the eyeball.*

Muscles which move the eyeball

Eyelid

Eye – in its socket

Skull

Choroid – layer containing the blood vessels which supply the eye with food and oxygen. Also produces a black pigment to prevent internal reflection

Tear gland

Ciliary muscle in ciliary body – changes the shape of the lens

Iris – a muscle to alter the size of the pupil

Lens – focuses light onto the retina

Conjunctiva

Pupil

Cornea – transparent front of the eyeball. Bends the light to focus it onto the retina

Aqueous humour – a transparent liquid

Suspensory ligaments – hold the lens in position

Vitreous humour – a jelly which helps maintain the shape of the eyeball

Retina – layer containing the light sensitive cells

Sclera – tough protective outer coat

Fovea – area of clearest vision because it contains the highest density of cone cells

Blind spot – no light sensitive cells

Optic nerve – takes nerve impulses from rods and cones to the brain

Figure 1 *A section through the eyeball.*

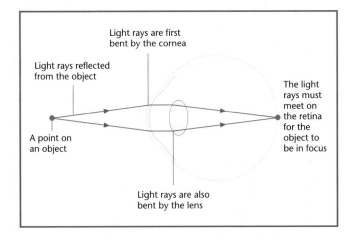

Light rays are first bent by the cornea

Light rays reflected from the object

A point on an object

The light rays must meet on the retina for the object to be in focus

Light rays are also bent by the lens

Figure 3 *How the eye focuses on an object.*

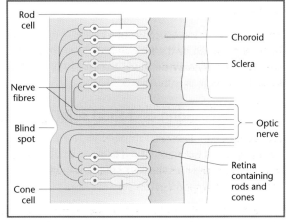

Rod cell

Nerve fibres

Blind spot

Cone cell

Choroid

Sclera

Optic nerve

Retina containing rods and cones

Figure 4 *Detail of the retina.*

6.3 Seeing clearly

How does your eye change its focus?

Your eye can bring light rays from a distant object into focus and then change to focus on a near object by altering the shape of its lens. In general, the fatter, more rounded a lens is, the more it bends the light rays. When your eye is focusing on a distant object, it will have a thinner, flatter lens. As the object moves closer, the lens keeps it in focus by getting more rounded. This automatic adjustment of the lens to keep an object in focus is called **accommodation.**

How is the lens shape altered?

The lens is held in position by **suspensory ligaments** attached to the **ciliary body**. The ciliary body contains a circular muscle called the **ciliary muscle**. This muscle can contract or relax, changing the tension on the suspensory ligaments and, in doing so, altering the shape of the lens. When the suspensory ligaments are taut, the lens is pulled into the thinner, flatter shape needed for distant vision. When the suspensory ligaments are slack, this allows the natural elasticity of the lens to change its shape and become fatter and more rounded for near vision (see figure 1).

As you get older, the elasticity of the lens often decreases, making accommodation difficult. This is called old sight (**presbyopia**) and is the stage when many people have to start wearing glasses for reading.

In some older people, the lens becomes clouded stopping light passing through it. This is known as a **cataract**. A cataract can be treated by replacing the lens with an artificial one, but you will still have to wear spectacles for reading.

Why does the size of the pupil alter?

The **pupil** is the opening through which light enters your eye. The size of it can be altered to allow more or less light into the eye as required by the surrounding conditions (see figure 1). This is altered automatically by the **iris**, a membranous structure containing two sets of opposing muscles and the pigment that provides your eye colour. Contraction of the **circular** muscle reduces the diameter of the pupil and contraction of the **radial** muscle increases it.

What causes long and short sight?

To see clearly, your eyeball must be perfectly formed and not too long or too short. The lens must be able to change shape easily. For many people, this is a problem which affects their vision:

- **Long sight** (hypermetropia). A long sighted person can see distant objects clearly, but has difficulty focusing on near objects. This is usually the result of a short eyeball, but can also be caused by a lens which is too weak (too thin). To correct long sight, the eye must be helped to bend the light rays more, so that they are brought into focus on the retina. This can be achieved by wearing spectacles containing **converging** (**convex**) **lenses**. A converging lens will bend the light rays inwards a little before they enter the eye (see figure 2).

- **Short sight** (myopia). A short sighted person can see near objects clearly, but has difficulty focusing on distant objects. This is usually the result of a long eyeball, but can also be caused by a lens which is too strong (too fat). To correct short sight, the light rays must be bent outwards before they enter the eye. This can be achieved by wearing glasses that contain **diverging** (**concave**) **lenses** (see figure 3).

Other eye defects

- **Astigmatism**. This describes the blurred vision and distorted images that some people suffer because the curvature across the front of the eye from side to side is not the same as that from top to bottom. As light rays pass through the **cornea**, some are bent more than others and this makes it impossible to focus all the rays at the same point on the retina.

  Astigmatism can be corrected by wearing specially prepared lenses. In very bad cases a corneal graft may be needed.

- **Glaucoma**. This describes a build up of pressure in the eye caused by a failure to drain away excess fluid. It commonly affects older people and is a major cause of blindness.

What do YOU know?

You should now be able to:

- Name the parts of the eye involved in changing the shape of the lens for accommodation.
- Describe how the shape of the lens differs for focusing on near and distant objects.
- Describe and explain what happens to the pupil when focused on near and distant objects.
- Explain how the ciliary muscle and suspensory ligaments alter the shape of the lens.
- Describe the causes and solutions to short sight.
- Describe the causes and solutions to long sight.
- Explain the difference between converging and diverging lenses.
- Describe what astigmatism and cataract are.

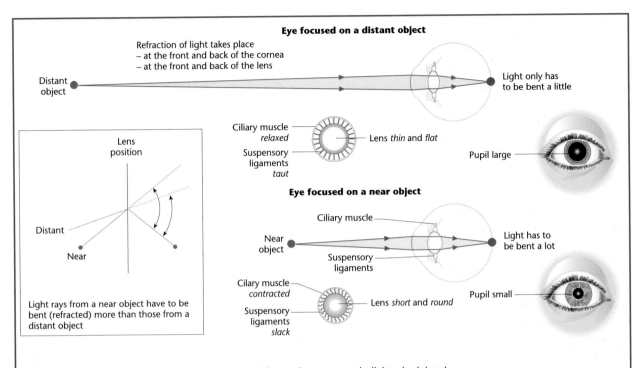

Eye focused on a distant object

Refraction of light takes place
– at the front and back of the cornea
– at the front and back of the lens

Distant object

Light only has to be bent a little

Lens position

Distant

Near

Light rays from a near object have to be bent (refracted) more than those from a distant object

Ciliary muscle *relaxed*

Suspensory ligaments *taut*

Lens *thin* and *flat*

Pupil large

Eye focused on a near object

Ciliary muscle

Near object

Suspensory ligaments

Light has to be bent a lot

Cilary muscle *contracted*

Suspensory ligaments *slack*

Lens *short* and *round*

Pupil small

Figure 1 *Changes in the eye when looking at near and distant objects.*

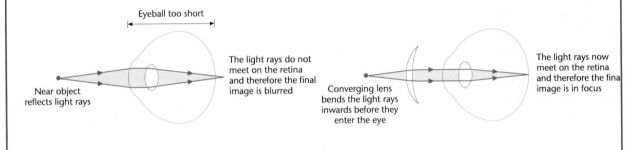

Eyeball too short

Near object reflects light rays

The light rays do not meet on the retina and therefore the final image is blurred

Converging lens bends the light rays inwards before they enter the eye

The light rays now meet on the retina and therefore the final image is in focus

Figure 2 *Long sight and its correction.*

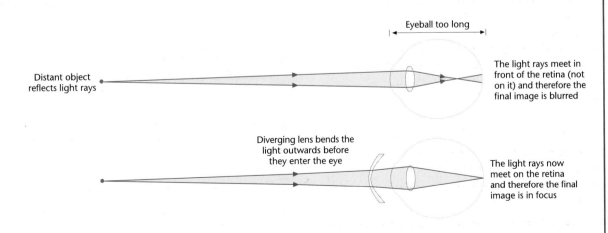

Eyeball too long

Distant object reflects light rays

The light rays meet in front of the retina (not on it) and therefore the final image is blurred

Diverging lens bends the light outwards before they enter the eye

The light rays now meet on the retina and therefore the final image is in focus

Figure 3 *Short sight and its correction.*

6.4 The ear and sound perception

Your ear as a sense organ

You use your ears to hear sound. The receptor cells are housed in a fluid filled part of the middle ear called the **cochlea**. The sound sensation heard by your ears is actually caused by vibrations in the air. These pass into the fluid within the cochlea and stimulate the receptors which generate a nerve impulse in the **auditory nerve** leading to the brain. It is your brain which translates this into sound.

The ear also contains the **semi-circular canals**, the organ which gives you your sense of balance.

The structure of the ear

The ear (see figure l) contains:

- The sound receptors called **sensory hair cells**. These form part of the **cochlea** within the inner ear.

- Structures to convert sound waves into mechanical vibrations, i.e. the **ear drum**, **ear ossicles** and **oval window**.

- Structures to direct sound waves into the ear and onto the ear drum, i.e. the **pinna** and **ear canal**.

- Receptors which are sensitive to movement of the head with respect to gravity. These are housed in the organs of balance, i.e. the **semi-circular canals**, **utriculus** and **sacculus**.

Messages are taken from the receptors in the ear to the brain via the **auditory nerve**.

How does the ear work?

Sound waves in the air are collected by the **pinna** (ear flap) and directed onto the **ear drum**, which is made to vibrate. These vibrations are intensified by the **ear ossicles**, three tiny bones in the middle ear, before being passed onto the **oval window** and then into the fluid within the **cochlea**. The vibrations within the cochlea stimulate the **sensory hair cells** which send a signal to the brain via the **auditory nerve** (see figure 2). Each sound creates a different pattern of signals. These signals arriving at the brain give us the sensation of hearing.

Loudness and pitch

A loud noise will cause large vibrations within the cochlea. When your brain gets the signal it will assign a loud sound. Noises of different pitch are picked up by different receptor cells in the ear. A high pitched noise stimulates the receptor cells near the oval window which then send the signal to the brain. A low pitched noise stimulates the receptors near the end of the cochlea.

Your brain can also tell you the direction the sound came from by using messages from both ears.

What gives you your sense of balance?

Your body maintains its balance and posture in a very complex process. Your brain receives messages from special receptors, mainly in your joints, muscles and tendons. Messages also come from the organs of balance in your inner ear. The semi-circular canals are three fluid-filled tubes at right angles to one another. At one end of each is a sense organ (**ampulla**). When the fluid moves as your head moves, this organ is stimulated. Dizziness is the feeling you get when your brain receives conflicting messages. If you suddenly stop moving, the fluid in the semi-circular canals continues to move and your brain thinks you are still moving, yet the messages from your eyes contradict this. The position of your head with respect to gravity and acceleration are detected in a similar way by the **utriculus** and **sacculus**.

Why do your ears pop?

The pressure on both sides of the ear drum must be the same for you to hear things clearly. If the external air pressure changes, the pressure in the middle ear is automatically adjusted to match this by air entering or leaving via the **eustachian tube**. As you ascend in an aeroplane, the external pressure goes down and if air is not free to leave the middle ear, the ear drum bulges outwards. When you swallow, this opens the eustachian tube and air rapidly exits the middle ear. The pop is caused by the ear drum quickly returning to its normal position.

Your eustachian tube may become blocked with mucus when you have a throat infection. This will affect your hearing as well as your ability to cope with pressure changes.

What do **you** know?

You should now be able to:

- Label a diagram of the ear.
- Annotate the diagram with functions of the ear canal, ear drum, ossicles, cochlea, semi-circular canals, auditory nerve and eustachian tube.
- Use a diagram to explain how you hear sound.
- Explain the role of the eustachian tube.
- Explain how you keep your balance.
- Explain why you sometimes feel dizzy.

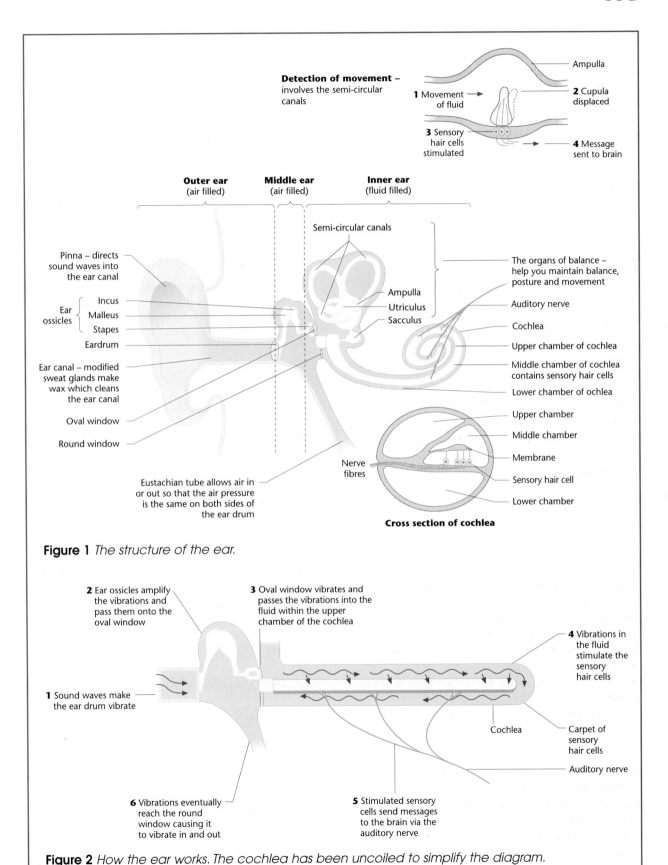

Detection of movement – involves the semi-circular canals

1 Movement of fluid

Ampulla

2 Cupula displaced

3 Sensory hair cells stimulated

4 Message sent to brain

Outer ear (air filled) **Middle ear** (air filled) **Inner ear** (fluid filled)

Semi-circular canals

Pinna – directs sound waves into the ear canal

Ear ossicles { Incus, Malleus, Stapes

Eardrum

Ear canal – modified sweat glands make wax which cleans the ear canal

Oval window

Round window

Eustachian tube allows air in or out so that the air pressure is the same on both sides of the ear drum

Ampulla
Utriculus
Sacculus

Nerve fibres

The organs of balance – help you maintain balance, posture and movement

Auditory nerve

Cochlea

Upper chamber of cochlea

Middle chamber of cochlea contains sensory hair cells

Lower chamber of ochlea

Upper chamber

Middle chamber

Membrane

Sensory hair cell

Lower chamber

Cross section of cochlea

Figure 1 *The structure of the ear.*

2 Ear ossicles amplify the vibrations and pass them onto the oval window

3 Oval window vibrates and passes the vibrations into the fluid within the upper chamber of the cochlea

4 Vibrations in the fluid stimulate the sensory hair cells

1 Sound waves make the ear drum vibrate

Cochlea

Carpet of sensory hair cells

Auditory nerve

6 Vibrations eventually reach the round window causing it to vibrate in and out

5 Stimulated sensory cells send messages to the brain via the auditory nerve

Figure 2 *How the ear works. The cochlea has been uncoiled to simplify the diagram.*

Chapter 6: Questions

1 The diagram shows a section through the skin.

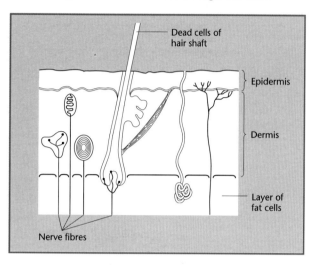

a How many different types of nerve endings are shown? *(1 mark)*

b Name a stimulus other than touch which can affect one of the receptors in the skin. *(1 mark)*

c Describe one way in which a named effector in the body could respond to this stimulus. *(1 mark)*
(SEG June 1990)

2 a Name the organ in the human body which is sensitive to
  i presure *(1 mark)*
  ii vibrations. *(1 mark)*
  The diagram shows a section of an eye.

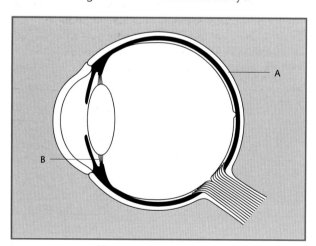

b Name the parts labelled A and B. *(2 marks)*

c Name one structure which
  i allows light to enter the eye; *(1 mark)*
  ii focuses light. *(1 mark)*

d i Name the part of the eye which contains light sensitive cells. *(1 mark)*
  ii Describe how the eye detects light and sends information to the brain. *(2 marks)*

e The diagram shows the part of the eye which controls the amount of light entering.

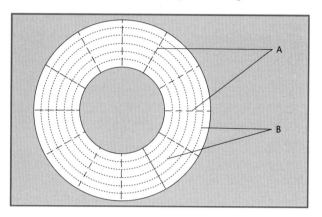

i Name the parts labelled A and B. *(2 marks)*

ii Name the part of the eye which controls the amount of light entering. *(1 mark)*

f Opticians sometimes use tropicamide to keep the pupil wide open while they examine the retina. This substance works by preventing muscle contraction.

i Which eye muscles would be affected by this drug? *(1 mark)*

ii After using tropicamide people are kept in a darkened room for a short time. Suggest why.
(1 mark)
(NEAB June 1999)

3 a The diagram shows a section through a human eye which is focusing light rays from a near object.

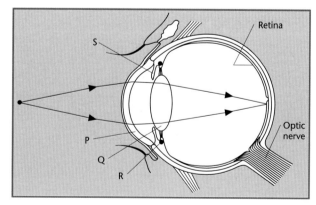

i Name structures P, Q, and R. *(3 marks)*

ii If the object were moved further away from the eye,
  1 What would happen to the shape of structure Q? *(1 mark)*
  2 What must structure R do to cause this change in the shape of Q? *(1 mark)*

iii How do changes in structure S help us to see clearly. *(2 marks)*

b The diagram shows the eye of a person who suffers from an eye defect. The light rays are shown coming from a very distant object.

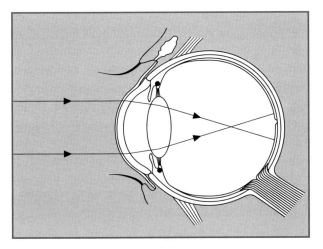

i Is this person long-sighted or short-sighted? *(1 mark)*

ii Explain why this person would not see the object clearly. *(2 marks)*

iii Draw a simplified diagram and add in front of the eye, the type of lens needed to correct this eye defect. *(1 mark)*

c What do the retina, the optic nerve and the brain each do to help a person to see? *(4 marks)*

(SEG June 1996)

4 The diagram shows a section through the ear.

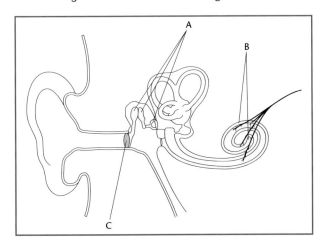

a Name the parts A, B and C. *(3 marks)*

b Name the part of the ear which contains the sound receptor cells. *(1 mark)*

c i Name the part of the ear which collects sound waves. *(1 mark)*

ii Draw a diagram with arrows to show the path followed by sound waves from the outside to the receptor cells. *(2 marks)*

d The diagram shows the path of sound waves from a sound source.

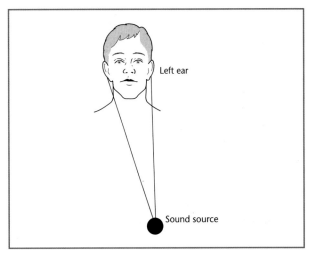

The sound is louder in the left ear than in the right ear. Suggest how this allows a person to work out the direction of a sound source. *(2 marks)*

e Each of the following is a possible cause of deafness. For each, suggest one reason why it may cause some loss of hearing:

i excess ear wax hardening and forming a lump in the external ear;

ii fluid building up inside the middle ear during an infection:

iii the auditory nerve from the ear to the brain is destroyed by a neurone disease. *(3 marks)*

f The diagram below is from the packaging of cotton wool buds which may be used to clean the ears. Suggest why using the cotton buds incorrectly may damage hearing. *(2 marks)*

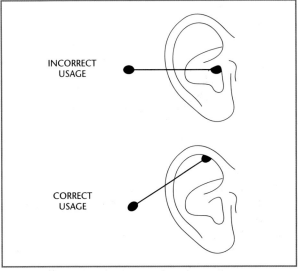

(NEAB June 1998)

7 Co-ordination

Classical pianists can make over 1000 movements a minute with their hands and fingers. Speaking involves precise co-ordination of breathing, mouth shape and the tension in the vocal cords. Neither of these would be possible without an overall control and communication system within your body. In this chapter you find out how the nervous system manages the other body systems.

After you have worked through this chapter, you should be able to:

- Explain the precise role of the nervous system in your body.
- Outline the organisation of the nervous system and describe the roles of the different components.
- Distinguish between reflex and voluntary actions.
- Describe the structures and functions of the three kinds of nerve cell.
- Show how neurones work together to co-ordinate reflex actions.
- Explain the nature and roles of the synapse and neurotransmitters.

- Label a diagram of the brain.
- Describe some of the main functions of the different areas.
- Outline the structure of the spinal cord.
- Explain how the central nervous system is protected from injury.
- Describe the location in the body of the main endocrine glands.
- Outline the actions of the main hormones these produce.
- Compare nervous and chemical co-ordination.

The brain

The human brain is an amazingly complex organ. It consists of over 20 billion nerve cells and billions of connections between them. It's difficult to imagine but it runs a complicated human body, apparently without any hitches. At this very moment, millions of messages about the state of your body are passing into your brain and it's sending out the appropriate responses. At the same time it can be responding to messages from external stimuli, forming pictures and sounds, creating mental images and feeling emotions. No wonder it receives about one fifth of the body's blood supply – it's doing a lot of work!

The whole brain is important, but in reviewing its functions we can select several parts. The largest and most prominent part is the **cerebrum**. This looks like a walnut (see figure 1) because the surface is wrinkled and folded to maximise the space available in the skull.

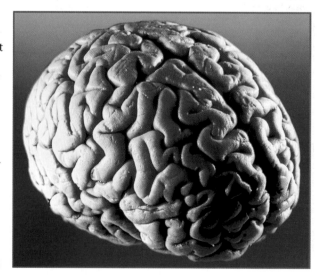

Figure 1 *The area of the brain called the cerebrum.*

The cerebrum is divided into two halves, the right and left cerebral hemispheres. It is in the outer layer of these, the **cerebral cortex**, that we do our thinking, feel sensations, store memories and feel emotions. Strangely, the left hemisphere receives messages from the right side of the body and vice versa. There is also evidence that the left hemisphere is more involved in spoken and written language, reading, reasoning and numerical and scientific skills. In contrast, the right hemisphere is responsible for the imagination, creating mental images, musical and artistic appreciation and our sense of humour.

The hemispheres are connected by groups of nerve fibres, which are called the **corpus callosum**. These connections are crucial to normal functioning and if anything disrupts them, such as brain damage or epilepsy, they operate as separate brains. This is called the split brain personality. Interestingly, if a person with this closes the left eye and looks at a familiar object, he will recognise it but will be unable to speak its name.

Each cerebral hemisphere has several lobes, the **frontal**, **parietal**, **temporal**, **limbic** and **occipital lobes**. Although the brain integrates all its parts to function, it is possible to assign specific functions to these lobes. For example, the frontal lobe is the area concerned with the conscious mind, intellect and emotion. Much of your individualised behaviour comes from here and it is because of this that surgical removal of part of this (frontal lobotomy) was a recognised medical treatment. These days it is more common to use drugs as a treatment.

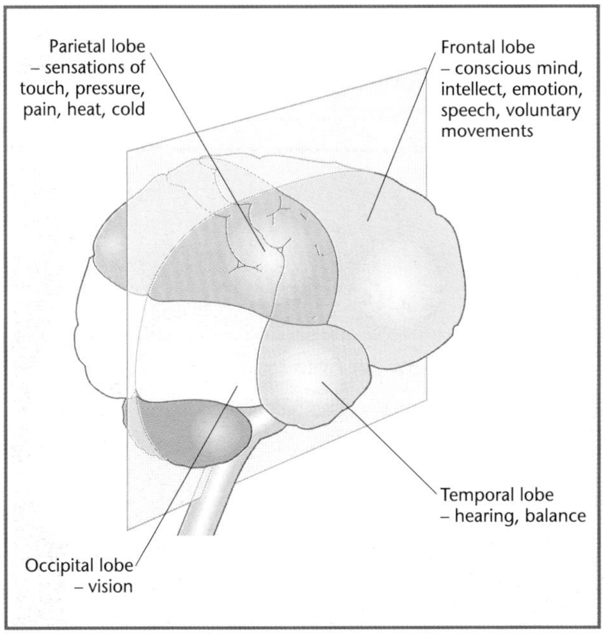

The limbic lobe is located below the other lobes and is thought to provide the link between thoughts and emotions. It forms part of the **limbic system**, which is partly responsible for emotions, sexual drive, motivation, pleasure thoughts and biological rhythms.

Different parts of the cerebral cortex interpret different kinds of information, and the **thalamus**, an area underneath the cerebrum, just above the brainstem, acts as a reliable relay centre to direct the sensory input to the relevant area. The thalamus first decodes the message before re-directing it. If emergency action to prevent tissue damage is required then it will also send out a response to the appropriate effectors, for example, to pull your hand away from something hot.

Part of your brain monitors and controls the internal environment of your body. This is the main role of the **brainstem** and **hypothalamus**. These collect information from other parts of the body and make appropriate responses by sending out messages via the **autonomic nervous system**. For instance, to slow the heart rate, increase the breathing rate or increase sweating to cool the body.

Does your brain sleep?

Your brain does not sleep, but it can alter its degree of alertness. In the brainstem is a complicated collection of nerve cells called the **reticular activating system** (RAS). This is linked to the cerebral cortex and by interfacing with this it maintains consciousness and a state of alertness. If it is continually stimulated then you are kept awake and messages are passed on to the cerebral cortex. If stimulation slows, you can drift into sleep. Intense stimulation such as pain will induce the RAS to arouse you from sleep. Many drugs, such as amphetamines and anaesthetics, work by stimulating or inhibiting the RAS.

Parietal lobe – sensations of touch, pressure, pain, heat, cold

Frontal lobe – conscious mind, intellect, emotion, speech, voluntary movements

Temporal lobe – hearing, balance

Occipital lobe – vision

Figure 2 *The cerebral hemispheres have several lobes.*

7.1 The nervous system

Why do you have a nervous system?

Your nervous system manages your body by:

- **collecting information** about changes in your internal and external environments, i.e. from receptors located at various places in your body

- **interpreting** this information, sometimes using memories of past experiences

- **initiating responses** to these changes, i.e. muscular contractions and glandular secretions.

By these actions, your nervous system co-ordinates muscles so you can do things like walking, swimming, writing and reading. It also helps to regulate your body's internal environment by, for example, making adjustments to your breathing and heart rate to meet the demands of exercise. This helps to maintain a constant environment around the cells, a process called homoeostasis (chapter 8.1). In short, it organises nearly everything that goes on in your body.

The organisation of the nervous system

The nervous system has two parts (see figure 1):

- The **central nervous system** (CNS) formed from the **brain** and **spinal cord**. All the messages from sensory receptors are first sent here. They are interpreted and responses initiated.

- The **peripheral nervous system** (PNS) formed from the **nerves** carrying messages from sensory receptors into the CNS and taking messages away from the CNS to the effectors.

The basic unit of both systems is the nerve cell. The brain alone consists of over ten thousand million nerve cells bound together by supportive tissue. Nerves are formed from bundles of nerve cells wrapped in a protective connective tissue.

How does the nervous system work?

You can compare your nervous system to a telephone system (see figure 2). In a telephone system, a person dials a number which is sent as an electrical signal to the exchange. The signal is relayed to the appropriate outgoing line and results in the ringing of a telephone at the end of it.

Your nervous system works in a similar way. The spinal cord is like the exchange, receiving messages from sensory receptors in all parts of the body, and sending out an appropriate response to the effectors. In our telephone system the receptors and effectors would be the telephones and the nerves would be the lines to and from the telephones.

The similarity does not stop there. If someone needs some extra help, such as finding a telephone number he can ring the operator at the exchange. A similar thing happens in your nervous system. Sometimes before a message is sent out from the spinal cord, it is relayed to the brain to be interpreted using the memories there, and then the most appropriate response sent out.

Reflex and voluntary actions

- **Reflex actions** are those actions that you do without any conscious thought. Blinking to clear dust from the surface of your eye, altering the size of your pupil when entering a dark room, and your mouth watering when you smell or see food are all examples of reflex actions. You have no control over these. They happen automatically.

- **Voluntary actions** are actions which you can control, that is, you decide to do them. You decide to run or walk, read or write, empty your bladder and so on. Some of these, such as emptying your bladder, start as reflex actions, but you learn to control them.

What is the autonomic nervous system?

The **autonomic nervous system** (ANS) is the part of your nervous system which controls all the things that you do not think about, but are necessary for life. For example, when you start exercising, to meet the demand for extra oxygen, your brain sends out messages, which result in an increase in your rate and depth of breathing. To speed up the delivery of this oxygen, a similar message is sent to your heart, resulting in an increase in the heart rate. These actions are involuntary; i.e. they happen automatically, as do all the actions involving the ANS.

What do **you** know?

You should now be able to:

- Explain the role of the NS in managing your body.
- Give an example of how the NS helps to maintain homeostasis.
- Outline the functions of the CNS.
- Describe the functions of the PNS.
- Explain the difference between a simple reflex and a voluntary reflex.
- Outline the role of the ANS in your body.

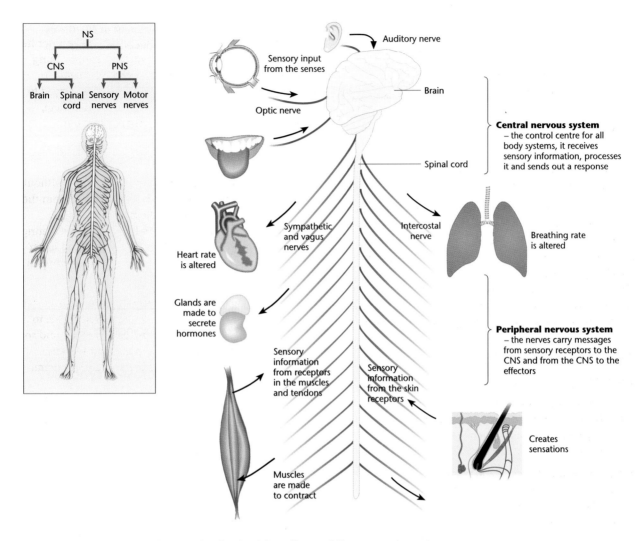

Figure 1 *The organisation and selected functions of the nervous system.*

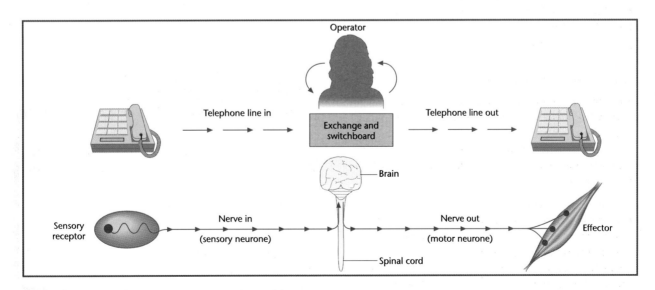

Figure 2 *The nervous system compared to a telephone system.*

7.2 Neurones and reflexes _____

What do nerve cells look like?

A nerve cell is usually referred to as a **neurone**. Neurones are highly specialised for carrying tiny electrical messages called **nerve impulses**. In addition to a nucleus and cyloplasm, they have long thread like processes called fibres, some of which can be over a metre long.

There are three basic kinds of neurone:

- **sensory neurones**. These carry messages from the sensory receptors into the CNS.

- **motor neurones**. These carry messages out of the CNS to the effectors (muscles and glands).

- **relay** (connecting) **neurones**. These carry messages around inside the CNS and link sensory and motor neurones together. They can also relay messages to and from the brain.

The full structure of sensory and motor neurones is shown in figure 2. Notice that the neurone fibre has two parts, the **dendron**, which carries the nerve impulse towards the cell body and the **axon**, which carries it away from the cell body. The fibres of neurones outside the CNS are covered in a fatty material called **myelin**. A **nerve** is formed from hundreds of these fibres and their myelin bundled together and enclosed in a connective tissue tube (see figure 1). Compare this to a telephone cable: the cable contains individual lines from the telephones just like a nerve contains individual neurones from receptors.

How do neurones work together?

The neurones form a link between a receptor and an effector. This can be illustrated by the simplest form of nervous activity, a **reflex action**. Figure 3 shows how the neurones link together when you prick your finger. This nerve pathway is called a **reflex arc**. Notice that the neurones are not physically joined together, but separated by a small gap called a **synapse**. Similar simple reflex arcs exist for all involuntary responses such as blinking, the production of saliva and altering the size of the pupil. Many are inbuilt survival mechanisms and present at birth. You can see this in the actions of a newborn baby (chapter 10.1).

The learning process involves setting up what are often called **conditioned reflexes**. Learning to walk for example, may be difficult to start with, but then you do it without thinking about it, i.e. it becomes a reflex action; a conditioned reflex. Conditioned reflex arcs often involve the brain and can be very complex.

What is a nerve impulse?

The message carried by neurones is called a **nerve impulse**. This takes the form of a small electrical

current and is created by the movement of chemicals, mainly sodium ions (Na^+) and potassium ions (K^+) in and out of the neurone fibre.

The myelin around the neurone fibres provides insulation, and so increases the speed of the nerve impulse along a fibre.

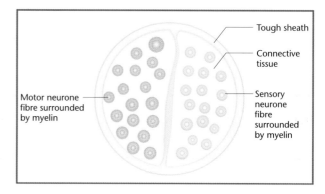

Figure 1 *A section through a spinal nerve.*

How do nerve impulses cross a synapse?

Nerve impulses are transferred from one neurone to another by chemicals called **neurotransmitters**. There are many examples, but the main one in your body is called **acetylcholine**. How this works is illustrated in figure 4. Many drugs, e.g. nicotine, mimic the action of these neurotransmitters and therefore stimulate or depress the nervous system (chapter 12.6).

Synapses are extremely important to the working of the nervous system because they act like gates and make sure messages only travel in one direction. They also help filter out weak or unwanted stimuli and enable information from different sources to interact.

What do **you** know?

You should now be able to:

- Describe the functions of the 3 types of neurone.
- Draw and label a sensory and a motor neurone.
- Explain the difference between a neurone and a nerve.
- Draw the reflex arc for pricking your finger. Annotate with the sequence of events.
- Explain the term conditioned reflex.
- Describe the nature of the nerve impulse.
- Describe how a nerve impulse crosses a synapse.
- Name a neurotransmitter.

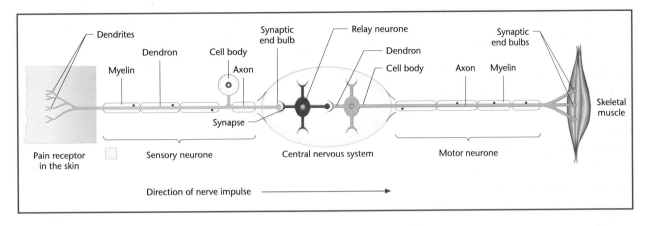

Figure 2 *Reflex arc showing the structure of the neurones.*

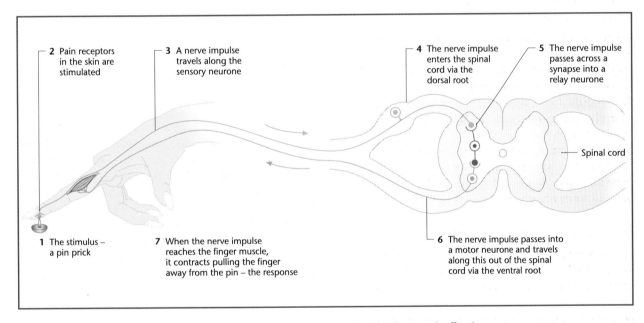

Figure 3 *A simple reflex action showing the link between receptor and effector.*

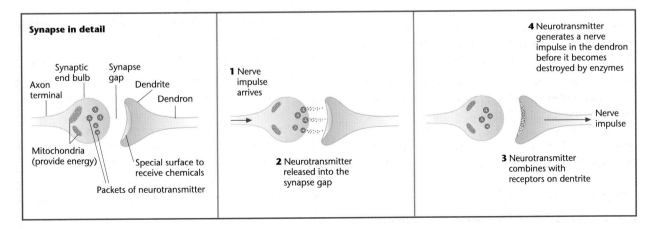

Figure 4 *How a nerve impulse crosses a synapse.*

7.3 The central nervous system

What does your brain do?

Your brain is an immensely powerful and complex organ that will probably never be fully understood. From what is known, it is thought to function very much like a computer. It is composed of circuits, not wires, transistors, etc., but circuits of neurones. Some of these circuits form a memory to store received information, whereas others are used to process the information and form a response.

The brain also acts as a monitoring device, making sure your body is functioning efficiently, and making adjustments, as necessary, by sending out messages to the effectors. But there are some important ways in which the brain differs from a computer. You use your brain to make conscious decisions, to make choices between good and bad and to register emotions. Computers have yet to achieve this.

It is possible to identify different areas of the brain which contain the **centres** that control these functions and emotions (see figure 1).

- The **cerebrum**. This is the largest part of the brain. It has two halves called the **cerebral hemispheres**. Each cerebral hemisphere contains three different types of area (see figure 2). **Sensory areas** receive messages from sense organs and use them to create the sensations of taste, smell, sight, sound, touch, and so on. **Motor areas** relay messages to the skeletal muscles to produce movements, and **association areas** integrate information from other areas and with stored information from the past. It is in the association areas that we memorise learned activities such as writing, and do much of our thinking. We feel emotions, reason, solve problems and make judgements here.

- The **cerebellum**. This helps to co-ordinate and control all the voluntary movements of your body, such as walking, cycling, chewing and typing. Walking alone requires the co-ordination of 27 muscles. The cerebellum also helps maintain balance and posture by managing muscle tone.

- The **medulla**. Located at the very base of your brain, the medulla forms part of the **brain stem**. It manages many of the automatic processes that take place inside your body, such as heart rate, blood pressure and breathing adjustments: all processes that are vital to life.

- The **hypothalamus**. This manages many more of the processes involved in **homeostasis** (chapter 8.0), such as body temperature and body fluid balance. It is located just above the pituitary gland and has some influence on this.

What does the spinal cord do?

Your spinal cord runs from the base of your brain to the lower part (lumbar region) of your back and is also made up of neurones. The spinal cord acts as an exchange, connecting incoming messages from the sensory receptors to the appropriate motor nerves and hence to the effector organs. It also relays messages to the brain.

A section through the spinal cord shows it to have two distinct regions (see figure 3). The outer **white matter** is made of nerve fibres (axons and dendrons) entering and leaving the cord. It appears white because of the colour of the myelin around the fibres. The inner 'H-shaped' area of **grey matter** is composed of the relay nerve cells, including those taking messages to the brain. A similar section through the brain would show that it also has white and grey matter.

What if the brain or spinal cord is damaged?

Unfortunately, if human nerve cells are damaged or destroyed, they are rarely repaired and never replaced. Fortunately, it is very difficult to physically damage the CNS because it is well protected by the skull and spinal column (see figure 1). In between the bone and nervous tissue are three membranes called the **meninges**. A fluid called **cerebrospinal fluid** circulates within these membranes. This fluid cushions the CNS and helps provide the nerve cells with nutrients.

Invading micro-organisms are the biggest threat to the CNS. **Polio** is one of the more serious infections. It is caused by a virus attacking the nerve cells at the base of the brain and top of the spinal cord. The damage can lead to paralysis of the limbs and of the breathing muscles. **Meningitis** is an inflammation of the meninges caused by viral or bacterial infections (chapter 13.4).

What do **you** know?

You should now be able to:

- Label a diagram of the brain.
- Summarise the functions of the cerebrum, cerebellum, medulla and hypothalamus.
- Explain the different roles of the sensory, motor and association areas of the cerebral hemispheres.
- Draw a diagram showing a section through the spinal cord and label the white and grey matter.
- Draw on your diagram the neurones forming a reflex arc.
- Describe how the CNS is protected from injury.

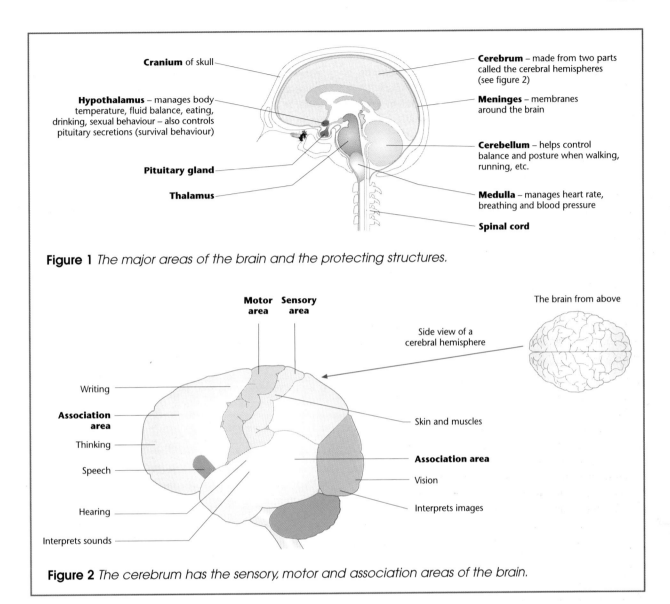

Figure 1 *The major areas of the brain and the protecting structures.*

Figure 2 *The cerebrum has the sensory, motor and association areas of the brain.*

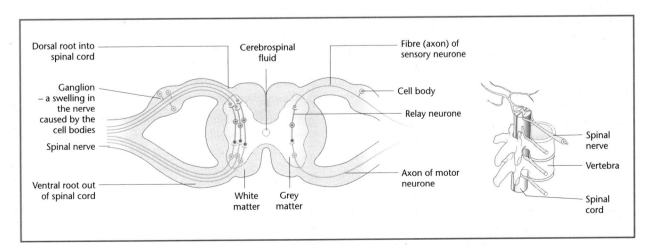

Figure 3 *A section through the spinal cord showing how the neurones link together.*

7.4 The endocrine system

Chemical co-ordination

The nervous system is not the only means by which your body can send messages from one part to another. The **endocrine system** produces chemical messengers called **hormones** which are released into your blood.

What are hormones?

Hormones are chemicals that make things happen inside your body. They are produced by glands, released directly into the blood and carried by this until they reach their place of action (i.e. the **target organ**). The cells of the target organ will have special receptors on their surface which the hormone can combine with and deliver its message. This message usually has an important modifying effect on the structure or function of that part of the body. For example, it may

- alter metabolism/energy production
- cause muscular contractions
- influence the immune responses
- influence growth and development.

There are over 30 hormones produced by 8 main glands. Each hormone has a different function, but generally they work with the nervous system to manage your body and maintain **homeostasis** (chapter 8.1). Over secretion or under secretion of many of these hormones can have very serious effects on the day-to-day working of your body and on the long term consequences for growth and development. **Negative feedback systems** (chapter 8.1) are used to prevent over and under secretion.

What are glands?

You have two kinds of gland in your body. Those which produce hormones are called **endocrine glands**. The main endocrine glands in your body and the hormones they produce are shown in figure 1.

The tear, sweat and salivary glands are **exocrine glands**. These do produce chemicals, but the chemicals are not hormones. Unlike hormones, they are delivered to their sites of action via tubes called ducts and not by the blood.

The pancreas is sometimes called a dual organ because it functions as both an endocrine and an exocrine gland. As an endocrine gland, it produces the hormones **insulin** and **glucagon**, which it secretes into the blood. As an exocrine gland, it produces **pancreatic juice**, which is secreted into the duodenum via the pancreatic duct.

The pituitary gland

The pituitary gland is often called the master gland because it produces several hormones which stimulate the secretions of other glands. For example, it produces **follicle stimulating hormone** (FSH), which controls the events in the ovaries including the production of the hormone **oestrogen**. The pituitary gland is located just underneath the **hypothalamus** in the brain which controls the secretion of many of its hormones.

Adrenaline – the 'fight or flight' hormone

Adrenaline is the hormone which is released in times of stress, for example when you are in a race or attending an interview. Its overall effect is to prepare your body for action. This is why it is called the 'fight or flight' hormone. Some of the ways in which it does this are:

- By making sure that some of the stored glycogen in your liver and muscles is converted back into glucose. This temporarily raises the blood sugar level enabling your body cells to release more energy.

- By increasing your rate and depth of breathing so that more oxygen is available to the blood.

- By constricting the blood vessels in your skin and gut and diverting the blood from these regions to your muscles and brain.

- By increasing your heart rate, thereby making your blood move more quickly and deliver more glucose and oxygen to the cells which require it.

You often know when extra adrenaline has been released into your blood because you will have a dry mouth, a pale face, a pounding heart, a sinking sensation in the stomach and clammy hands.

What do **you** know?

You should now be able to:
- Label the main endocrine glands on a diagram.
- Name the main hormones these glands produce.
- Explain why the pituitary gland is often called the master gland.
- Name 2 of the control hormones.
- Summarise the main effects of adrenaline.
- Explain the differences between exocrine and endocrine glands and name 3 exocrine glands.
- Explain why the pancreas is a dual organ.

Nervous system	Endocrine system
Message is fast	Message is slower
Response is immediate and over quickly	Response takes longer but acts longer
Delivers to a precise area	Acts over a larger area

Table 1 *The nervous and endocrine systems compared.*

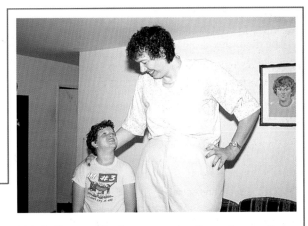

This is the result of overproduction of growth hormone by the pituitary gland.

This goitre in the neck is the result of an overactive thyroid gland.

Hypothalamus influences the secretion of some of the pituitary hormones

Pituitary gland produces many hormones some of which are:
- **Growth hormone** (HGH) to control the growth of bones and muscles
- **Anti-diurectic hormone** (ADH) controls the amount of urine produced (chapter 8.4)
- **Follicle stimulating hormone** (FSH) and **luteinising hormone** (LH) which control the female cycle (chapter 9.3)

Thyroid gland produces **thyroxine** which controls cellular metabolism

Adrenal glands produce several hormones –
- **Adrenaline** prepares your body for action by increasing blood sugar, heart rate and breathing rate
- Various **steroids** which help your body manage stress and control blood volume and pressure

Pancreas produces **insulin** and **glucagon** which control your blood sugar levels (chapter 8.2)

Ovaries produce two hormones, **oestrogen** and **progesterone**, which produce female characteristics, including egg production (chapter 9.5)

Testes produce **testosterone** which produces male characteristics, including sperm production (chapter 9.2)

Figure 1 *The endocrine glands in the body.*

Chapter 7: Questions

1 The body is controlled and co-ordinated by the nervous system and by the endocrine (hormone) system. The diagrams show the main features of these two systems.

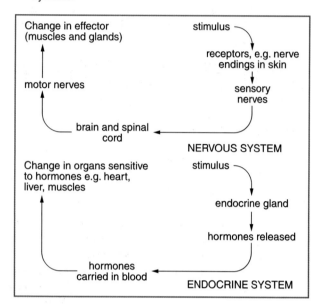

a Using information from the diagrams only:
  i give two ways in which these systems are similar; *(2 marks)*
  ii give one way in which these systems are different. *(1 mark)*
  (SEG June 1990)

2 The diagram shows a motor neurone (a type of nerve cell).

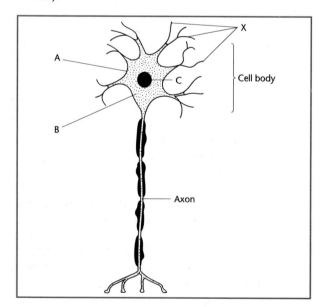

a Name structures A, B and C. *(3 marks)*
b The cell has many tiny branches, labelled X. Suggest the function of these. *(1 mark)*

c Where, in a human, would the cell body of a motor neurone be found? *(1 mark)*
d Draw a simple diagram with an arrow to show the usual direction a nerve impulse would travel. *(1 mark)*
  (SEG June 1998)

3 Most human actions may be classified as either voluntary actions or reflex actions.
  a What is meant by the term 'reflex action'?
  b The diagram shows a cross-section through the spinal cord and the nervous pathway involved in withdrawal of the hand from a hot object by reflex action.

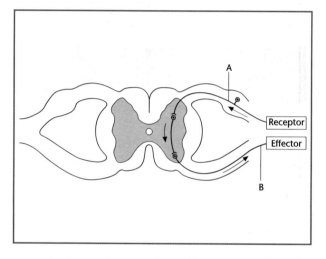

  i Name structures A and B. *(2 marks)*
  ii In this example of a reflex action:
    1 where would the receptor be found;
    2 what structure would act as the effector? *(2 marks)*
  iii The hand may also be raised by voluntary action. This will be controlled by the brain. Name the part of the brain responsible for the control of voluntary actions. *(1 mark)*
  iv Briefly describe one reflex action which is co-ordinated by the brain and not by the spinal cord. *(1 mark)*
c An experiment was performed to test the effect of drinking alcohol on the speed of response. One person held the top of a ruler. The thumb and forefinger of a second person were positioned alongside the bottom of the ruler as shown in diagram 1. The first person released the ruler and the second person caught it as quickly as possible. The position of the second person's thumb and forefinger on the scale of the ruler was recorded (see diagram 2). This was done 3 times. The experiment was repeated 20 minutes after the second person had drunk a litre of beer.

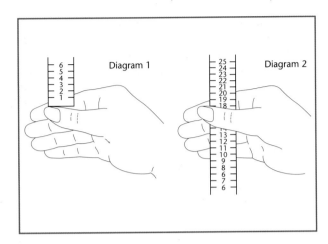

Diagram 1

Diagram 2

The results are shown in the table.

Attempt number	Distance ruler dropped before being caught in mm	
	Before drinking beer	After drinking beer
1	141	182
2	123	146
3	156	224
Average		

i Copy and complete the table by writing in the two average distances. *(2 marks)*

ii From these results, suggest why a person should not drink alcohol before driving a car *(1 mark)*
(SEG June 1998)

4 The diagram shows a side view of the human brain.

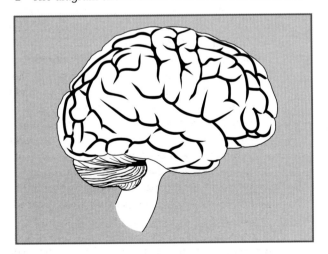

a Sketch the diagram. Write the letters X, Y and Z to show which part controls each of the following.
X: voluntary actions
Y: balance
Z: heart rate and breathing rate *(3 marks)*

b Most human actions are either reflex or voluntary actions.
i What is a reflex action? *(2 marks)*
ii Copy and complete the table by putting a tick (✓) in either the reflex or voluntary column. (One line has been completed for you as an example.)

Action	Reflex	Voluntary
Releasing saliva when food is smelled	✓	
Applying a car's brakes quickly in an emergency		
Blinking when a small insect touches the eyeball		
Dropping a hot dinner plate		

c Some drugs affect how the brain works. Caffeine is a stimulant found in tea and coffee. Alcohol, found in beer and wine, is a depressant.
Explain the difference between a stimulant and a depressant. *(2 marks)*
(SEG June 1998)

5 a The diagram shows a reflex pathway in the spinal cord.

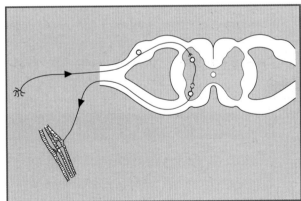

Copy the diagram and label
i the sensory neurone;
ii the motor neurone;
iii a synapse. *(3 marks)*
b On your diagram, draw in and label the receptor.
c i Give one example of a learned response. *(1 mark)*
ii Give one way in which a spinal reflex differs from a learned response. *(1 mark)*
iii In some diseases the motor neurones are damaged.
Suggest one way in which this might affect reflex actions. *(1 mark)*
(NEAB June 1997)

CHAPTER

8 Homeostasis

We live in an environment which is always changing, yet inside our bodies the conditions remain relatively constant. In this chapter you will learn how your body manages to maintain this constant environment, even though the external environment is unpredictable and constantly changing. You will learn how it copes with the stresses of exercise and illness and the central role the blood plays in this.

After you have worked through this chapter, you should be able to:

- Define the term homeostasis and explain the importance of maintaining a relatively constant internal environment.
- Name the five things which have to be carefully managed and which organs are involved.
- Explain the process of feedback control in the management of homeostasis.
- Describe the specific roles of the liver in regulating the composition of blood.
- Describe the causes, symptoms and control of diabetes mellitus.
- List the main waste products produced by cells and name the organs responsible for excreting them.

- Describe the structure and functions of the urinary system.
- Explain how urine is formed.
- Describe the processes involved in osmoregulation.
- Outline dialysis.
- Describe the structure and functions of your skin.
- Explain how body temperature is managed and controlled by your brain.
- Describe your body responses to overheating and overcooling.

Diabetes mellitus

What is diabetes mellitus?

Cells need glucose as an energy source. There is always a supply of glucose in your blood, but to access it your cells require the hormone **insulin**. Insulin combines with **receptors** on the cell membrane and in doing so, opens channels through which glucose can enter the cell.

After a meal your blood glucose level will usually rise to a level which is dangerous. This must be quickly reduced. Insulin released by the pancreas enables liver cells to take up the excess glucose from the blood and convert it into **glycogen**, which can be stored for use later. Details about the control of blood glucose levels can be found in chapter 8.3.

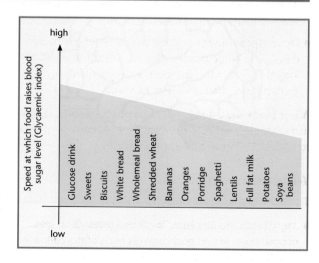

Figure 1 *Different foods raise the blood glucose level at different speeds.*

People with **diabetes mellitus** have no insulin control, either due to:

- a failure to produce enough insulin, or
- a failure of the cells to respond to insulin.

Without this insulin control, glucose can build up in the blood to levels which are dangerous or fall to levels which are insufficient to meet the needs of the cells.

How is diabetes mellitus detected?

Normally no glucose is excreted, but when the blood glucose level is very high, the kidneys are unable to reabsorb all of it and some appears in the urine. This can be detected using a **clinistix** (see chapter 14.7).

Confirmation is usually by blood tests. Blood glucose levels are measured before and after a glucose drink. A high blood sugar level is called **hyperglycaemia**.

What are the symptoms of diabetes?

- Your cells are unable to use glucose so they start to use fats and proteins to provide energy. This results in weight loss. The amount of fat in your blood increases, raising your risk of coronary heart disease (chapter 3.5). The use of fatty acids for energy also forms toxic waste substances (ketone bodies) which alter the pH of your blood. The first sign of this is breath which smells of pear drops. A low pH can affect your brain resulting in unconsciousness.

- The excretion of glucose uses water leaving you dehydrated and thirsty. Severe dehydration can result in brain damage.

- Hyperglycaemia over a long period of time can cause damage to blood vessels. This may result in blindness, kidney failure and peripheral vascular disease. Amputations are sometimes necessary.

A low blood sugar level, called **hypoglycaemia** can be just as damaging. Your brain cannot get enough glucose resulting in a coma and eventual death.

What causes diabetes?

There are two forms of diabetes mellitus:

- **Type 1**, also called **insulin dependent diabetes**, occurs when the body cannot make insulin. This is usually due to the insulin producing cells of the pancreas being destroyed by your own immune system. It is an **auto-immune disease**.

Type 1 develops early in life, usually before the age of 20 and accounts for about one quarter of the cases. It is thought to have a genetic cause, but needs an environmental trigger such as a viral infection.

- **Type 2**, also called **non-insulin dependent diabetes**, develops later in life, usually 40 years of age, because insulin production slows down or the body cells stop responding to the circulating insulin.

Type 2 probably has a genetic basis, but develops as a result of lifestyle. The risk factors include poor diet, obesity, age, low levels of physical activity and smoking.

The management of diabetes

All diabetics must monitor their blood glucose levels very carefully. The aim is to maintain a blood glucose level of between 4–8 mmol per litre of blood.

For Type 1 diabetes this is achieved by eating foods which raise the blood sugar level slowly (figure 1) and by regular injections of insulin to match the sugar intake. Insulin used to be extracted from pigs, but human insulin can now be produced by biotechnology (chapter 14.7).

Type 2 diabetes is controlled by altering the diet and lifestyle. Again, sugary foods which raise blood glucose levels quickly need to be replaced by more unrefined carbohydrates such as wholemeal bread, cereals and potatoes (see figure 1). Alcohol intake should be cut and regular exercise taken.

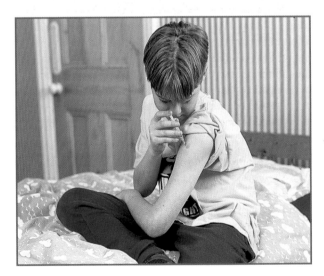

Figure 2 *Type 1 diabetics have to learn to inject themselves with insulin.*

8.1 Homeostasis

What is homeostasis?

When you exercise, the release of the extra energy places many stresses on your body. Some of these have the potential to be very damaging. For example:

- Extra **glucose** is removed from your blood depleting the blood glucose supply. Unless this is restored from glucose stores, other cells in your body will be starved of glucose and may die.

- Extra **oxygen** is required to release the stored energy. If your breathing rate is not increased to supply this, an oxygen debt may follow and cause cramp.

- More **carbon dioxide** is produced, which, if allowed to build up, could affect the pH of your blood and thereby affect many blood proteins, especially enzymes. Vital processes, such as blood clotting, could be affected.

- Extra **heat** is produced, which could raise your body temperature and affect the enzymes involved in metabolism.

- Extra heat is removed by sweating. This may lead to **dehydration** and your blood becoming too concentrated, therefore drawing water from your body cells and causing damage.

Your body must try and minimise these stresses to prevent any damage to its cells. The process of managing the internal environment to meet the ever-changing needs of your body systems is called **homeostasis**.

How does homeostasis work?

Homeostasis may be defined as *the maintenance of a constant internal environment*. For your cells, the internal environment is the **tissue fluid** formed from the blood. Cells are very delicate structures and will only function properly if suitable conditions are maintained in these fluids. Large changes in conditions can damage or kill them. In particular, the five conditions that need to be carefully managed in the blood and tissue fluid are:

- **glucose** content

- **water** content

- **salt** content

- **temperature**

- and **oxygen** content.

There are working levels for most of these which your body tries to maintain, i.e. normal body temperature is

37 °C. If conditions alter, mechanisms are used to remove or reduce the threat, i.e. when you exercise, you produce extra heat, which could raise your body temperature above 37 °C. To prevent this happenening you start sweating to remove the extra heat. This has a knock on effect on some of the working levels. Sweating will use up water from your blood, so your body adjusts and, for example, the amount of urine you produce is less.

Homeostasis also includes adjustments to meet the needs of the body, not only in supplying substances, but in managing waste substances such as **carbon dioxide** and **urea**, so they do not build up to dangerous levels.

Which organs are involved in homeostasis?

Homeostasis is a whole body process, involving the co-operation of many organs (see figure 1). In particular:

- the **liver** and **pancreas** work on maintaining a suitable glucose level in your blood (chapter 8.2)

- the **kidneys** remove metabolic waste products such as urea, and maintain suitable salt and water levels in the blood (chapter 8.3)

- the **skin** and **liver** help to maintain your body at a suitable temperature (chapters 8.5 and 8.6)

- the **lungs** are involved in controlling the oxygen and carbon dioxide content of your blood (chapter 4.3)

- the **blood** plays a central role in transporting the materials around the body (chapter 3.2).

The work of these organs is co-ordinated by your **brain**, which must be continually informed of both the internal and external conditions so that it can direct changes if necessary. Much of the information comes from your blood as it passes through the **hypothalamus** of the brain. There are sensory receptors here which monitor blood temperature, water and salt content, and carbon dioxide content. Other information comes from receptors located in other parts of the body. For example, receptors in the pancreas monitor blood glucose levels and receptors in the skin monitor changes in the outside environmental temperature. All this information is fed back to the brain via nerve connections. The brain therefore bases its decisions on the needs of the body.

The same receptors will tell your brain when the conditions are back to normal. This is called a **feedback control system** (see figure 2).

In feedback control systems the output is used to adjust the input. Most systems are negative feedback systems whereby the end result of the feedback is to bring the level back to normal.

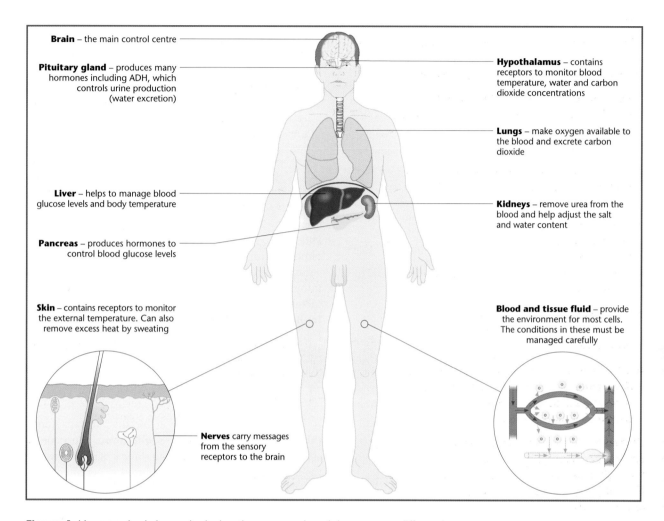

Brain – the main control centre

Pituitary gland – produces many hormones including ADH, which controls urine production (water excretion)

Liver – helps to manage blood glucose levels and body temperature

Pancreas – produces hormones to control blood glucose levels

Skin – contains receptors to monitor the external temperature. Can also remove excess heat by sweating

Nerves carry messages from the sensory receptors to the brain

Hypothalamus – contains receptors to monitor blood temperature, water and carbon dioxide concentrations

Lungs – make oxygen available to the blood and excrete carbon dioxide

Kidneys – remove urea from the blood and help adjust the salt and water content

Blood and tissue fluid – provide the environment for most cells. The conditions in these must be managed carefully

Figure 1 *Homeostasis is a whole body process involving many different organs.*

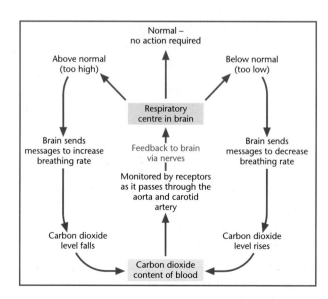

Normal – no action required

Above normal (too high)

Below normal (too low)

Respiratory centre in brain

Brain sends messages to increase breathing rate

Feedback to brain via nerves

Brain sends messages to decrease breathing rate

Monitored by receptors as it passes through the aorta and carotid artery

Carbon dioxide level falls

Carbon dioxide level rises

Carbon dioxide content of blood

Figure 2 *Feedback control systems are essential to homeostasis.*

What do **you** know?

You should now be able to:

- Explain the term homeostasis.
- Using the changes which take place during a run, explain why homeostasis is so important.
- List 5 things in the blood and tissue fluid which need to be carefully managed.
- Name the main organs involved in homeostasis and outline what they do.
- Explain with examples, why the blood is crucial to homeostasis.
- Explain the role of the brain and nerves in homeostasis.
- Explain what a negative feedback control system is and give an example.

8.2 Blood sugar regulation

What is blood sugar?

Blood sugar is **glucose** in the blood, which is the main source of energy your cells use. Some body cells can also use other energy sources, such as fatty acids, but the cells of your brain can only use glucose. It is therefore crucial that there is always glucose in your blood. This is called the **blood sugar level**.

The blood sugar level is usually maintained at about 5 mmol of glucose per litre of blood. If it falls too low, many cells, including those of your brain, are deprived of energy. If it is too high, it can poison the cells. The main organs responsible for maintaining your blood sugar level, regardless of supply or demand, are the **liver** and the **pancreas**, although hormones produced by several other endocrine glands can also alter your blood sugar level.

The liver

The liver is the largest organ inside your body, weighing about 1.5 kg in the average adult. It is also the most metabolically active organ in your body and in a resting adult, it receives about one third of the blood supply. The blood which flows in is very variable in composition, but the blood leaving is always fairly constant.

A healthy functioning liver is critical to homeostasis in many ways:

- **Food processing**. All nutrients (except some fats) absorbed from the small intestine are carried to the liver by the blood in the hepatic portal vein. Here they are processed and the blood levels adjusted.

- **Storage**. Many of the excess nutrients are stored in the liver. Glucose is stored as glycogen, vitamins A, D and B_{12} and iron are also stored in large quantities. Excess amino acids are **deaminated** (chapter 2.7) in the liver with the production of urea.

- **Detoxification**. Circulating drugs such as alcohol, and hormones like oestrogen are chemically altered in the liver, ready for excreting.

- **Heat production**. A great deal of heat is produced from the metabolic activities of the liver cells. At rest, this accounts for about 70% of the heat needed to keep your body warm.

In addition to these, your liver has many more functions, some of which are shown in figure 1.

The pancreas

The pancreas (see figure 3) is often called a dual organ because it:

- Produces a digestive juice containing enzymes. This juice, called **pancreatic juice** is secreted into the duodenum.

- Produces two hormones involved in blood sugar regulation. These hormones, **insulin** and **glucagon** are produced by groups of special cells known as the **islets of Langerhans**. The hormones are released into the blood as it flows through the pancreas.

How is your blood sugar level regulated?

This is a good example of a negative feedback system (see figure 2) and homeostasis. The amount of glucose in your blood, is checked as your blood passes through the pancreas. If it is too high, as will happen every time you eat a meal, your pancreas secretes the hormone insulin into the blood. Insulin increases the permeability of cell membranes to glucose so more glucose can enter them. In the liver and muscle cells, it activates enzymes to convert the glucose into the storage molecule **glycogen**. Insulin also promotes the removal of other potential glucose sources, such as fatty acids and amino acids from the blood. Together the liver and pancreas therefore reduce the blood sugar level.

If the blood sugar level falls too low, the pancreas stops producing insulin and produces **glucagon**. Glucagon stimulates the reconversion of the stores of glycogen in the liver and muscles back into glucose. This enters the blood bringing the sugar level back to normal. If this is not enough then other hormones convert fatty acids, glycerol and amino acids into glucose. During periods of intense exercise, blood sugar levels are also raised by the hormone **adrenaline**, which causes the conversion of glycogen into glucose.

What is diabetes?

People with **diabetes mellitus** cannot regulate their blood sugar levels usually because the pancreas fails to produce enough insulin. This has a number of effects on the body (see page 98).

The symptoms of diabetes are itchiness of the skin, weight loss, tiredness, irritability and more frequent urination. When the blood sugar level reaches such a level, glucose starts to appear in the urine. This is how diabetes is usually first detected. If it is not treated immediately the patient may lose consciousness and die. The usual treatment is to inject insulin into the blood before a meal. Insulin cannot be taken orally because it is a protein and will be digested. Diabetics usually have to learn how to give themselves regular injections of insulin to match their carbohydrate intake.

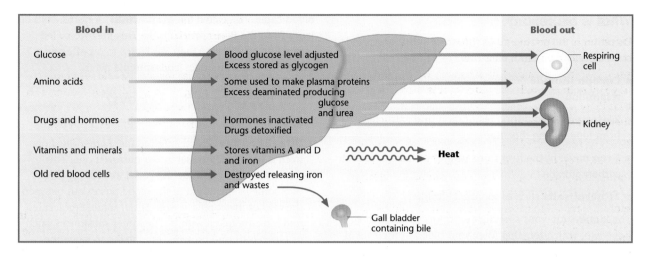

Figure 1 *The liver regulates the composition of your blood in many ways.*

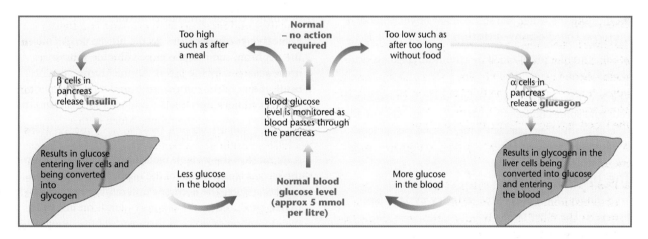

Figure 2 *The control of blood sugar levels is an example of homeostasis.*

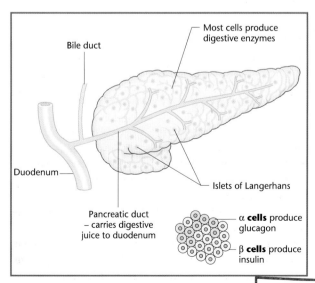

Figure 3 *The pancreas is a dual organ.*

What do **you** know?

You should now be able to:

● Explain what blood sugar is and why you always need some in the blood.

● Explain why your blood sugar level can go up and down.

● Draw a flow diagram to explain what happens when your blood sugar level is too high or too low.

● Describe how you could tell if your blood sugar levels were too high.

● Explain the causes and symptoms of diabetes mellitus. Suggest how it might be controlled.

● Outline the roles of the liver in regulating the composition of your blood.

The kidneys and excretion

What is excretion?

Excretion is the getting rid of the waste substances made by your cells. The main ones are:

- **Carbon dioxide** produced by the cells during respiration.

- **Water** produced during respiration and extracted from food during digestion.

- **Urea** made in the liver from surplus amino acids and carbon dioxide.

- **Mineral salts** such as sodium chloride.

The kidneys are your specialist excretory organs. You have two, which together filter your blood at the rate of 1200 cm^3 every minute, removing wastes and other harmful substances, together with a lot of water. This is the mixture we call **urine**. Your kidneys are also involved in:

- adjusting the water and salt content of your blood: a process called **osmoregulation** (see chapter 8.4).

- adjusting the pH of blood by eliminating excess acids and bases.

The liver also excretes breakdown products of red blood cells and some cholesterol. These pass with bile into the intestines and then pass out with the undigested food residues in the faeces.

The urinary system

Your kidneys form part of the **urinary system** (see figure 1). The other parts are:

- The **bladder** to store the urine. When this is full it holds about half a litre.

- Two muscular tubes which take the urine from the kidneys to the bladder. These are the **ureters**.

- A tube through which your bladder can be emptied. This is called the **urethra**. In men this runs through the penis.

Each kidney is supplied with blood directly from the aorta via a **renal artery**. Filtered blood is returned to the vena cava via a **renal vein**.

What is in a kidney?

The inside of a kidney has three regions, the outer **cortex**, the inner **medulla** and the **pelvis**. Urine is made in the cortex and medulla, collects in the pelvis before passing into the ureter on its way to the bladder.

The functional unit of a kidney is the **nephron** (see figure 2). Each of your kidneys contains over a million of these. A nephron consists of a cup shaped end, called the **Bowman's capsule** which surrounds a small knot of blood capillaries called the **glomerulus**. A narrow tubule leads from the Bowman's capsule. This has two coiled regions separated by a loop, and joins to a **collecting duct**. The collecting duct leads into the pelvis.

What happens in the kidneys?

Urine is produced in the nephrons by two processes:

1 **Ultrafiltration**. Blood entering the glomerulus flows from a wide blood vessel into a narrower one. This raises the pressure inside the vessel to such an extent that some of the liquid in the blood passes out between the cells of the capillary wall. Small soluble molecules and ions are taken with it. The larger substances, such as blood cells and proteins, are too big to leave the blood capillary. The filtrate formed, therefore, consists mainly of water, glucose, amino acids, various mineral salts and urea. This drains through pores in the Bowman's capsule and enters the tubule.

2 **Selective reabsorbtion.** As the filtrate passes along the nephron, some of the more valuable substances are reabsorbed by the blood. All the glucose, amino acids, many of the mineral salts and a lot of water are reabsorbed back into blood capillaries surrounding the first coiled region of the tubule. Much of this reabsorbtion is by active transport (chapter 1.5).

A lot more of the water is reabsorbed by osmosis, from the second coiled region of the nephron and the collecting duct. The hormone anti-diuretic hormone (**ADH**) produced by the pituitary gland can influence the absorption of water in these parts of the tubule. This is described in the next section. By the time it arrives at the pelvis, the filtrate has been converted into urine.

What do **you** know?

You should now be able to:

- List the main waste products produced by your body.
- Outline how your body gets rid of these wastes.
- Outline how a kidney is involved in homeostasis.
- Label a diagram of the urinary system and state the functions of the kidneys, ureters, bladder and urethra.
- Draw the blood supply to a kidney.
- Draw an enlarged nephron and use it to explain how a kidney makes urine.
- Draw a table to compare the composition of blood and urine.
- Explain why there is usually no glucose or protein in urine.

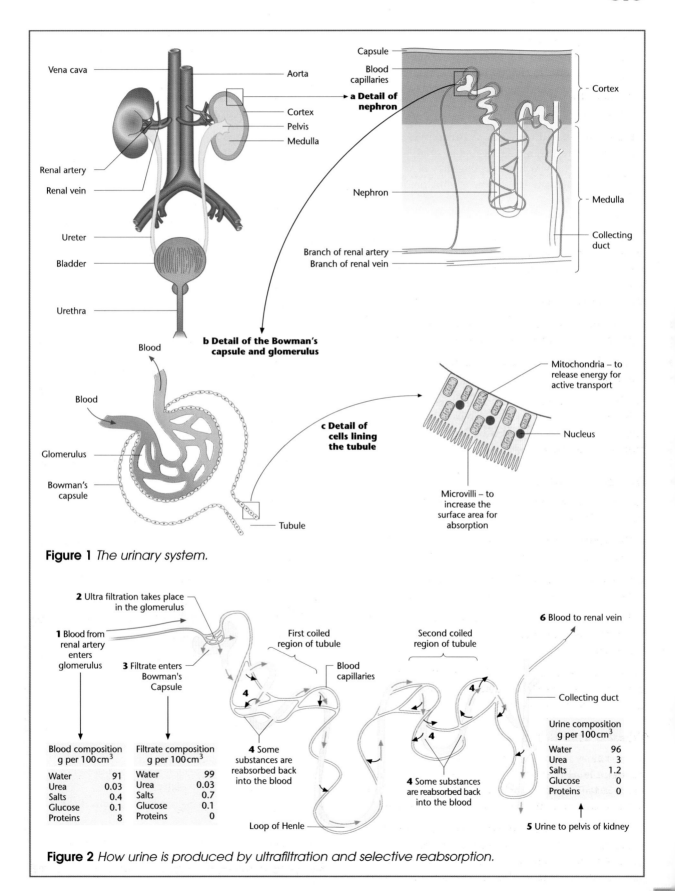

Figure 1 *The urinary system.*

Figure 2 *How urine is produced by ultrafiltration and selective reabsorption.*

8.4 The kidneys and osmoregulation

What does urine contain?

The final composition of typical urine compared to blood is given in figure 2 in chapter 8.3. The amount of most of the substances can vary quite considerably. For example, the amount of urea will depend on how much meat (protein) you have eaten. Water and salt will depend on how much you have sweated. Water content can also be affected by caffeine and alcohol. These have a **diuretic** effect, which means that they increase the amount of water you excrete, thereby the amount of urine you produce.

The presence of other substances in your urine is a good indication of the state of health of your body. Urine tests are often used to diagnose disorders. For example, if your urine contains glucose, this could mean you have diabetes, and protein in your urine could indicate that your kidneys are failing.

Urine tests can be used to confirm a pregnancy. A fertilised egg releases a hormone (human chorionic gonodotrophin: HCG) which the mother excretes in her urine. This can usually be detected from about 14 days after conception and is the basis of most pregnancy tests.

How is the water and salt content adjusted?

Having the right amount of water in the blood is crucial to the normal functioning of your body cells. Too much water and your tissue fluid will be too dilute and may result in the cells taking up water and swelling or even bursting. Too little water could lead to cell dehydration. Fortunately, this rarely happens due to the homeostasitic process outlined in figure 1. The antidiruetic hormone (ADH) released by the hypothalamus acts on the second coiled region of the kidney tubule and the collecting duct altering their permeability to water.

The kidneys also maintain the correct blood salt level by a similar process involving a hormone (aldosterone) produced by the adrenal glands. To maintain the correct blood volume, and therefore blood pressure, the water/salt balance must be correct. The management of blood water and salt concentrations is called **osmoregulation**.

What if your kidneys stop working?

If one kidney fails, the other can usually cope well with the extra burden. If both kidneys fail the build up of waste substances they normally filter out of your blood may prove fatal. There are several approaches to compensating for kidney failure:

- **Haemodialysis** uses a machine to do the work of the kidneys (see figure 2). Blood is taken from an artery

and passed through an artificial capillary made from a special porous membrane called a **dialysis membrane**. On the other side of this membrane is a special fluid called **dialysing fluid**. In the dialysis machine **diffusion gradients** are set up so that when the patients blood is passed through it

i)   all the waste substances such as urea diffuse out

ii) all the glucose is retained in the blood

iii) the water and salt levels are adjusted.

Other blood components such as blood cells and proteins are held back because they are too large to pass through the pores in the dialysis membrane. The treatment is continued until the blood has an acceptable concentration of constituents. This could take up to 12 hours, two or three times a week.

- **Peritoneal dialysis** uses one of the patient's own vascular membranes, the **peritoneum**. The peritoneum lines the abdomen. Dialysing fluid is introduced through a catheter (a tube) into the abdomen and left there for 5–6 hours before being drained away.

- A **kidney transplant** involves transplanting a working kidney from a doner. These transplants are difficult and costly to arrange because the kidneys have to be perfectly matched to prevent rejection (chapter 13.9).

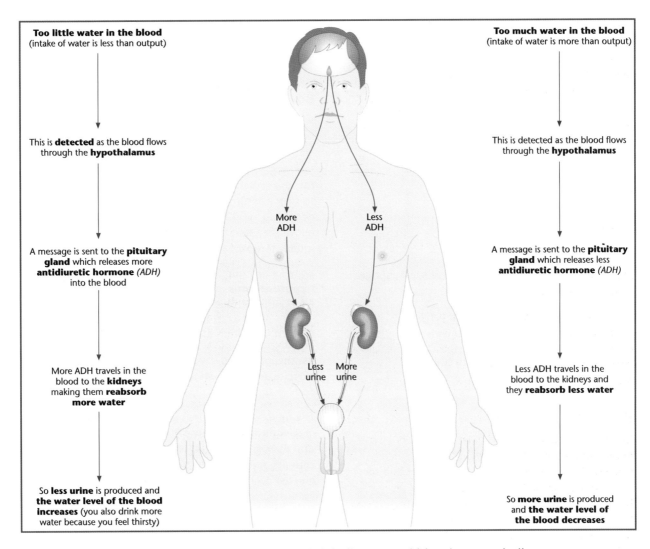

Too little water in the blood
(intake of water is less than output)

This is **detected** as the blood flows through the **hypothalamus**

A message is sent to the **pituitary gland** which releases more **antidiuretic hormone** (ADH) into the blood

More ADH travels in the blood to the **kidneys** making them **reabsorb more water**

So **less urine** is produced and **the water level of the blood increases** (you also drink more water because you feel thirsty)

Too much water in the blood
(intake of water is more than output)

This is detected as the blood flows through the **hypothalamus**

A message is sent to the **pituitary gland** which releases less **antidiuretic hormone** (ADH)

Less ADH travels in the blood to the kidneys and they **reabsorb less water**

So **more urine** is produced and **the water level of the blood decreases**

More ADH   Less ADH

Less urine   More urine

Figure 1 *A feedback system helps your body maintain the correct blood concentration.*

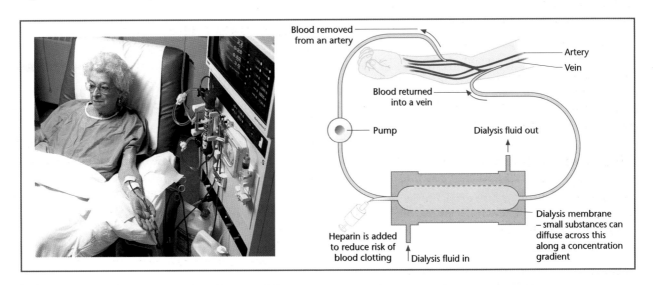

Blood removed from an artery

Artery

Vein

Blood returned into a vein

Pump

Dialysis fluid out

Heparin is added to reduce risk of blood clotting

Dialysis fluid in

Dialysis membrane – small substances can diffuse across this along a concentration gradient

Figure 2 *Most patients have to visit a hospital to undergo haemodialysis.*

8.5 The skin and body temperature

What does your skin do?

Your skin is the boundary between the harsh outside world in which you live and the delicate, precise world inside your body. As well as helping to maintain a constant body temperature, it also:

- protects the tissues beneath it from injury
- stops the entry into your body of poisonous chemicals and germs
- acts as a waterproof barrier stopping water getting in and, if necessary, out
- protects your body from the effects of ultraviolet radiation in sunlight by producing the blocking pigment melanin
- contains sense organs which help us detect changes in the outside world
- makes vitamin D in the presence of sunlight
- stores food in the form of fat
- excretes excess salt and water in sweat
- is modified to form teeth, nails and mammary glands
- makes hair.

Skin structure

The skin has three parts:

1 The surface layers form the **epidermis**. The cells of the outermost layers contain the protein **keratin** and provide a tough protective barrier, resisting heat, and entry of germs and chemicals. These are constantly worn away and replaced by new cells from below. Some of these living cells can produce the pigment **melanin**, which protects against the entry of damaging ultra violet light.

2 Below the epidermis is the **dermis**. This is a much thicker layer of connective tissue. It contains elastic proteins and tough **collagen** fibres as well as various types of cells. Within the dermis are several types of **receptor** cells to detect changes in the outside environment. It also contains **sweat glands** and **sebaceous glands**; the latter produce the waterproofing oils (**sebum**) that cover the surface and hairs of the skin. The blood supply serving your skin is in the dermis. Nutrients have to diffuse into the epidermis from these capillaries.

3 Below the dermis is **adipose tissue**. Fat, which can be used for energy, is stored in the cells of this tissue. It is a useful place to store fat because it also cushions the body from mechanical damage and acts as an insulating layer.

The full structure of the skin is shown in figure 2.

Body temperature regulation

We need to keep our **core body temperature** at 37 °C because this is the optimum working temperature for the enzymes involved in metabolism. At temperatures below this, enzymes work much more slowly. At 27 °C enzymes are only working half as fast and this rate is not enough to keep you alive. If your body temperature rises a few degrees above 37 °C, the enzymes speed up. At 41 °C and above they start to become denatured by the heat and unable to work.

Body temperature is set by a thermostat in the **hypothalamus** of your brain. This needs to balance heat gains with heat losses.

Most heat is produced when living cells release energy. The muscles and liver produce most heat because they use the most energy. You will produce heat when you exercise and can even absorb it from external sources, such as sunlamps or other hot objects.

The main ways you lose heat are by the **evaporation** of sweat from the surface of your skin and by **radiation** into the air. Heat is also lost by convection (into cold air currents) and by conduction (when you sit or touch cold objects). You even lose some heat when you breathe out and when you excrete urine. The amount of heat you lose will depend on the external temperature (the **heat gradient**) and your **surface area to volume ratio** (see figure 3).

Your body can use a range of **physiological mechanisms**, many involving the skin, to conserve or help lose heat. It also uses **behavioural responses**. These are described in chapter 8.6.

What is brown fat?

Brown fat is a special kind of fat that only produces heat energy when metabolised. It is found in babies and young children who still have a large surface area to volume ratio and therefore lose a lot of heat. Animals which hibernate use it to raise their body temperature quickly at the end of the hibernating period.

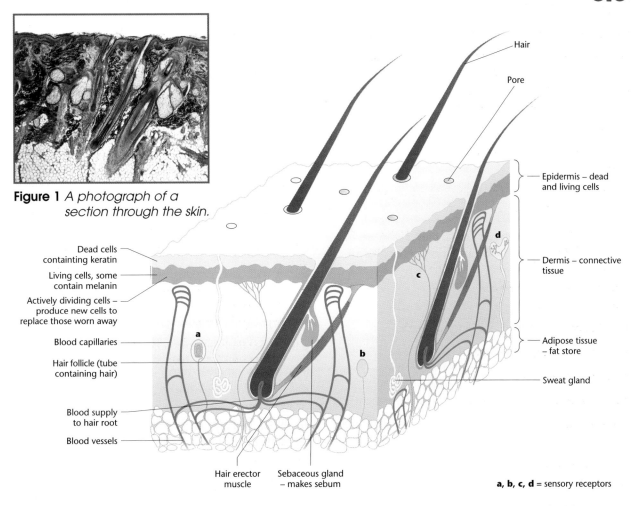

Figure 1 *A photograph of a section through the skin.*

Hair

Pore

Epidermis – dead and living cells

Dermis – connective tissue

Adipose tissue – fat store

Sweat gland

Dead cells containting keratin

Living cells, some contain melanin

Actively dividing cells – produce new cells to replace those worn away

Blood capillaries

Hair follicle (tube containing hair)

Blood supply to hair root

Blood vessels

Hair erector muscle

Sebaceous gland – makes sebum

a, b, c, d = sensory receptors

Figure 2 *The skin is your body's largest organ. It contains many different structures all with specific functions.*

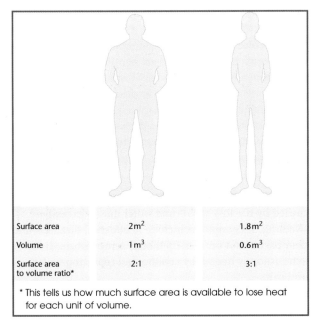

Surface area	2m²	1.8m²
Volume	1m³	0.6m³
Surface area to volume ratio*	2:1	3:1

* This tells us how much surface area is available to lose heat for each unit of volume.

Figure 3 *The amount of heat lost depends on the surface area to volume ratio.*

What do **you** know?

You should now be able to:

- Label a diagram of the skin.
- Annotate your diagram with details of the composition of the epidermis and dermis.
- Write a list of skin functions.
- Explain why 37 °C is the most suitable body temperature and outline the consequences of it going up or down.
- List the 4 main ways of losing heat.
- Describe where your body heat comes from.
- Explain the importance of surface area to volume ratio in heat loss.

8.6 Overheating and overcooling

How is body temperature regulated?

Your blood temperature is checked as the blood passes through the **hypothalamus** in the brain. If it rises or falls then your body tries to make adjustments.

Overheating

If your blood temperature is too high, your body will use homeostatic mechanisms to:

- increase heat loss

- reduce heat production.

Some of the immediate responses to prevent overheating are shown in figure 1. These mechanisms are only effective between 37 °C and 41 °C. Above 41 °C, they start to fail and your body goes into shock, followed by death.

Longer term responses include:

- Cellular metabolism slows down so less heat is produced. This is controlled by the hormone **thyroxine**.

Overcooling

If your blood temperature is too low, your body will use homeostatic mechanisms to:

- reduce heat loss

- generate more heat.

Some of the immediate mechanisms to prevent overcooling are shown in figure 1. These mechanisms start to fail at 29 °C and your body goes into a coma, followed by death.

Longer term responses include:

- Under the control of thyroxine, cellular metabolism increases, producing more heat for the blood to distribute around your body.

- More fat is deposited under the dermis of the skin. This provides an insulating layer.

What is the role of the skin senses?

Your skin temperature receptors monitor changes in the external temperature. For example, if the temperature falls, the cold receptors will be stimulated and a message will be sent to your brain. The brain will initiate behavioural changes, such as putting on more clothing or having something warm to drink.

The receptors in the skin also protect your skin from damage. For example, when you pick up something hot they are stimulated and form part of a reflex action that results in you dropping the hot object (chapter 7.3).

What is hypothermia?

Hypothermia (exposure) is the condition which develops when your body temperature falls below 35 °C because the heat generated is too little to replace the heat lost. The young and old are particularly susceptible. Young babies are at risk because they have a large **surface area to volume ratio** and lose a lot of heat. Older people are susceptible because they are less able to regulate their body temperature. Also, many live in unheated surroundings and do not get enough food or do not move around sufficiently to generate heat.

The symptoms of hypothermia are:

- shivering in the early stages

- cold, pale and dry skin

- low body temperature

- slow pulse and breathing rates

- irrational and confused behaviour.

If not treated immediately, the body temperature may continue to fall. Once it gets below 29 °C, the patient may lose consciousness and die.

Treating a hypothermic person involves preventing further heat loss and raising their temperature at the same speed as it fell. Recovery is unlikely if body temperature has fallen below 26 °C

Extreme cold may also damage the skin and result in **frostbite**.

What is heat stroke?

Heat stroke is the result of your body being unable to shed enough heat to stop its temperature rising. This may happen if you are in a very hot atmosphere for long periods or have a fever. Occasionally, it is due to a failure of your body's thermostat. Body temperature rises and you start to feel dizzy and develop a headache. Your pulse rate will rise and start bounding. Eventually you will lose consciousness. If your body is not cooled immediately, you may die.

A milder form of heat stress is **heat exhaustion**. This is caused by the loss of salt and water due to excessive sweating. Its symptoms include headaches, dizziness and cramps, but not an increased body temperature. Heat exhaustion is treated by cooling and replacing water and salt.

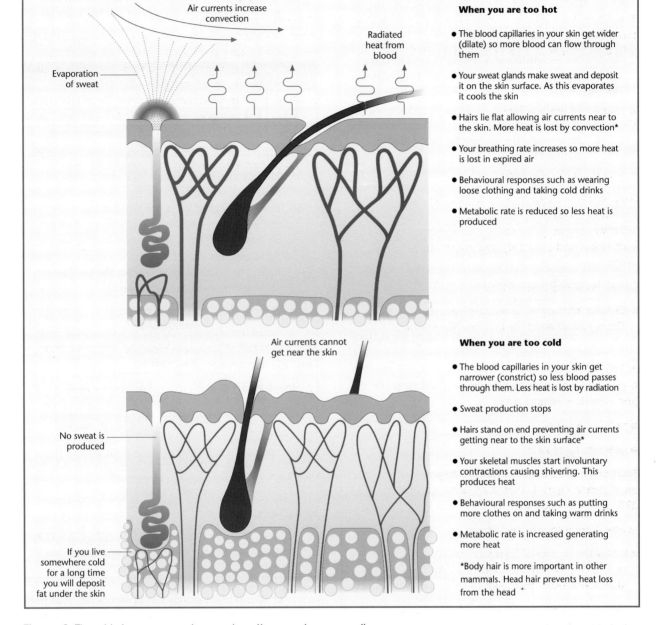

Figure 1 *The skin's response to overheating and overcooling.*

Text from the figure:

When you are too hot

- The blood capillaries in your skin get wider (dilate) so more blood can flow through them

- Your sweat glands make sweat and deposit it on the skin surface. As this evaporates it cools the skin

- Hairs lie flat allowing air currents near to the skin. More heat is lost by convection*

- Your breathing rate increases so more heat is lost in expired air

- Behavioural responses such as wearing loose clothing and taking cold drinks

- Metabolic rate is reduced so less heat is produced

Air currents increase convection
Radiated heat from blood
Evaporation of sweat

When you are too cold

- The blood capillaries in your skin get narrower (constrict) so less blood passes through them. Less heat is lost by radiation

- Sweat production stops

- Hairs stand on end preventing air currents getting near to the skin surface*

- Your skeletal muscles start involuntary contractions causing shivering. This produces heat

- Behavioural responses such as putting more clothes on and taking warm drinks

- Metabolic rate is increased generating more heat

*Body hair is more important in other mammals. Head hair prevents heat loss from the head

Air currents cannot get near the skin
No sweat is produced
If you live somewhere cold for a long time you will deposit fat under the skin

What do **you** know?

You should now be able to:

- Generate a diagram to show the changes in the skin in response to being too hot.

- Use another diagram to show how your skin responds when your blood is too cold.

- Explain the role of the skin senses.

- List some of the behavioural responses.

- Explain how you would recognise and treat hypothermia.

- Explain the different cause of heat stroke and heat exhaustion.

Chapter 8: Questions

1 Ray Swinner was training hard. He went for a long run. It was a hot day and sweat poured down his face. He could feel his heart beating faster and hear the sound of his deep breathing. Every 20 minutes he took a few mouthfuls of a special 'Sportade' drink, containing glucose and mineral salts. Even so, when he tried to increase his pace, his muscles hurt and he soon had to drop back.

a Ray's drink contained glucose and mineral salts.

i How would the glucose be useful to Ray during his run? *(1 mark)*

ii Why would Ray need extra mineral salts in his drink? *(1 mark)*

b In the above account, Ray's body changed in three ways to help him during the run.
Give each of these changes and explain how each of these changes would help. *(9 marks)*

c Ray's muscles hurt when he increases his pace because they produce lactic acid.
Explain why lactic acid is produced. *(2 marks)*

(NEAB Sample Assessment)

2 a The diagram shows a way of finding the surface area of a person. A ruler line joining the figures for body mass and height is drawn. The reading where this line crosses the central axis is the surface area of the body.

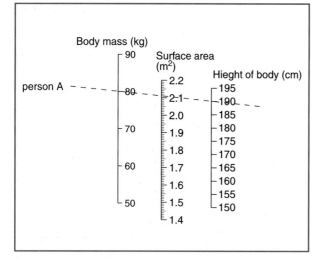

i Person A has a body mass of 80 kg and a height of 190 cm. The dotted line between these readings crosses the central axis to indicate a surface area of 2.11 m². What is the surface area of Person B who has the same body mass as Person A, but is 180 cm tall? *(1 mark)*

ii If all other conditions are the same (such as external temperature and amount of clothing) which person will lose body heat the faster? Explain the reason for your answer. *(1 mark)*

b Briefly describe one way in which human skin helps to reduce the heat lost from the body on a cold day. *(1 mark)*

(SEG June 1992)

Gland	Description
X	Gland attached to the base of the brain.
Y	Pair of organs that secrete progesterone.
Z	Pair of glands found at the anterior end of each kidney.

3 a Identify endocrine glands X, Y and Z from their descriptions: *(3 marks)*

b The level of glucose in the blood is controlled by two hormones (insulin and glucagon) that have an opposite effect to each other. Insulin lowers the blood sugar level. Glucagon raises the blood sugar level. The diagram shows the mechanism by which these hormones operate:

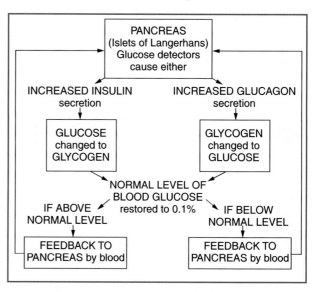

i What is the normal level of glucose in the blood? *(1 mark)*

ii How do these two hormones raise and lower the blood sugar level? *(4 marks)*

iii Explain what is meant by the term 'feedback' as shown in the diagram. *(3 marks)*

iv Sketch a graph to show what happens within an hour to the glucose level in the blood of a diabetic who, after eating a meal containing glucose, is in need of an insulin injection. Label both axes of your graph. *(3 marks)*

v Describe what would happen to the glucose level if the diabetic was injected with the correct dose of insulin in the next hour.

(1 mark)

(SEG June 1993)

4 The diagram shows a kidney tubule.

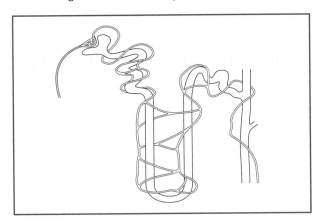

a Draw a simplified diagram and label it with the letters X, Y and Z to show the following:

X: where filtration occurs;

Y: the blood vessel containing the highest concentration of oxygen;

Z: a tube containing the fluid most similar to urine. *(3 marks)*

b The table shows some of the substances present in blood plasma and in the filtrate formed directly from the blood plasma in the kidney tubule.

| Substance | Concentration in g per dm³ | |
	Plasma	Filtrate
Water	900.0	900.0
Protein	80.0	0.0
Glucose	1.0	1.0
Amino acids	0.5	0.5
Urea	0.3	0.3
Inorganic ions	7.2	7.2

i 1 Give the name of one substance in the table which does not pass out of the blood during filtration. *(1 mark)*

2 Explain why this substance cannot filter out of the blood. *(1 mark)*

ii 180 g of glucose and 550 g of sodium ions may be filtered out of a person's blood each day by the kidneys. Normally, however, no glucose and only 5 g of sodium ions are lost in the urine. Explain these observations.

(3 marks)

c A person with kidney failure may be treated by using a kidney machine. The process is called dialysis. A dialysis session may last up to 8 hours and the patient undergoes dialysis every 3 to 4 days. The diagram shows the principles of dialysis.

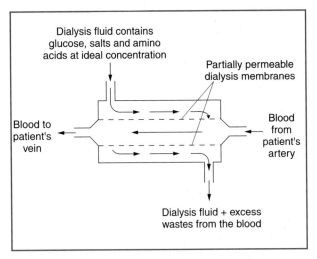

i Why is it important that the dialysis fluid should have ideal concentrations of dissolved substances? *(3 marks)*

ii One danger of using a kidney machine is that blood clotting is more likely to occur and an anti-clotting drug is usually added to the patient's blood to prevent this.

1 Explain why blood clotting is more likely to occur. *(1 mark)*

2 Why is it important that blood clots do not re-enter the patient's body? *(3 marks)*

(SEG June 1997)

5 a The diagram shows a section of the skin.

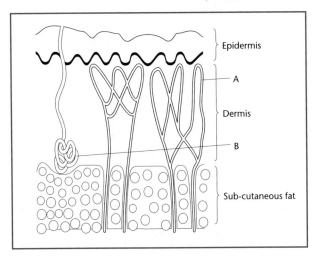

i Name parts A and B. *(2 marks)*

ii Explain how the product of B helps the body to lose heat. *(2 marks)*

b After waiting outside on a cold day a person may look pale and start to shiver.

i Why may the skin look pale?

ii What causes shivering? *(2 marks)*

(NEAB June 1997)

9 Reproduction

One of the most wonderful moments in a couple's life is the arrival of a new baby. In this chapter, you will learn about the events leading up to this, from the production of the sex cells through to the birth itself. You will also find out about the changes which take place in the mother's body and how her pregnancy is monitored.

After you have worked through this chapter, you should be able to:

- Describe the male and female reproductive organs and show how they are organised for their functions.
- Describe the male and female gametes and outline their importance in the reproductive process.
- Describe and explain the changes in a female body in preparation for pregnancy.
- Outline the roles of the sex hormones testosterone, oestrogen and progesterone.
- Describe the events leading up to pregnancy.

- Describe and comment on the relative effectiveness of the main methods of birth control.
- Outline the structure and role of the placenta during pregnancy.
- Describe the healthy development of a foetus.
- Explain why a pregnant woman needs to look after herself.
- Outline the changes in the reproductive organs during birth.
- Discuss the needs of a lactating woman.

Infertility

What are the causes of infertility?

Infertility describes the situation of a couple who are unable to achieve a pregnancy after trying for more than a year. The reasons for this can be physical, emotional or psychological. The factors may be present from birth or develop later due to other influences such as prolonged stress, illness, alcohol or drug abuse, trauma or obesity. Figure 1 illustrates some possible physical problems.

How can couples be helped?

Before doctors can offer help for infertility they need to know the nature of the problem. The couple are referred to a clinic for tests.

The sperm test is always carried out first as 30 to 40% of all infertility problems are due to sperm deficiencies. The doctors are looking for a sperm count of at least 20 million per cm^3 of semen, of which 60% of the sperms are normal. If the sperm count proves acceptable then tests are directed towards the woman.

Diagnosing the problem may take some time but once it is known, treatment can begin. The following treatments may be recommended:

- **Surgery** to clear a blocked Fallopian tube or remove an ovarian cyst.
- **Drugs** to clear up an infection.
- **Hormone treatment** to correct an inadequacy/ imbalance.
- **Artificial insemination** (AI) to get past the cervix.
- **In vitro fertilisation** (IVF) followed by implantation.

What is artificial insemination?

Artificial insemination involves placing healthy sperm into a woman's uterus at the time of ovulation. The chances are that one sperm will fertilise the ovum. Most women become pregnant within three months of starting this procedure.

The sperm used for artificial insemination can either be donated by a woman's partner or by any other male. Sperm banks have now been set up where sperm can be stored for up to three years. This of course, opens up the possibility of selective breeding as women can choose to have a baby by any man who has donated a sperm sample to the sperm bank.

What is *in vitro* fertilisation?

When all other possible procedures for infertility have failed both the egg and sperm can be removed and fertilisation encouraged in a suitable receptacle outside a human body (*in vitro*). It is even possible to inject a sperm into the egg to ensure fertilisation takes place. The resulting embryo can be kept alive and in a very healthy state for a few days giving the doctors a chance to re-implant it into the woman's receptive uterus.

This has now been done successfully on many occasions and produced many normal healthy babies, the so called 'test tube babies'.

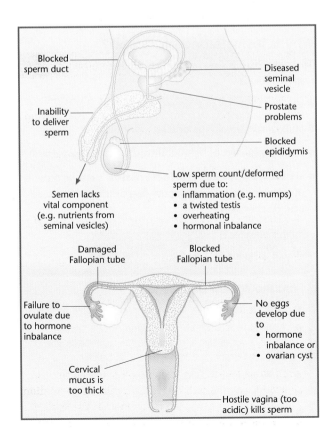

Figure 1 *Some of the reasons for infertility.*

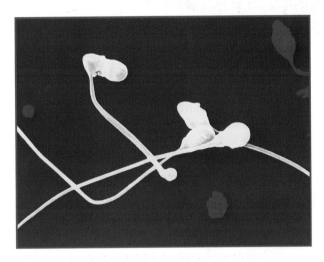

Figure 2 *Not all sperm are healthy.*

Substituting genes

Many diseases are known to be caused by a single defective gene which is passed on from parents to their offspring. About one hundred of these have been detected, including **muscular dystrophy**, **cystic fibrosis** and **haemophilia**. *In vitro* fertilisation opens up the possibility of checking for any of these. The procedure involves removing a cell from a two-day-old embryo and checking the chromosomes for a defective gene. If no defective gene is present then the embryo can be implanted into the female uterus. It will grow as normal.

This type of **gene therapy** could also help couples who, until now, have chosen not to have children because of the possibility of 'bad' genes coming together. It must be said, however, that there are very strict regulations governing the practice of gene therapy.

When are fertility drugs used?

Fertility drugs are used when a woman is not releasing eggs from her ovaries, or eggs are failing to develop due to a hormone inbalance in her blood. These drugs, many of which are hormones themselves, correct the problem, resulting in a normal cycle of events. For example, drugs can be given to increase the production of **follicle stimulation hormone** (FSH) by the pituitary gland and **human chorionic gonadotrophic hormone** (HCG) can be given to induce ovulation.

Occasionally this drug treatment may result in a multiple birth, but this is rare.

Sexual reproduction

Sexual reproduction in humans involves the production of special cells, the sex cells called **gametes** (eggs and sperms). It is in these gametes that the characteristics of the parents are transferred to their offspring. This hereditary information is stored in the **genes** on the **chromosomes** within the nucleus of a gamete.

The gametes are produced by a special kind of cell division called meiosis (chapter 11.3). During meiosis, some of the genes are moved around between chromosomes and then half the chromosomes are transferred into each gamete. When a male and female gamete fuse during **fertilisation**, the cell produced is called a **zygote**. This cell contains a full set of chromosomes, half of which carry genes from the male partner and half of which carry genes from the female partner. This results in the offspring having some characteristics from the male parent and some from the female parent.

The parts of the human body concerned with reproduction form the **reproductive system**. This system in the male differs from the female system, because (apart from the production of gametes) it performs different functions.

The male reproductive system

The male reproductive system has three main functions and its structure is organised to fulfil these:

- the **testes** produce the male gametes (**sperm**)
- the **penis** deposits the sperm inside the female's reproductive system.
- the testes produce the male hormone **testosterone**.

Additional structures, the **seminal vesicles** and **prostate gland**, supply nutrients for the sperm to use after it has been released inside the female (see figure 1).

Sperm production

The male gamete is the sperm cell (see figure 2). Male individuals produce these from **puberty** for the rest of their lives. This production is controlled by hormones (follicle stimulating hormone, FSH and luteinising hormone, LH) secreted by the pituitary gland (chapter 10.4).

The sperms are produced in tiny tubes, the **seminiferous tubules** within the testes. They are stored until ejaculation in another tube called the **epididymis** (see figure 1). Those not used are broken down, reabsorbed and replaced. The testes are held in sacs (the **scrotal sacs**) outside the body, because the best temperature for sperm production is 33–34 °C, a few degrees lower than body temperature. Too much heat can result in a low sperm count.

What does semen contain?

The release of sperms from the epididymis is called **ejaculation**. During sexual excitement, the erectile tissue in the penis fills with blood making it hard and erect. This makes it easier to insert into the female's vagina. At the climax of intercourse, the epididymis, **vas deferens** and muscles at the base of the penis contract expelling the sperms out of the penis. Also expelled are secretions of the **seminal vesicles** and **prostate gland**.

The seminal vesicles provide nutrients (fructose and vitamins) for energy for the sperms and the prostate gland produces alkaline substances, proteins, minerals and enzymes to provide a suitable physical environment for the sperms – the female vagina even releases an antibiotic to inhibit growth of bacteria. This mixture of sperms and glandular secretions is called **semen**.

What is a normal sperm count?

An ejaculate, on average, contains about 2 to 3 cm^3 of semen. A normal sperm count is about 110 million sperm per cm^3. A sperm count of 60 to 70 million per cm^3 is low and below 20 million per cm^3 is considered infertile (page 115). The main reasons for a low sperm count include failure of the testes to develop properly, over heating in the scotal area, or contraction of a disease such as mumps.

Why is testosterone produced?

Testosterone is the male sex hormone and is responsible for:

- the development and maintenace of the sex organs
- changes in the shape and size of the body
- changes in sexual behaviour and attitude (sex drive)
- **secondary sexual characteristics**, such as growth of hair on the face and body, deepening of the voice and thicker skin.

What do **you** know?

You should now be able to:

- Label a diagram of the male reproductive system.
- Annotate it with the functions of the testes, penis, scotal sacs, sperm ducts, prostate gland and urethra.
- Draw and label a diagram of a sperm cell.
- Explain what semen contains.
- Outline the roles of testosterone.

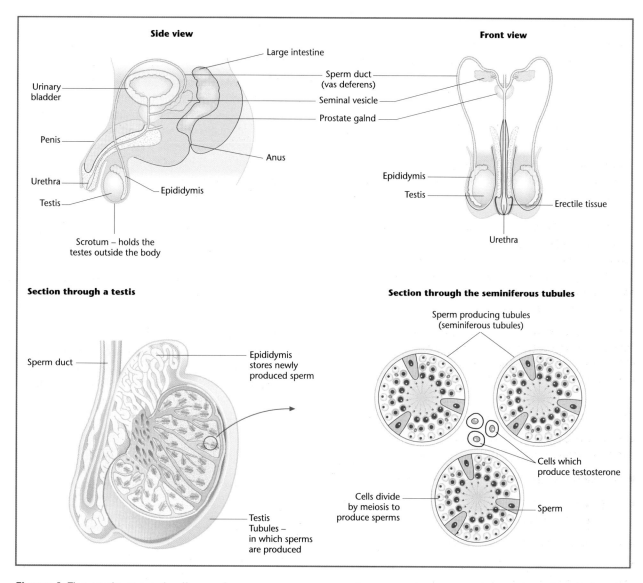

Figure 1 *The male reproductive system.*

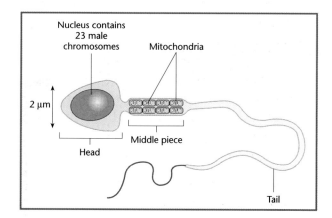

Figure 2 *A sperm cell.*

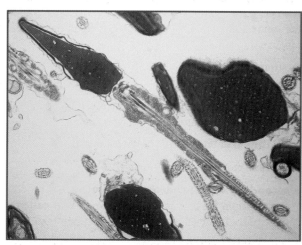

Figure 3 *A single sperm showing the head, middle piece and tail regions.*

9.2 The female reproductive system

The female reproductive system

The female reproductive system has four main functions and its structure (see figure 1) is organised to fulfil these:

- the **ovaries** produce the female gametes (**eggs**)
- the **uterus** provides a safe home for the developing baby and aids the transfer of food
- the ovaries produce the hormones **oestrogen** and **progesterone**
- the **mammary glands** (breasts) provide food for the newly-born baby

Egg production

The female gamete is the egg, more correctly called an **ovum**. It is produced by the ovary (see figure 1). When a girl is born, each ovary contains all (and more) of the eggs it will ever produce, but these are in an immature state. When a girl starts her periods (menstruation), around the age of 12 to 13 years, the eggs start to mature. Under the direction of hormones produced by the pituitary gland, one of these eggs ripens about every 4 weeks around the age of 50 years until menopause. This period, from puberty to **menopause**, is the fertile period of a female's life.

An egg matures as part of a fluid filled capsule called a **Graafian follicle**. The cells forming the follicle both feed the egg and produce oestrogen. After about two weeks, the egg is mature and ready to be released into the oviduct. The follicle ruptures and the egg is 'blown' out, taking a few follicle cells with it. The remains of the follicle form a 'scar tissue' known as the **corpus luteum** (or yellow body). This continues to produce small amounts of oestrogen, but mostly produces large amounts of **progesterone**.

What are oestrogen and progesterone?

Both oestrogen and progesterone are hormones involved in the control and changes that take place during the female menstrual cycle. These are described in chapter 9.3.

Oestrogen, together with other hormones, is also responsible for:

- the development and maintenance of the female reproductive structures
- the control of body fluid/salt balance
- calcium/protein balance in bones
- **secondary sexual characteristics**, such as fat distibution in the breasts and hips, female hair pattern, voice pitch, broadening of the pelvis and skin texture.

The amount of oestrogen produced declines after menopause and this can have noticeable affects on the female body (chapter 10.4).

Female cancers

There are two main cancers affecting the female reproductive structures:

- **Cervical cancer** accounts for between 2–3% of all female cancer deaths in the UK, but this is falling, partly because of an effective screening programme. All women over the age of 35 years are encouraged to have regular cervical smear tests. Most of the deaths from cervical cancer are of women who have not had these tests.
- **Breast cancer** affects about 1 in every 14 women. Its causes still remain a mystery, but if detected early, it can often be treated successfully. Women should get into a routine of examining their breasts for lumps.

Sperm	Egg
Very small ≈1/500 mm	Very large ≈1/10 mm
Nucleus contains half of the male's chromosomes	Nucleus contains half of the female's chromosomes
Cytoplasm contains lots of mitochondria to release energy	Cytoplasm contains lots of yolk as food for the initial stages of embryo development
Can move on their own	Cannot move on their own
Several hundred million produced every day from puberty onwards	Present from birth and one matures about every 4 weeks from puberty to menopause
Each ejaculate contains about 200–400 million	One released about every 4 weeks

Table 1 *A comparison of the male and female gametes.*

What do **you** know?

You should now be able to:

- Label a diagram of the female reproductive system.
- Annotate it with the functions of the ovary, oviduct, uterus, cervix and vagina.
- Draw and label a diagram of an egg cell.
- Draw a series of diagrams to show the changes that take place in an ovary as an egg matures.
- Describe what happens in an ovary after ovulation.
- Outline the roles of oestrogen and progesterone.

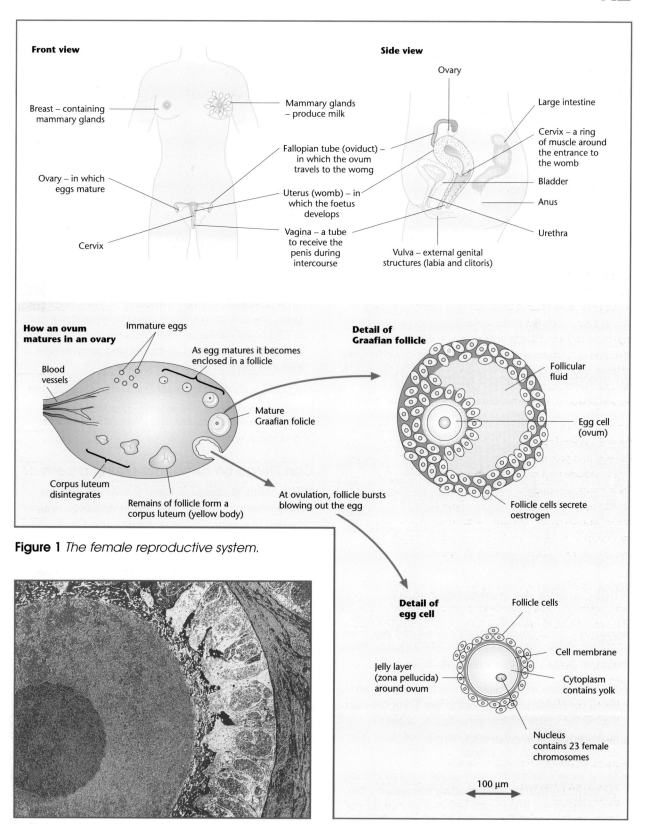

Front view

Breast – containing mammary glands

Ovary – in which eggs mature

Cervix

Mammary glands – produce milk

Fallopian tube (oviduct) – in which the ovum travels to the womg

Uterus (womb) – in which the foetus develops

Vagina – a tube to receive the penis during intercourse

Side view

Ovary

Large intestine

Cervix – a ring of muscle around the entrance to the womb

Bladder

Anus

Urethra

Vulva – external genital structures (labia and clitoris)

How an ovum matures in an ovary

Immature eggs

Blood vessels

As egg matures it becomes enclosed in a follicle

Mature Graafian folicle

Corpus luteum disintegrates

Remains of follicle form a corpus luteum (yellow body)

At ovulation, follicle bursts blowing out the egg

Detail of Graafian follicle

Follicular fluid

Egg cell (ovum)

Follicle cells secrete oestrogen

Figure 1 *The female reproductive system.*

Detail of egg cell

Follicle cells

Cell membrane

Cytoplasm contains yolk

Jelly layer (zona pellucida) around ovum

Nucleus contains 23 female chromosomes

100 μm

Figure 2 *A photograph of part of a mature egg with the cytoplasm shown in pink and nucleus shown in red.*

9.3 The female cycle

What is the female cycle?

At **puberty**, a female becomes sexually mature and starts producing mature eggs. She is capable of having a baby and her body prepares for this every time a new egg is released from an ovary. This happens about once a month, and the cycle of events is called the **menstrual cycle**.

The menstrual cycle continues throughout a female's fertile period. This fertile period ends with the **menopause** (chapter 10.4), at, on average, age 52 years. The cycle stops during pregnancy and it is this that is often taken as the first sign of a pregnancy.

When does the menstrual cycle start?

At the start of puberty, a girl will experience her first '**period**'. This is a discharge of blood from her vagina which shows that her menstrual cycles have begun. The periods may be irregular at first, but will eventually happen approximately every 28 days. The discharge usually lasts for the first 5 days.

Where does this blood come from?

To understand where this blood comes from you need to understand how the female body prepares itself for pregnancy. This involves cyclic changes in both the ovary and the uterus. The aim is to produce a mature egg and to prepare the uterus for the implantation of the egg if is fertilised. The changes in the ovary are described in chapter 9.2. The preparation of the uterus involves the development of an extra layer lining the uterus wall (endometrium) which contains lots of blood spaces. The blood discharged during the period is from the breakdown of this layer.

What controls the menstrual cycle?

The cyclic changes are co-ordinated and controlled by **hormones**, two from the pituitary gland and two from the ovary. The main stages are summarised below. These should be studied in conjunction with figure 1.

- The cycle starts at the beginning of the period (also called the menstrual flow). This is day 1. For the next 5 days, the unused extra uterus lining, called the **endometrium**, together with some blood, is discharged through the vagina.
- At the same time the pituitary gland starts producing the hormone **follicle stimulating hormone** (FSH). This initiates the maturation of a new egg within the ovary and the production of oestrogen by the follicle cells around the egg. The oestrogen builds up in the blood and at the end of the period, directs the uterus to start repairing the uterus lining and preparing a

new layer once again. The high level of oestrogen in the blood also has a negative feedback on the production of FSH and its production ceases.

- A high oestrogen level also triggers the release of another pituitary hormone called **luteinising hormone** (LH). This causes **ovulation** and the development of a **corpus luteum** (yellow body) from the remains of the follicle. The corpus luteum continues to produce small amounts of oestrogen and starts to produce a second hormone, called **progesterone**. The build up of progesterone in the blood, indicates to the uterus that an egg is on its way and therefore, it completes its preparations. It also continues to inhibit the production of FSH.
- If, by day 24, a fertilised egg has not arrived at the uterus, the corpus luteum degenerates and therefore stops producing the two hormones. In the absence of these, the new uterus lining starts to break down and is discharged on day 29. This becomes day 1 of the next cycle. In the absence of oestrogen and progesterone, FSH also starts to be produced again.

The timings given here are for the average female. The length of a cycle can vary considerably and in some cases can be very irregular. Not every female has her period every 28 days.

Can life go on as normal during a period?

This monthly discharge of blood should not interfere with any normal activity. However, it does require more attention to personal hygiene. An absorbent pad can be worn to catch the flow of blood. This pad can be worn externally as a **sanitary towel** or internally in the form of a **tampon**. It must be changed regularly and disposed of hygienically.

What happens if the egg is fertilised?

If the egg is fertilised, the corpus luteum persists and continues to produce oestrogen and progesterone for a further three months. By this time, the placenta has formed and this takes over the work of producing the two hormones for the rest of the pregnancy. The presence of these hormones in the blood ensures that the uterus lining remains intact and continues to develop, and inhibits the production of FSH so that no more eggs mature in the ovaries. The high levels of oestrogen and progesterone present in the blood also stimulate breast development.

Just before the birth the progesterone level in a mother falls and this signals the pituitary gland to produce two more hormones: **prolactin** and **oxytocin**. Prolactin triggers the breasts to start producing milk and oxytocin initiates labour.

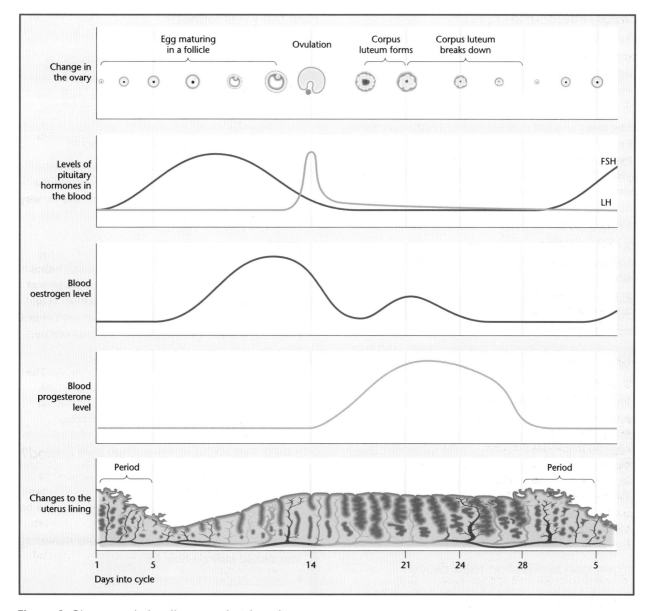

Figure 1 *Changes during the menstrual cycle.*

What do **you** know?

You should now be able to:

- Explain what FSH is and what it does.
- Outline the changes which take place in the ovary as a result of the presence of FSH.
- Explain why ovulation takes place.
- Describe the changes in the ovary after ovulation.
- Explain the role of the corpus luteum.

- Outline the structural changes in the uterus due to the presence of oestrogen and progsterone.
- Explain why the endometrium starts to break down.
- Explain why FSH production stops before ovulation and starts again on day 1 of the cycle.
- Outline what happens if a fertilised egg implants in the uterus.

9.4 Fertilisation and implantation

Sexual intercourse

During **sexual intercourse**, semen is deposited into the vagina. The vagina is a very acid and hostile place and immediately kills many of the sperms. The survivors make their way through the cervix and to the oviduct at an average rate of 3 mm per minute.

After being released from the ovary (**ovulation**), the egg is moved along the oviduct by the beating cilia on the lining cells. For a successful pregnancy, the egg and sperm need to meet well into the oviduct. This gives the fertilised egg time to develop before it has to implant in the uterus wall. Only a few thousand of the sperms will reach the oviduct and only a small proportion of these will reach the egg.

How do the egg and sperm meet?

In order to fertilise the egg, the sperm head must undergo a change called **capacitation**. Only when this has happened will it be able to release the enzymes necessary to penetrate the outer layers surrounding the egg, bind to the egg cell membrane, and enter the cell. Once a sperm is in an egg cell the membrane thickens to prevent the entry of any more sperms.

Inside the egg, the sperm nucleus, containing the 23 chromosomes from the father, and the egg nucleus containing the 23 chromosomes from the mother fuse together. **Fertilisation** is now complete and the resulting cell is called a **zygote**. This contains all the instructions for a new life, but for a pregnancy to develop, a lot more changes have to take place before this reaches the uterus.

When can fertilisation take place?

Sperms are usually capable of fertilising an egg for up to 3 days after ejaculation. However, eggs are only receptive for about 24 hours. The most successful fertilisations take place within 12 hours of ovulation.

What happens after fertilisation?

After fertilisation, the zygote continues to be pushed along the oviduct towards the uterus. It uses the stored food in the cytoplasm of the egg to divide several times. By the time it reaches the uterus some 4 days later, it consists of a ball of cells and is called an **embryo**. The embryo now uses enzymes to penetrate the specially prepared soft uterine lining and 2 days later is completely engulfed. This process is called **implantation**. The female is now technically pregnant. From this moment on, the embryo will grow by receiving food from its mother's blood. To aid this transfer of food a special organ called the **placenta** develops.

How are twins formed?

There are two kinds of twins:

- **Identical twins** are produced when a fertilised egg divides into two and each new cell develops into a full embryo. Identical twins will have the same genes and will, therefore, be alike in everything controlled by the genes. **Siamese twins** are identical twins resulting from the incomplete separation of the divided zygote.

- **Fraternal twins** result from two separate eggs being fertilised at the same time. Because they are the products of completely different eggs and spems, they can be very different, even different sexes.

How do pregnancy tests work?

An implanted embryo produces a hormone called **human chorionic gonadotrophin** (HCG), to trigger the ovaries to continue producing oestrogen and progesterone. This hormone can be detected in the mother's urine soon after implantation and is one of the first signs of pregnancy.

What are the signs of pregnancy?

The first sign of pregnancy is usually a missed period, but there are other signs, such as feeling nauseous (at any time of day, not just in the morning), having enlarged and tender breasts, feeling tired and needing to pass water more often. Some women just know in their own mind when they are pregnant.

What do **you** know?

You should now be able to:
- Explain how sperms reach the egg.
- Explain why capacitation is necessary prior to fertilisation.
- Explain why only one sperm can fertilise an egg.
- Draw some diagrams to explain the full process of fertilisation.
- State how many chromosomes are in a zygote and where they came from.
- Explain the difference between a zygote, embryo and foetus.
- Explain the process of implantation and why it is so crucial to the continued development of the embryo.
- Outline how fraternal and identical twins can be produced.
- Outline how you can tell if you are pregnant.

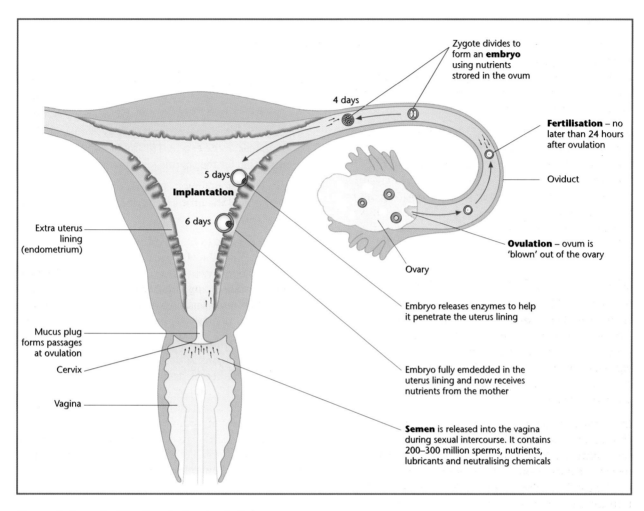

Figure 1 *From fertilisation to implantation.*

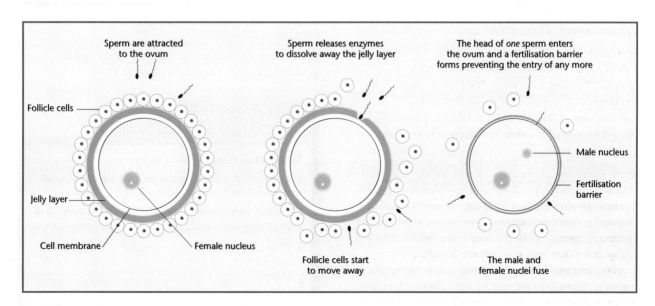

Figure 2 *The stages leading to fertilisation.*

Not all couples want children, some want to limit the size of their family and others find it difficult to produce children. There are now a variety of methods available to help all categories.

Preventing pregnancy

There are many methods of preventing an unwanted pregnancy. Some of these **contraceptive methods** are more reliable than others and some even carry health risks (see table 1).

1 **Natural methods** involve no artificial devices and fall into two categories:

- The **withdrawal method** requires the man to withdraw his penis immediately before ejaculation so no sperms enter the vagina.

- The **safe period** requires a woman to predict when ovulation will take place each month by monitoring her body temperature and cervical mucus. She must avoid intercourse for the five days before the predicted ovulation date and the five days after. This is known as the **fertile period**. The remaining days of the cycle are known as the safe period and it is only during this time that intercourse should take place (see figure 1).

  It is now possible to measure the level of hormones in the urine using an electronic monitoring device. This makes it easier to predict ovulation (chapter 9.4).

2 **Barrier methods** are used to prevent the egg and sperms meeting. This can be achieved by using a condom or diaphragm.

- The **condom** is a very thin sheath of rubber which is rolled over the penis, or fitted into the vagina (**femidom**), before intercourse. On ejaculation, the sperms are caught in the sheath (see figure 2). A **spermicidal cream** should always be used with a condom. This is the only form of contraception which gives protection against sexually transmitted diseases.

- The **cap** or **diaphragm** is a dome shaped piece of rubber which fits over the entrance to the uterus (cervix). It should be fitted before intercourse and left in position for six hours afterwards (see figure 3). A spermicidal cream should be used with it.

3 **Intra-uterine devices** (IUD/coil) are small pieces of carefully shaped plastic or copper, which when inserted through the cervix into the uterus stop the fertilised egg implanting (see figure 4). Some now contain progesterone to thicken the mucus plug in the cervix and prevent the sperms passing through. Another variation of this is the **morning after coil** which can provide protection if inserted up to 72 hours after intercourse.

4 **Contraceptive pills** make use of hormones. There are two main kinds of contraceptive pill, the combined pill and the progesterone only pill (mini-pill).

- The **combined pill** contains the hormones oestrogen and progesterone. It works by preventing the release of an egg from the ovary.

- The **progesterone only pill** works by thickening the mucus in the cervix. This makes it almost impossible for the sperms to get through.

  Both types of pill must be taken regularly and according to the instructions if contraception is to be successful.

It is now possible to have synthetic progesterone injections under the skin just four times a year. This works by preventing ovulation. A variation is provided by six flexible matchstick sized capsules, which when inserted under the skin can prevent ovulation for up to five years.

5 **Surgical methods** can be used to alter the reproductive organs so that it is impossible for eggs and sperms to meet, effectively creating sterility.

- Male sterilisation is called **vasectomy**. It involves cutting and tying the sperm (vas deferens) duct so that no sperms can be released during ejaculation (see figure 5).

- Females can be sterilised by a similar operation to cut the Fallopian tubes (see figure 5). This is called **tubal ligation**.

Sterilisation techniques are usually irreversible.

Why do some couples find it difficult to produce children?

There are many reasons for this and many possible solutions. These are discussed on page 114.

What do **you** know?

You should now be able to:

- Describe the advantages and disadvantages of natural methods of birth control.
- Explain why barrier methods and IUD's work.
- Compare the different forms of contraceptive pill.
- Draw diagrams to show surgical sterilisation methods.
- Produce a table to compare the effectiveness of different birth control methods.

Method	Approx. pregnancies per 100 users	Some disadvantages
No contraception	40+	
Withdrawal	10+	May not withdraw in time.
Safe period	15+	Only suitable for women who have regular cycles. Needs careful record keeping.
Condoms + spermicidal cream	4	May slip off.
Cap + spermicidal cream	3 / 15 without cream	Needs to be the correct size and inserted before intercourse and left in place for 6 hrs after intercourse.
IUD	3	Must be fitted by a doctor. Sometimes causes heavier periods.
Combined pill	0	Pill must be taken daily. Can have some side effects such as high blood pressure.
Mini-pill	2	Pill must be taken at the same time every day – there is no margin for error.
Sterilisation	0	Usually irreversible.

Table 1 *The success/failure rate of contraceptives.*

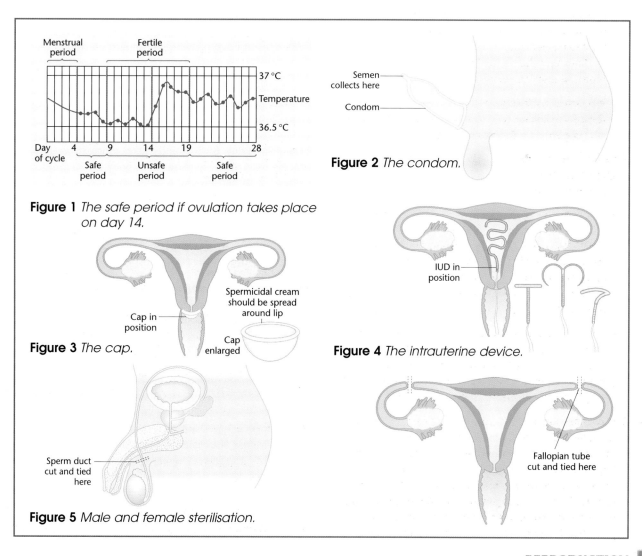

Figure 1 *The safe period if ovulation takes place on day 14.*

Figure 2 *The condom.*

Figure 3 *The cap.*

Figure 4 *The intrauterine device.*

Figure 5 *Male and female sterilisation.*

What is the placenta?

The **placenta** is part of the support system which develops around the embryo. It is necessary for the growth of a healthy baby while it is in the mother's uterus. The placenta develops from some of the cells of the embryo and some of the cells from the uterus lining. It develops from a few finger-like projections which penetrate the uterus lining into a complex organ in just three months. The functions of the placenta are:

- To allow **the diffusion of food substances**, such as glucose, amino acids, minerals and vitamins, from the mother's blood into the foetal blood. Some can even be stored in the placenta for a short while.

- To allow **the diffusion of waste substances**, including urea, from the foetal blood into the mother's blood so that she can excrete them.

- **Gas exchange** takes place over the placenta. Oxygen diffuses into the foetal blood and carbon dioxide diffuses out into the mother's blood. The foetus contains a special kind of haemoglobin to facilitate the exchange of oxygen.

- Initially **to produce human chorionic gonadotrophin** (HCG), which directs the ovaries to continue to secrete oestrogen and progesterone. These hormones are necessary for the continuation of pregnancy because they help maintain the lining (endometrium) of the uterus wall. The placenta eventually takes over the **production of oestrogen and progesterone**.

- To **provide a protective barrier** which many disease causing micro-organisms cannot cross. Unfortunately there are still many, such as those for **HIV**, **German measles**, **chickenpox** and **polio** which can cross the placenta, sometimes with dreadful consequences. If the foetus is infected with German measles (rubella) for example, especially during the first few months of pregnancy, it may develop deafness, heart problems and even mental handicap. Most **drugs**, including **alcohol** and many of the **chemicals** in **cigarette smoke**, can also cross the placenta (chapters 4.4, 9.7, 12.6)

A simplified version of the placenta, along with the additional structures that develop to house and protect the embryo, are shown in figure 1.

How long from zygote to baby?

It takes 38 weeks (from **conception**) for a zygote to become a baby. This is known as the **gestation period**. Considering the zygote starts off as one cell about the size of a full stop, and grows to a fully formed baby consisting of about 30 million million cells, its growth and development has to proceed very rapidly.

After only 4 weeks in the uterus it is already 4 mm long and has a beating heart. After 5 weeks it has grown to about 12 mm and has the beginnings of its arms and legs. At 8 weeks it has a recognisable human form, and is now known as a foetus (see figure 3). It is now about 46 mm long from its head to its bottom. In week 9 it is possible to tell whether a baby is going to be a boy or a girl.

It is during these first few weeks of development that tissues are formed and organs take shape. At this stage a baby is particularly susceptible to the effects of drugs (chapter 12.7).

After 12 weeks, the foetus is 92 mm long and has all its internal organs (see figure 2). About 2 weeks later its kidneys actually start working. The foetus will be about 120 mm long.

The first kicking movements are usually felt by the mother after 16 weeks. After 20 weeks the foetus is fully formed, even having eyebrows, fingernails and fingerprints. It is now about 185 mm long and weighs approximately 700 g.

By week 26 of the pregnancy the foetus has grown to about 250 mm (1500 g) and has a reasonable chance of surviving if born. From week 35 the foetus takes on 14 g of fat a day. Birth usually takes place 38 weeks after conception. The average full term baby is 360 mm from its head to its bottom and weighs 3400 g.

What do **you** know?

You should now be able to:
- Label a diagram of a foetus inside the womb.
- Describe 2 functions of the amnion and 2 functions of the amniotic fluid.
- Explain the role of the umbilical cord.
- List 5 functions of the placenta.
- Name 3 useful substances which can cross the placenta into the foetus and 2 substances which pass into the mother.
- Produce a table to summarise the main changes to the foetus during pregnancy.
- Name 2 harmful substances which can cross the placenta.

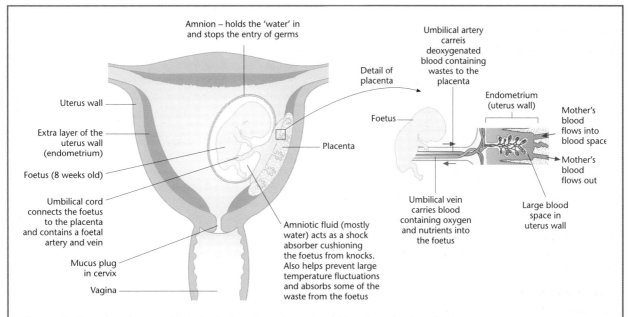

Amnion – holds the 'water' in and stops the entry of germs

Uterus wall

Extra layer of the uterus wall (endometrium)

Foetus (8 weeks old)

Umbilical cord connects the foetus to the placenta and contains a foetal artery and vein

Mucus plug in cervix

Vagina

Detail of placenta

Placenta

Amniotic fluid (mostly water) acts as a shock absorber cushioning the foetus from knocks. Also helps prevent large temperature fluctuations and absorbs some of the waste from the foetus

Umbilical artery carreis deoxygenated blood containing wastes to the placenta

Foetus

Endometrium (uterus wall)

Mother's blood flows into blood space

Mother's blood flows out

Umbilical vein carries blood containing oxygen and nutrients into the foetus

Large blood space in uterus wall

Figure 1 *The structures which help feed and protect the developing foetus.*

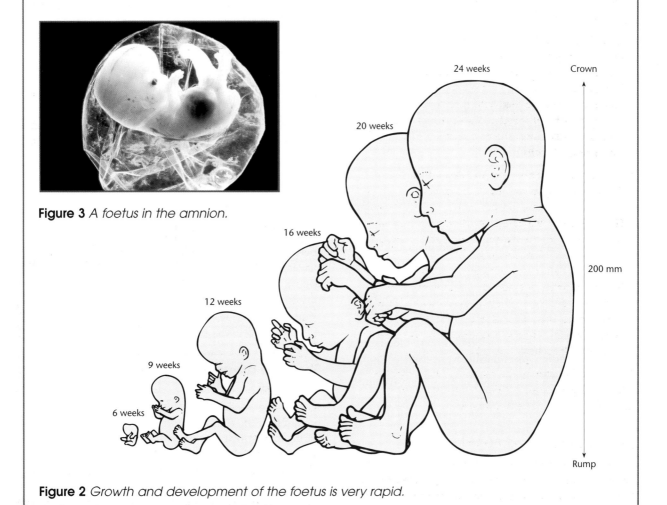

Figure 3 *A foetus in the amnion.*

24 weeks — Crown

20 weeks

16 weeks

12 weeks

9 weeks

6 weeks

200 mm

Rump

Figure 2 *Growth and development of the foetus is very rapid.*

Taking care

Having a baby puts an enormous strain on a mother emotionally and physically (see figure 1). During her pregnancy, a mother needs to take good care of herself by staying as healthy as possible and receiving care and support from her partner, friends and family. Usually, as soon as pregnancy is confirmed, a mother will be referred by her doctor to an **antenatal clinic** where her health and that of the growing foetus will be checked throughout the pregnancy.

What happens at an antenatal clinic?

The first visit to the clinic is by far the longest. The doctors and midwives have to find out the state of health of any prospective mother. Later visits are shorter. On the first visit, a mother will be:

- Asked many questions about her health, past and present, in order to build up a **full medical history**. Her personal circumstances may be discussed so that any other problems can be foreseen.

- Given a **full physical examination** including measurements of height, weight and blood pressure. These are checked at every visit, as they can be good indicators of possible problems.

- Given an **internal examination** to check on the size of the womb. A **cervical smear** may be taken so that changes can be monitored.

- Given **urine** and **blood tests**. A urine sample is checked for glucose, protein and infections. The presence of glucose is usually an indication of **diabetes**. The presence of protein usually indicates that the kidneys are not coping with the extra load. The urine is also checked for placental hormones. The blood sample is used to check **blood group** (ABO and **rhesus** group), for **antibodies** to German measles, and to test for **anaemia**. It can also show up infections like syphilis, hepatitis B and AIDS. Any of these will certainly complicate the pregnancy and may even give rise to the very difficult question of terminating the pregnancy (an abortion). Blood and urine samples are taken during every visit.

Around the 16th to 18th week of pregnancy, a routine **ultrasound scan** will be carried out to confirm the age of the foetus and indicate the position of the placenta. It can also show up any problems in growth.

A mother over 35 years old, or those with a family history of **Down's syndrome**, **spina bifida** or **muscular dystrophy**, will be given the chance of an **amniocentesis** (see figure 2). This is a special test, which can indicate whether a child is likely to develop abnormally.

A similar test called **chorionic villus sampling** (CVS) can now be carried out after 8 weeks of pregnancy, enabling an earlier decision on termination to be made.

Weight gain during pregnancy

A pregnant woman will need to supply nutrients and energy for the growth and development of her baby. She will also require extra energy for herself as she carries the foetus. The main changes to her diet are shown in table 1. The extra nutrients can be supplied as part of a **well balanced diet**. More protein can be obtained from meat and fish, more vitamins from fresh fruit and vegetables, and more energy from carbohydrates and fats. The antenatal clinic will supply a diet sheet to help. An average weight gain during pregnancy is about 12.5 kg.

Should a pregnant woman smoke and drink?

There is a lot of evidence to suggest that a mother who smokes during pregnancy will produce a smaller, under-developed baby. This is because chemicals in the cigarettes cause the placental blood vessels to constrict, reducing the flow of blood and so reducing the amount of food available to the baby. The carbon monoxide taken in reduces the amount of oxygen in the mother's blood, and nicotine actually crosses the placenta and can directly affect the baby. Nicotine is a stimulant and makes the baby's heart beat too quickly, putting great stress on its circulation.

There is also evidence available which suggests that if there is alcohol in the mother's blood, it can cross the placenta and enter the foetus, resulting in **foetal alcohol syndrome**. The baby can be born with physical disabilities and may even be mentally retarded. Some researchers have also linked drinking alcohol with a higher incidence of miscarriage.

Should a pregnant woman take medicines?

A number of medicines, including some which can be bought over the counter, can harm the developing foetus particularly early on in pregnancy (chapter 12.7). To be safe, all medicines and other drugs should be avoided during pregnancy unless prescribed or taken with the consent of a doctor.

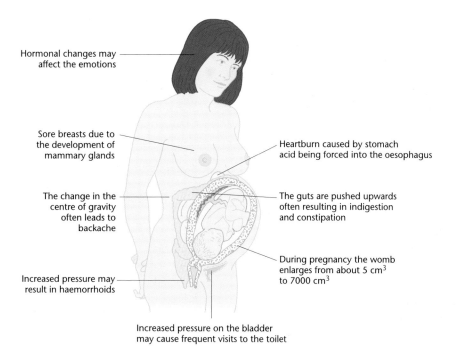

Hormonal changes may affect the emotions

Sore breasts due to the development of mammary glands

Heartburn caused by stomach acid being forced into the oesophagus

The change in the centre of gravity often leads to backache

The guts are pushed upwards often resulting in indigestion and constipation

During pregnancy the womb enlarges from about 5 cm^3 to 7000 cm^3

Increased pressure may result in haemorrhoids

Increased pressure on the bladder may cause frequent visits to the toilet

Figure 1 *Some minor problems are associated with pregnancy.*

Nutrient	Non-pregnant (19–50 year old)	Pregnant (19–50 year old)
Energy (kJ)	8100	8900
Protein (g)	45	51
Calcium (mg)	700	700
Iron (mg)	14.8	14.8
Vitamin A (µg)	600	700
Vitamin C (mg)	40	50
Vitamin D (µg)	No RNI	10
Folic Acid (µg)	200	300

Table 1 *How a woman's diet should change during pregnancy (last 3 months).*

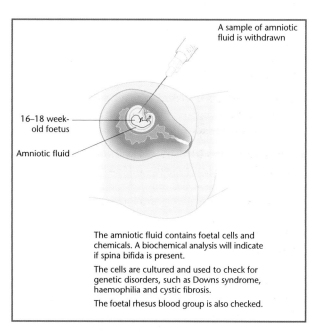

A sample of amniotic fluid is withdrawn

16–18 week-old foetus

Amniotic fluid

The amniotic fluid contains foetal cells and chemicals. A biochemical analysis will indicate if spina bifida is present.

The cells are cultured and used to check for genetic disorders, such as Downs syndrome, haemophilia and cystic fibrosis.

The foetal rhesus blood group is also checked.

Figure 2 *Testing for abnormalities using amniocentesis.*

What do **you** know?

You should now be able to:

- Outline what happens at an antenatal clinic and what problems may be discovered.
- Explain why a pregnant woman has an ultrasound test after 16 weeks.
- Explain why an amniocentesis may be required and describe the procedure.
- Suggest how and why a mother's diet should change during pregnancy.

9.8 Birth

When does birth take place?

Birth usually takes place in the 38th week of pregnancy. Mothers can get a good idea of the expected date of the birth by counting on 40 weeks from the first day of their last period. The foetus starts to get ready for birth from about the 32nd week by moving into the **birth position**, that is, turning so its head is nearest the cervix (see figure 1).

What happens during birth?

Birth begins with **labour**. This is the term used to describe the regular contractions of the muscles in the uterus wall brought on by hormonal changes in the blood (chapter 9.3). Labour consists of three stages:

- **Dilation**. The time from the onset of labour to the complete dilation of the cervix, this typically lasts between 6 to 12 hours. It starts with weak labour contractions and the dislodging of the mucus plug from the cervix. The passing of this plug is often called a '**show**' indicating that the birth is about to start. The contractions gradually get stronger, and eventually the cervix opening expands to about 10 cm. The head of the baby now breaks the amnion and the fluid is released. The female will suddenly pass a lot of watery fluid and this is a sign that the birth of her baby is not far off. This is sometimes called the '**waters breaking**'.

- **Delivery**. The expulsion of the baby usually lasts between one and two hours. Strong contractions of the uterus wall force the baby through the cervix and vagina and out into the world. As soon as the baby has started breathing, the umbilical cord is tied and cut, separating the baby from the placenta, and the mother.

- **Afterbirth**. The labour contractions may stop for a short period, but eventually start up again, forcing the placenta out. This is called the **afterbirth**.

Is labour ever induced?

Labour will occasionally be induced if the baby is well overdue and there is a threat to the health of the mother or the baby. The first attempt is often to break the amnion, but if this fails, the hormone **oxytocin** is fed through a drip into a vein in the mother's arm.

What if the foetus is not in the birth position?

If the foetus fails to get into the birth position, it may have to be delivered bottom-first. This is called a **breech birth**. Breech births need more care and therefore often take longer. Sometimes **forceps** need to be used so that the doctor can guide and pull the baby's head safely through the pelvis. This use of forceps is quite common, especially during awkward births or when the labour contractions are not sufficiently strong.

Occasionally, rather than perform a very difficult breech birth or for other health reasons, the doctor may do a **Caesarean birth**. This is the delivery of the baby through a cut in the abdomen wall. It can be done under general anaesthetic or with an **epidural** anaesthetic. This is a local anaesthetic that is injected into the space around the spinal cord in the lumbar region of the back. Here it numbs the nerves that carry the feelings of pain from the lower abdomen to the brain. Many mothers prefer an epidural Caesarean so they will be conscious and involved when their baby is born.

What is a premature baby?

A baby born before it is due is said to be **premature**. It is not uncommon for babies to be born soon after the 7th month of pregnancy and survive. Babies who have a birth weight of less than 2.5 kg are also described as premature.

Many premature babies are not fully developed and will need extra care and attention. For example, they may not be able to control their body temperature, breathe easily or be able to suck and therefore may have feeding difficulties. These babies will need help, and must be kept in a controlled environment, such as in an **incubator**, until they can survive on their own.

Many premature babies are jaundiced and need **phototherapy** treatment. This involves using blue light to help break down bile pigments, which build up in the blood because the liver is not yet fully developed and functioning. Sometimes a blood transfusion will be necessary.

What is a miscarriage?

Technically, a miscarriage is the ending of a pregnancy before the 28th week, that is before the baby is able to survive outside the womb. Miscarriages are frequent and about one in six pregnancies end this way. Most miscarriages happen before the 12th week, often due to a fault developing in the foetus or the mother contracting an infection such as German measles. Miscarriages later in pregnancy are often due to the placenta not working correctly or sometimes due to a weak cervix.

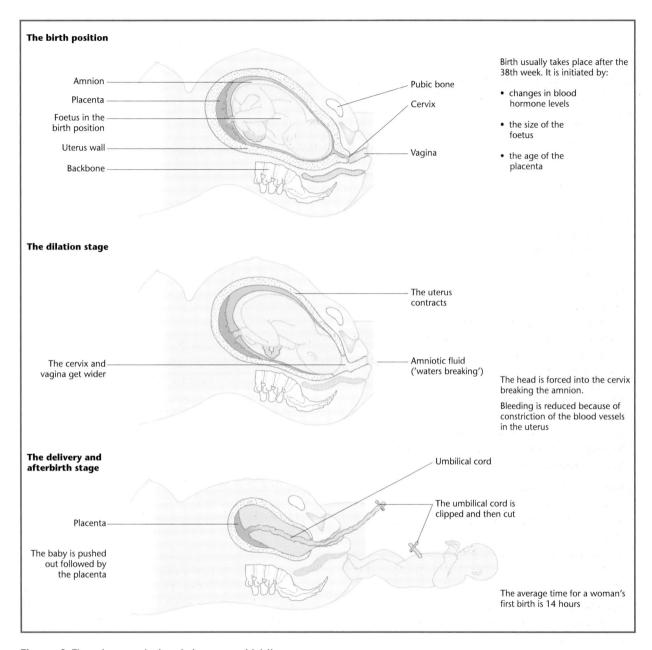

The birth position

Amnion
Placenta
Foetus in the birth position
Uterus wall
Backbone

Pubic bone
Cervix
Vagina

Birth usually takes place after the 38th week. It is initiated by:

- changes in blood hormone levels

- the size of the foetus

- the age of the placenta

The dilation stage

The cervix and vagina get wider

The uterus contracts

Amniotic fluid ('waters breaking')

The head is forced into the cervix breaking the amnion.

Bleeding is reduced because of constriction of the blood vessels in the uterus

The delivery and afterbirth stage

Umbilical cord

The umbilical cord is clipped and then cut

Placenta

The baby is pushed out followed by the placenta

The average time for a woman's first birth is 14 hours

Figure 1 *The stages during labour and birth.*

What do **you** know?

You should now be able to:

- State how long a normal pregnancy is and what initiates birth.

- Explain what a premature baby is and why it will need extra attention and care.

- Explain what happens during the 3 stages of birth.

- Describe 3 changes to the females reproductive organs during birth.

- Explain what an epidural is and when it would be used.

Examination of the new baby

Immediately after birth, all babies are given an **Apgar** score as a standard way of monitoring their condition. This is outlined in table 1. A total score of 5 or less indicates problems.

The newly born baby is also examined very carefully for any physical abnormalities, such as a cleft palate, number of toes, and so on. Its joints are tested for mobility and any dislocations caused by the birth. The umbilical cord is clamped and cut near the skin. Over the next week this will dry out and drop off leaving the navel scar (belly button).

During the next 24 hours, the baby will have several medical tests to establish it's state of health and development. For example, babies are incapable of producing voluntary movements, but they do have several simple survival reflexes (chapter 10.1). These are checked.

After six days, a small amount of blood is taken from the heel and used to check for the inherited disorder **phenylketonuria** (PKU). PKU is caused by the absence of an enzyme which breaks down an amino acid present in milk. If this amino acid builds up in the baby, it will interfere with the development of the nervous system. If PKU is discovered, the baby will have to be put on a special diet.

The blood is also used to check for **thyroxine** levels. This hormone is necessary for normal growth and development.

What happens to the mother after birth?

The mother will be emotional, sore and very tired. She will probably have stitches, especially if forceps were used and an **episiotomy** was necessary. During birth, the vaginal opening is stretched to its limit but may not be wide enough to deliver the baby's head, and the skin between the vagina and anus has to be cut a little. This is an episiotomy. This can make walking and visiting the toilet painful. Some mothers also suffer from piles due to all the pushing required during labour. These should soon heal, but plenty of fibre in the diet can help.

The most noticeable change will be the stretched skin around the abdomen. This should also disappear over the next few weeks and again a good healthy diet and plenty of light exercise, such as walking and stretching will help.

If the mother was **rhesus negative** and the father was **rhesus positive**, the mother will be given an injection to protect her next baby from anaemia. The rhesus blood group is due to the presence of an antigen 'D' on the surface of the red blood cells. About 85% of the UK population have this D antigen and are described as rhesus positive. The remaining 15% are rhesus negative.

If a rhesus negative person is given rhesus positive blood, the body will make antibodies to destroy it. This could happen if during late pregnancy some Rhesus positive blood from the foetus leaked across the placenta into a rhesus negative mother. The resulting antibodies could enter the foetus and clot its blood.

The postnatal check-up

Every new mother is given a full check up 4 to 6 weeks after the birth of her baby. This includes:

- a check on her weight to moniter change
- a urine test to see if the kidneys are working properly
- a check on blood pressure and on a sample of blood to test for rubella antibodies
- an examination of any stitched area to check for healing and possible infection
- an internal examination to check the size of the womb and to take a cervical smear.

She will also have the opportunity to discuss her emotional situation and any problems that have arisen.

Feeding the baby

Within 24 hours of its birth, the baby will need feeding. For the first four months of its life, its food consists entirely of milk. During pregnancy the woman's breasts will have grown more milk glands (**mammary glands**) in preparation for this. By the end of pregnancy they will be about one third larger than normal.

The production of milk by the mammary glands is controlled by the pituitary hormone **prolactin**. The expulsion of the milk from the glands is due to another pituitary hormone called **oxytocin**. The production of this is increased as the baby sucks on the nipple, and is an example of a positive feedback system (see figure 1).

It is important for a new mother to eat correctly, especially if she is breast feeding her baby. Producing milk requires a lot of energy, calcium and protein. A lactating woman must make sure her diet contains all of these (see table 2).

Function	Response	Score
Breathing	Regular, crying	2
	Slow, irregular	1
	Absent	0
Heart rate	Over 100	2
	Slow, below 100	1
	Absent	0
Colour	Pink	2
	Body pink, extremities blue	1
	Blue, pale	0
Muscle tone	Moving actively	2
	Moving extremities only	1
	Limp	0
Reflexes	Cough or sneeze	2
	Grimace	1
	None	0

Table 1 *All new babies are given an Apgar score immediately after birth.*

Nutrient	Normal	Breastfeeding
Energy (kJ)	8100	10500
Protein (g)	45	56
Calcium (mg)	700	1250
Iron (mg)	14.8	14.8
Vitamin A (μg)	600	950
Vitamin C (mg)	40	70
Vitamin D (μg)	No RNI	10

Table 2 *How a woman's diet should alter when lactating.*

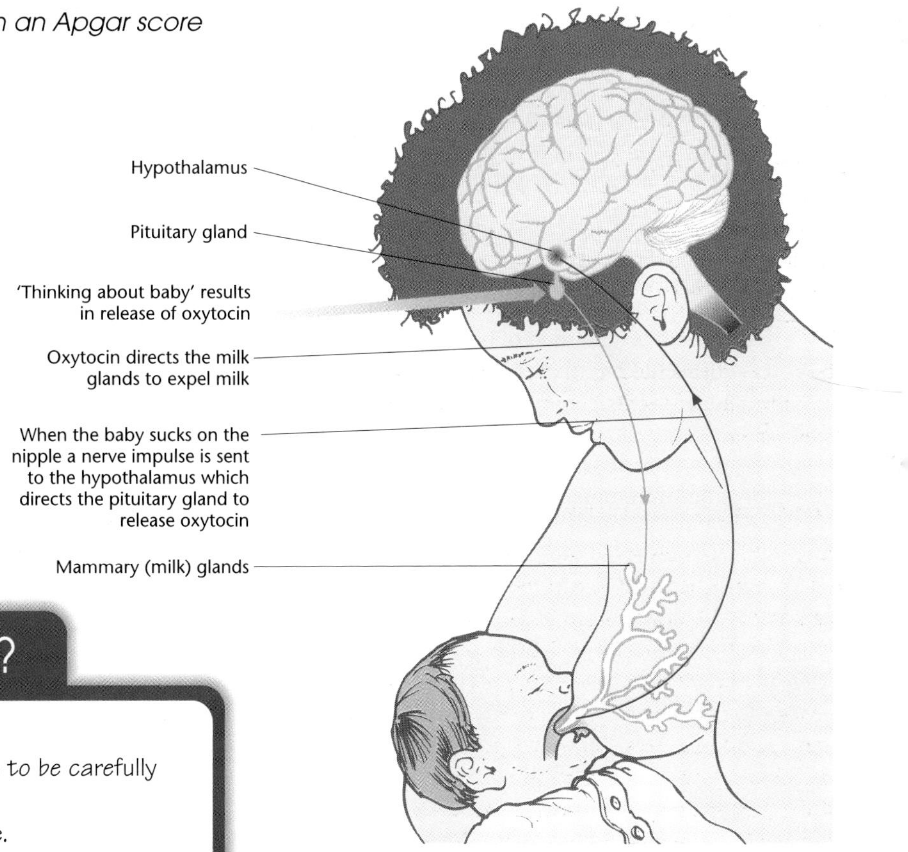

Hypothalamus

Pituitary gland

'Thinking about baby' results in release of oxytocin

Oxytocin directs the milk glands to expel milk

When the baby sucks on the nipple a nerve impulse is sent to the hypothalamus which directs the pituitary gland to release oxytocin

Mammary (milk) glands

Figure 1 *The release of milk is a reflex action involving a positive feedback system.*

What do **you** know?

You should now be able to:

- Explain why all new babies have to be carefully examined.
- Explain why a PKU test is done.
- Suggest how a mother's diet should alter when she is breastfeeding.
- Describe the changes in the breasts during pregnancy.
- State which 2 hormones are involved in milk production and flow.
- Explain the reflex action involved in milk flow from the mammary glands.

Chapter 9: Questions

1 a The diagram shows a human egg cell.

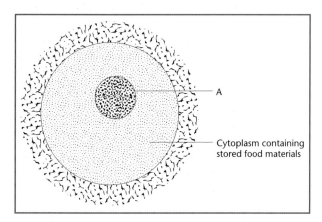

A

Cytoplasm containing stored food materials

   i Where are egg cells made? *(1 mark)*
   ii Name the part labelled A on the diagram.
       (1 mark)
   iii What is the function of the part labelled A?
       (1 mark)
   iv What is the function of the stored food materials in the cytoplasm? *(1 mark)*
b Name one feature of a sperm cell which helps it to reach an egg. *(1 mark)*
c i One method of birth control involves cutting and tying the Fallopian tubes. Explain how this prevents conception. *(1 mark)*
   ii The coil is a method of birth control which affects the lining of the uterus. Explain how this prevents pregnancy. *(1 mark)*
       (NEAB June 1997)

2 a The diagram shows the reproductive organs of a pregnant human female.

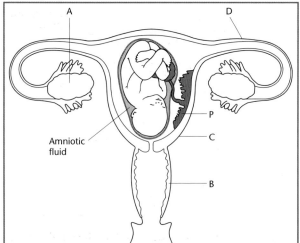

A   D

P

C

Amniotic fluid

B

   i Name structures A, B, C and D. *(4 marks)*
   ii What is meant by fertilisation? Make a sketch and label it to show where fertilisation normally occurs. *(2 marks)*

   iii The structure labelled P is the placenta. Give three functions of the placenta. *(3 marks)*
   iv Give one function of the amniotic fluid. *(1 mark)*
   v If structure D became blocked, this would cause infertility. Why is this? *(1 mark)*
b The table shows some of the dietary needs of a woman in different circumstances.

Different circumstances	Energy in MJ	Protein in g	Calcium in mg
Most jobs	9.0	54	500
Pregnant	10.0	60	1200
Breast-feeding	11.5	69	1200

   i When compared with the level for most jobs, what happens to the amounts of energy, protein and calcium needed by a woman when she becomes pregnant? *(1 mark)*
   ii Explain the change in the need for calcium when a woman becomes pregnant. *(1 mark)*
   iii Why should a woman breast-feeding her baby need to eat more protein than a woman in most jobs? *(2 marks)*
       (SEG June 1995)

3 a Explain what is meat by the terms **fertilisation** and **implantation**.
   i Fertilisation.
   ii Implantation. *(4 marks)*
b There are two types of contraceptive pill. One contains only progesterone. The other type is called the combined pill because it contains both progesterone and oestrogen.
The progesterone-only pill causes changes in the uterus which make it difficult for sperm to swim to an oviduct. The combined pill stops ovulation. The progesterone-only pill may result in about two pregnancies in every hundred users. The combined pill is almost 100% effective. Suggest the reasons for the different numbers of pregnancies. *(2 marks)*
       (SEG June 1992)

4 Suggest an explanation for each of the following.
a The alimentary canal of a very young baby does not contain any starch-digesting enzyme such as amylase. *(1 mark)*
b The mother's milk which feeds a baby does not contain iron, but the baby does not suffer anaemia. *(1 mark)*
c A baby's stomach produces an enzyme which makes the soluble proteins of milk into solids. The stomach of adults does not produce this enzyme. *(1 mark)*
       (SEG June 1992)

5 The diagram shows part of the placenta from a pregnant woman.

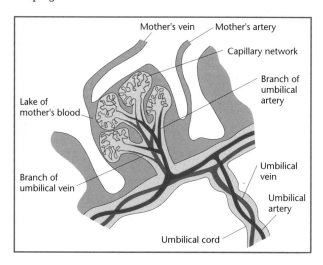

a **i** In what organ of the pregnant woman's body is the placenta found? *(1 mark)*

ii Describe two ways, that you can see in the diagram, in which the placenta is adapted to transport substances across it. *(2 marks)*

b **i** Draw and complete the table by naming two substances which pass across the placenta from the mother to the foetus and two substances which pass from the foetus to the mother. *(4 marks)*

Substances which pass from mother to foetus	Substances which pass from foetus to mother
1	1
2	2

ii Substances which cross the placenta pass from a region where they are in high concentration to a region where they are in low concentration. Name the process by which this can happen. *(1 mark)*

c **i** Explain why the German measles (rubella) virus can pass from mother to foetus across the placenta but the mother's blood cells cannot. *(1 mark)*

ii Suggest why it is important that the mother's white blood cells do not pass across the placenta to the foetus. *(1 mark)*
(SEG June 1997)

6 **a** Briefly describe what happens to each of the following at the birth of a baby:
i cervix
ii placenta
iii amnion. *(3 marks)*

b **i** Give two advantages gained by a baby who is fed on milk produced by the mother's breasts. *(2 marks)*

ii Give one advantage of bottle-feeding a baby. *(1 mark)*
(SEG June 1990)

7 **a** **i** In humans, describe briefly how a sperm cell reaches an egg cell to fertilise it. *(2 marks)*

ii There are 46 chromosomes in a body cell. How many chromosomes would you expect to find in the nucleus of the egg cell? *(1 mark)*

b What sex chromosomes(s) is/are present in:
i an egg cell
ii a sperm cell
iii a body cell of male foetus? *(3 marks)*

c Explain how identical twins are produced. *(2 marks)*

d **i** Explain how the uterus is prepared to receive a fertilised egg. *(3 marks)*

ii The coil is a method of birth control which affects the lining of the uterus causing constant irritation. Suggest how this prevents pregnancy. *(1 mark)*

e **i** A woman has blocked Fallopian tubes. Suggest why this causes infertility. *(1 mark)*

ii The blockages in her Fallopian tubes cannot be treated. Describe, in detail, how embryo transplantation could be used to help the woman become pregnant. *(4 marks)*
(NEAB June 1997)

8 The diagram shows a sperm.

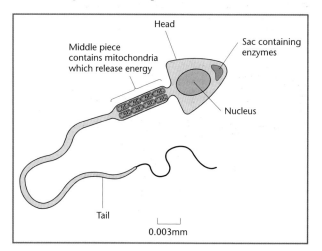

a **i** What is the actual length of the middle piece? *(1 mark)*

ii Suggest why the sperm needs a large number of mitochondria. *(1 mark)*

b Suggest one function for the enzymes. *(1 mark)*
(SEG June 1992)

10 Growth and development

Although every baby contains a blueprint for its future growth and development, this can be influenced by many factors. A child needs a stable, supportive environment for normal growth and development. The parents play a crucial part in this.

This chapter looks at the role of parents in providing for their child and follows the pattern of normal growth and development through childhood and into adulthood. It also looks at the natural, and some not so natural, changes which can take place as you age.

After you have worked through this chapter, you should be able to:

- Discuss the role of the parents in providing for the physical and emotional needs of their child.
- Outline the changes to a babies circulatory system at birth.
- Use graphical representations to describe patterns of growth and development after birth.
- Outline the main stages in the motor, emotional, social and mental development of a child.
- Describe the changes during adolescence including the development of the secondary sexual characteristics.
- Discuss the theories of ageing and the importance of remaining physically and mentally active into your old age.

New parts for old

For years the story of Frankenstein has both fascinated and frightened many people of all ages – because he was made from bits of human body, some dead and some alive. At the time the story was written, even minor surgery was difficult and to put someone together from body parts was a total fantasy. But now, in the 21st century, it is *almost* possible. What is more, if transplant parts or organs are not forthcoming from donors then there are many artificial replacements now available. It is even possible to grow new parts. Figure 1 shows some of the transplants that can be achieved by medical science.

Growing new parts

Modern **tissue culture** techniques have made it possible to grow many different types of body cells. The procedure involves extracting the cells and then growing them in an artificial medium containing all the required nutrients. Human blood serum may be added to promote growth. The most successful use of tissue culture

has been to grow skin to treat patients with severe burns. Connective tissue for use in repairing ligaments has also been grown and, very recently, scientists have even grown nerve cells from rats. This raises hopes of repairing nerve damage in the near future.

Using animal parts

The drawback in transplant surgery is the availability of human organs and parts. An alternative is to use animal parts. So far, collagen from the intestines of pigs has been used as a temporary skin. The collagen seems to stimulate the growth of new human skin cells over a wound. Collagen from cows has also been used for heart valves and a pioneering procedure was recently carried out when human cartilage cells were grown in the shape of an ear on the back of a mouse. Using parts from other animals will still create rejection problems because of the surface markers of cells. This could be overcome in the future by transferring human genes into animals, so they produce human tissue.

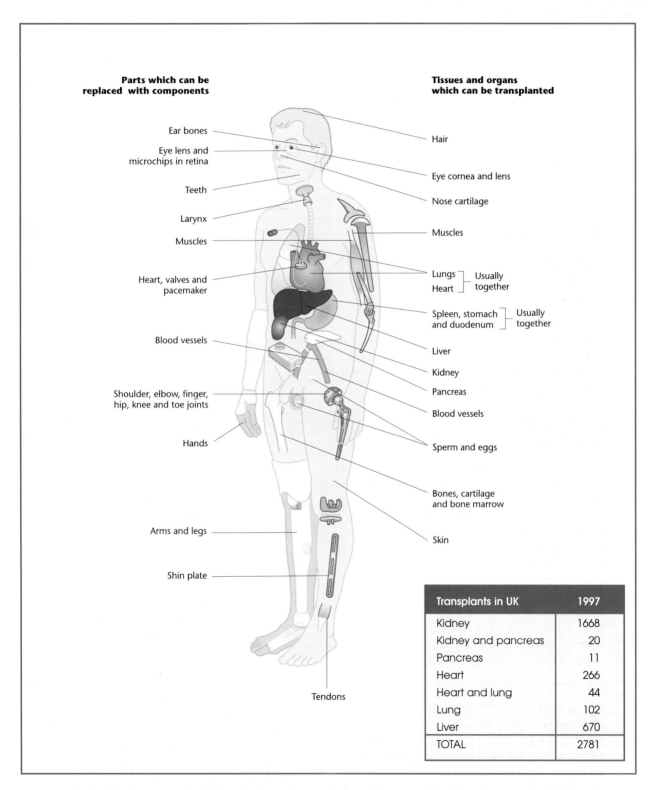

Parts which can be replaced with components

Ear bones

Eye lens and microchips in retina

Teeth

Larynx

Muscles

Heart, valves and pacemaker

Blood vessels

Shoulder, elbow, finger, hip, knee and toe joints

Hands

Arms and legs

Shin plate

Tendons

Tissues and organs which can be transplanted

Hair

Eye cornea and lens

Nose cartilage

Muscles

Lungs ⎤ Usually
Heart ⎦ together

Spleen, stomach ⎤ Usually
and duodenum ⎦ together

Liver

Kidney

Pancreas

Blood vessels

Sperm and eggs

Bones, cartilage and bone marrow

Skin

Transplants in UK	1997
Kidney	1668
Kidney and pancreas	20
Pancreas	11
Heart	266
Heart and lung	44
Lung	102
Liver	670
TOTAL	2781

Figure 1 *Parts of the human body which can be replaced.*

10.1 The newborn baby

The birth of a baby

Birth for a baby is a 'shocking' experience. Its whole environment suddenly changes. There are people, lights, noises – all very different from the stable, watery rhythm of the womb. The baby now has to start surviving on its own. When the umbilical cord is cut the baby's only source of oxygen is the air, so it must use its own lungs to breathe. This involves some major adjustments to the baby's circulatory system (see figure 1). Until birth the lungs only need to receive enough blood to supply them with food for growth and development. After birth, the lungs receive all the blood from the body. Similar changes must take place to bring the digestive system into full operation.

What can a newborn baby do?

Although the major organs of a healthy newborn baby are all fully formed and most are functioning, some are not yet 100 per cent efficient. Compared to many other animals, a human baby is quite helpless. It struggles to communicate, cannot walk, has few, if any, of its homeostatic mechanisms working at maximum efficiency and has no fully developed senses and a partially developed nervous system. For example, the eyes have only a small field of vision and cannot focus beyond 20 cm or so. The sense of hearing is worse, but quickly improves. The most developed sense is smell, and it is through smell that the baby first learns to recognise its mother and father.

A newborn baby has little control over its muscles, but does show several survival reflexes (see figure 2). These are soon replaced by deliberate movements as the baby gains control.

After birth the baby continues to grow into a child and its organs continue to develop until they are working at maximum efficiency. As the organs develop, so do its **sensory functions**, **motor skills**, and **intellectual abilities**. These are described in chapter 10.3.

At about 18 years of age a child becomes a fully formed adult and growth stops. Development, of course, goes on for life.

The importance of the parents

The parents have to do a lot for their baby. They have to feed it, protect it and care for it. They must provide a suitable environment in which their baby can grow and develop. They need to help it learn to talk, walk and eventually how to look after itself so it can become an independent and productive member of society. No other animal takes care of its young quite so well or for as long as the human animal.

What does a baby eat?

At first, a baby feeds on nothing but milk. Human breast milk supplies all the nutrients a baby needs, in the right amounts and in an easily absorbable form. Iron is not present in breast milk but a baby can draw on its own supplies stored up during pregnancy. Most women can breast feed their baby, but if this is not possible, there are many commercially produced infant milks which aim to provide the same nutrients (see table 1). Most women will be encouraged to try and breastfeed their baby for at least the first three days of life, because it is over this period that breasts produce a creamy nutritive liquid called **colostrum**. This contains many **antibodies** which will help the baby resist infection over the first few months of its life.

After four months or so, a baby is able to feed on 'solids'. The gradual transfer to solid food is known as **weaning**. It is very important that a good diet for normal growth and development is established and overfeeding avoided. As a general guide, a baby's diet must supply:

- enough energy – growing children require a lot of energy even though they are quite small

- enough protein for growth – this must contain all the essential amino acids

- adequate minerals for growth – calcium for bones and iron for blood

- a selection of vitamins and minerals to maintain healthy growth – vitamin C for healthy skin.

A baby's food should be in an easily absorbed form, free from added salt and sugar and whole milk (not skimmed), should replace breast or formula milk. By about 18 months, a toddler can be eating a mixed diet similar most other older children.

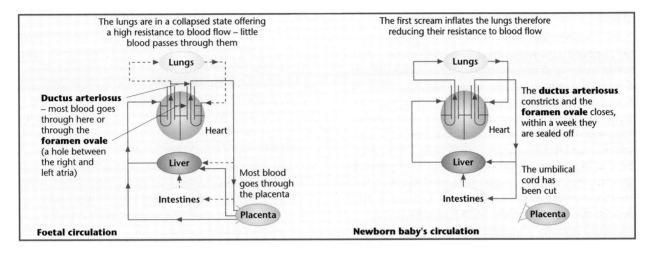

Figure 1 *The circulatory system of a newborn baby has to make some major adjustments in the first few moments after birth.*

Nutrients per 100 cm³	Human milk	Typical formula milk
Energy (kJ)	293	280
Carbohydrates (g)	7.4	7.2
Proteins (g)	1.3	1.5
Fats (g)	4.2	3.6
Calcium (mg)	35	46
Vitamin A (µg)	60	75
C (mg)	3.8	9
D (µg)	0.01	1.1

Table 1 *Formula milks are very similar in composition to human breast milk.*

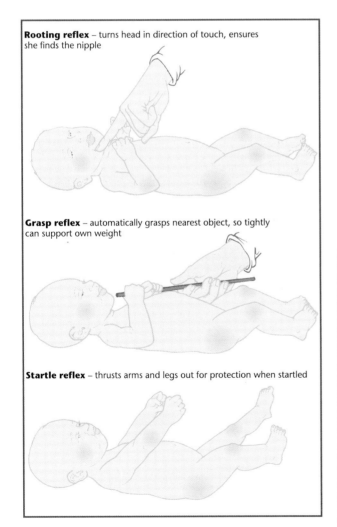

Rooting reflex – turns head in direction of touch, ensures she finds the nipple

Grasp reflex – automatically grasps nearest object, so tightly can support own weight

Startle reflex – thrusts arms and legs out for protection when startled

Figure 2 *Newborn babies have several survival reflexes.*

What do **you** know?

You should now be able to:

- Explain why the first scream for a baby is so important.
- Describe with the help of a diagram, the changes that take place in the foetal blood circulation at the time of birth and explain why these are necessary.
- Outline what a newborn baby can do and explain the reasons for the 3 survival reflexes.
- Draw up a table of advantages and disadvantages of breast and bottle feeding.
- Describe the diet of a typical 12 month old baby. List the guidelines you would use.
- Explain why a baby's life is only as good as its parents make it.

10.2 The growing child

What makes every child different?

Every newborn baby contains an inbuilt programme for its future growth and development, that is, a predetermined set of instructions. These instructions are contained within its **genes**. Some of the instructions will be the same in every baby, in that they are a basic recipe for a typical human (as opposed to any other organism). Others are very specific instructions which make a child a unique individual with characteristics from both parents. For example, a child may grow tall like its father, but have curly hair like its mother. The exact features he or she displays from each parent will depend upon the genes that were passed on in the respective gametes (chapter 11.4).

What influences the growth and development of a child?

Although the genes are very important, they are not the only things that influence growth and development of a child. Some of the others are:

● **Food intake**. Both quantity and quality of food can affect growth and development. Overeating can lead to obesity and its related problems (chapter 12.4), whereas an inadequate intake of food may produce stunted growth and development. For example, if a baby does not get enough energy foods (**malnutrition**), its nervous system often fails to develop fully. Eating the wrong foods will lead to **deficiency diseases**, many of which are growth-related (chapter 2.2).

● **Hormones**. There are many hormones which affect the growth and development of a child. Some of the main ones are:

1 **Human growth hormone** (HGH), produced by the pituitary gland. This influences the rate at which tissues grow, especially bone and muscle tissue. A child who overproduces growth hormone during childhood will grow too much and too quickly. This may result in **giantism**. Underproduction results in **dwarfism**. Children with these conditions will be normal, just larger or smaller than normal.

2 **Thyroxine**, produced by the thyroid gland. This influences metabolic rate (energy production), and protein synthesis. A child who overproduces thyroxine during childhood will have a very high metabolic rate and may not put on weight in a normal way. Underproduction results in poor physical and mental growth, even retardation and a condition known as **cretinism**.

3 The **oestrogens** and **androgens**, sex hormones of the females and males, respectively. Small amounts of these hormones are produced throughout life by the adrenal glands. These are especially important during the **growth spurts** of life. From puberty, the ovaries also produce oestrogen, which is responsible for many of the changes which take place during a growth spurt and for maintaining the female secondary sexual characteristics.

The main androgen is **testosterone**. From the onset of puberty, this is produced by the testes and controls the further development of the male secondary sexual characteristics (chapter 10.4).

4 **Insulin**, produced by the pancreas. This regulates the amount of glucose in the blood and therefore indirectly affects growth and development. It is as crucial as the other hormones as it affects carbohydrate metabolism, fat mobilisation and protein synthesis.

All these hormones must work together for normal growth and development.

● The **environment**. Light, pollution and disease are just some of the environmental factors that can affect growth and development. For example, light is needed for your skin to make vitamin D. Vitamin D is essential for the absorption of calcium, which itself is needed for proper growth of bones. The environmental influences on growth and development are dealt with more fully in other chapters.

What do **you** know?

You should now be able to:

● Explain why children look like their parents and brothers and sisters.
● Outline how food intake can influence growth and development.
● Outline the roles of the growth hormone, thyroxine, sex hormones and insulin on growth and development.
● Draw a graph to compare the normal growth of boys and girls.
● Indicate on your graph the ages at which the growth spurts occur.
● Use data and graphs to explain how the body proportions (head, trunk and legs) change during development.
● Explain why different organs grow at different rates.

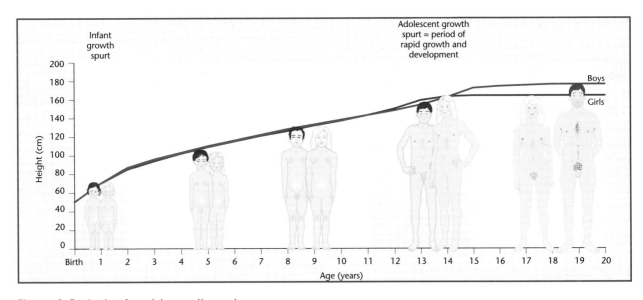

Figure 1 *Periods of rapid growth and development in children.*

	Newborn	Adult
Fat	16	12
Skeletal muscle	25	40
Skeleton	18	14
Liver	5	2
Kidney	1	0.5
Brain	12	2
Overall water	75	60

Table 1 *A comparison of percentage body weight of organs in newborn babies and adults.*

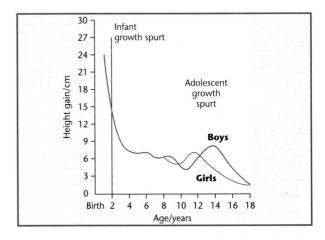

Figure 2 *Height gain per year from birth to 18 years.*

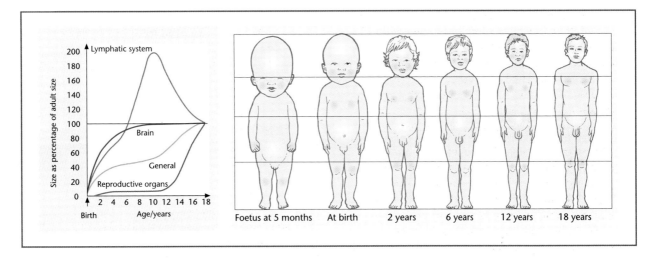

Figure 3 *Different parts of the body grow at different rates. The diagram above shows how the body proportions change.*

GROWTH AND DEVELOPMENT

When does a child start walking?

As a child grows in size and the parts of its body mature, it begins to lose its helplessness and to feed itself, walk and talk.

Walking requires very strong muscles and the ability to co-ordinate them all. Much practice is needed and the child who experiments and is encouraged will usually progress well. However, few children start walking before the end of their first year, simply because their muscles are not strong enough. For some children, learning to walk can take as long as 20 months.

The development of co-ordinated movement is called **motor development** (see figure 1).

When does a child start talking?

Young babies make quite a lot of different sounds. When only a few months old, they gurgle, laugh and cry to show pleasure, displeasure or other emotions. This is a way of **communicating** without words. Later, between 10 and 18 months most children will start to copy sounds and say and understand simple words. A two year-old child can usually join words together and a three year-old will usually have a vocabulary of more than 500 words. Of course, this varies from child to child.

Why do some children throw tantrums?

Tantrums are a normal part of growing up. They are a part of every child's **emotional development**. Probably the first emotions to be displayed are love and affection, closely followed by anger and frustration. Children often start to have tantrums at about 18 months, sometimes described as the 'terrible twos'. They are the child's way of getting attention. The normal sequence of mental, emotional and social development is outlined in figure 3. It is important to realise that these can be seriously affected by early 'bad' experiences, such as constantly being smacked, and greatly helped by good supportive parental attitudes.

How important is play?

All children like to play and this should be encouraged as much as possible. Play helps the child's physical, mental, emotional and social development.

- **Physical development**. The activity of play, e.g. building bricks or pulling a toy, helps the child develop strong muscles and better co-ordination.

- **Mental development**. Children learn through their senses. Play can stimulate all senses and give children new chances to learn. It also helps develop intellect and encourages creativity. Having to talk to others during play helps with communication skills.

- **Emotional development**. Play can provide a necessary outlet for emotions such as anger and aggression.

- **Social development**. Play with parents and other children encourages co-operation, communication and friendship. It helps children understand that they have responsibilities, as well as helping understand the roles of others with themselves.

When does a child start school?

In the UK formal schooling begins when a child is five years old, but parents can, if they wish, send their child to school well before this. Nursery schools are available to children from the age of two and in some areas the Social Services provide playgroups and nursery classes for even younger children. All children are entitled to a state education up to the age of 19 years.

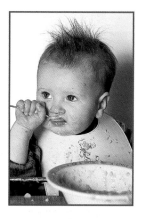

Figure 1 *This child is developing its motor skills*

What do **you** know?

You should now be able to:

- Describe motor development and draw or explain two pieces of equipment which will help a child with its motor development.
- Draw up a table which shows when the main changes in mental, emotional and social development take place in a pre-school child.
- Suggest some ways in which parents can help with a child's mental, emotional and social development.
- Briefly describe why play is so important for young children.
- Draw or describe suitable toys for (a) a 2 year-old, and (b) a 4 year-old child.
- Plan a day's nursery schooling for a 3 year old stating your reasons for including each activity.

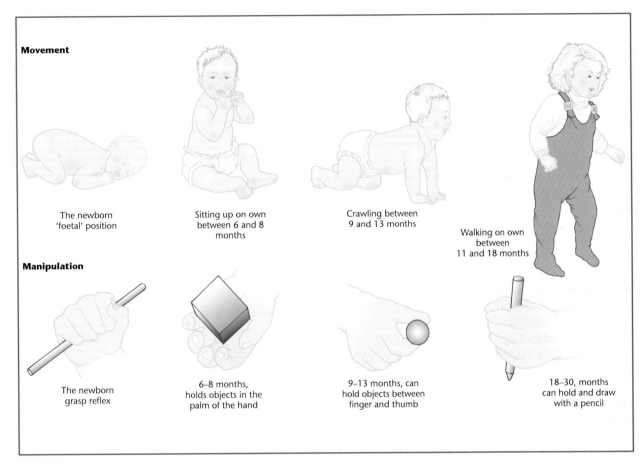

Figure 2 *There are well recognised stages in the physical development of a child.*

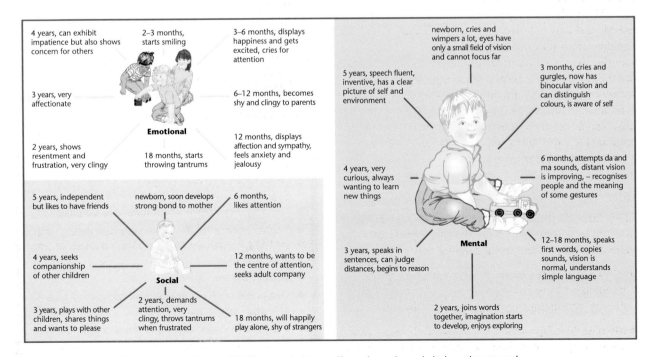

Figure 3 *Some of the stages in a child's mental emotional and social development.*

10.4 Into adulthood

What is adolescence?

The early teenage years can be a very difficult time for a young person. Many changes take place in the body and teenagers may feel emotionally different. This stage, called **adolescence**, is the time during which a young person passes from childhood to a sexually mature adult. It is a period of rapid physical growth and development and includes the period over which the sex organs mature, called **puberty**.

Some teenagers go through adolescence without experiencing any major problems. Unfortunately, there are many more who do not. A lot suffer from mild depression, worrying about rapid increases in height and weight, spots, disagreements with parents and any number of problems. For a few these can be so serious as to threaten life itself. Teenage suicide rates are one hundred times higher than pre-teenage rates. Girls in particular suffer from eating disorders such as **anorexia nervosa** and **bulimia**. Many adolescent boys become aggressive. Statistics suggest that drug taking and criminal offences increase.

What causes puberty?

The actual trigger for puberty is unknown, but the changes that occur are caused by hormones put into action by the brain.

Some time during your teens, the **hypothalamus** of the brain instructs the **pituitary gland** to start releasing the hormones **leuteinising hormone** and **follicle stimulating hormone** (chapter 9.3). These travel in the blood to your gonads (testes or ovaries), and cause the changes outlined in figure 1.

In general, girls start puberty on average 18 months before boys. In the UK the average age for girls reaching puberty has dropped. At the turn of the 19th century, the average age for a girl to have her first period was 15, while in the 21st century it is 13 years.

The adolescent growth spurt

Height is a great worry to many teenagers. It is difficult to understand why your friend has suddenly got taller and you have not, or vice versa. During adolescence, everyone will have a period of rapid growth. This is brought on by changes in hormone levels, especially **growth hormone** (HGH) and adrenal **androgens**. Boys, on average, grow 7 cm per year during this period and the overall growth accounts for up to 15% of their final height.

What can you expect as an adult?

You have survived adolescence and now you are an adult. The beginning of adulthood is considered to be when the irreversible growth stops. For most women this happens by the age of 18, and for most men by the age of 20. From now on you don't grow but may put on weight, but you can just as easily lose it. Development of your body organs continues, usually into your mid- to late-twenties. And then it is, to a large extent, up to you how quickly you age.

What is the menopause?

The **menopause** is the stage of a woman's life when menstruation ceases. It represents the end of a woman's fertile period and is often called the 'change of life'. In some women it may be a gradual process, lasting several years or it may just last a few months. It can be a difficult time for a woman as she comes to terms with the physical and mental changes that are associated with the menopause. By the age of 55, most women will have experienced the menopause.

The menopause is the result of hormonal changes within the body. In particular, the ovaries stop producing oestrogen and as the blood oestrogen level falls, some of the female characteristics maintained by this hormone disappear. Some of the possible changes to the female body are shown in figure 2.

One of the more worrying effects of the menopause is the increased risk of **osteoporosis** (chapter 5.2). Many women use **hormone replacement therapy** (HRT) to help with menopausal symptoms. HRT makes up the loss of oestrogen and thereby delays many of the menopausal changes.

What do **you** know?

You should now be able to:

- State 2 changes that normally occur during adolescence.
- Explain what causes these changes.
- List the similarities and differences at puberty between boys and girls.
- List the secondary sexual characteristics of boys and girls.
- Explain the menopause.
- List some of the changes a woman can expect after her menopause.
- Suggest why oestrogen can delay the onset of some of the changes after menopause.

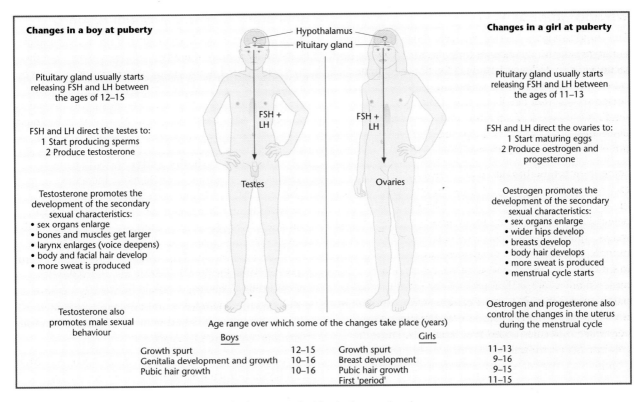

Figure 1 *Many changes take place in boys and girls during puberty.*

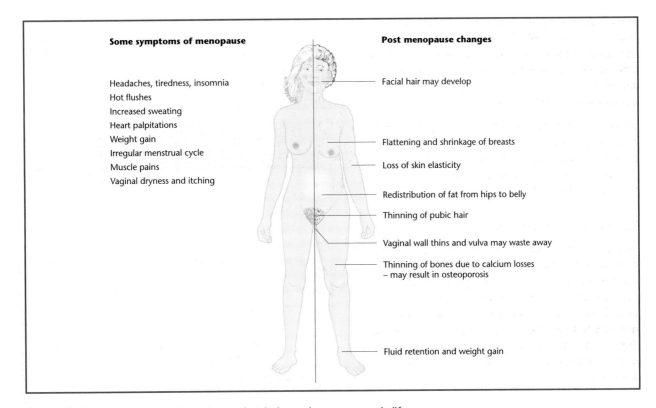

Figure 2 *The menopause is an important stage in a woman's life.*

GROWTH AND DEVELOPMENT

10.5 Senescence

Why do we age?

You begin to age as soon as you have finished growing. For years scientists have been trying to find out why, and so far have come up with some clues, but no definite reason. Current knowledge suggests:

- Your **genes are involved**. Evidence shows that long life seems to run in families and all animals, including humans, have a maximum life span. It is also known that cells have a programmed maximum number of divisions before they die.

- Many **whole body processes are involved**. For example, as you age the immune system stops working as efficiently and faulty cells, such as cancer cells, are no longer destroyed. Many cells also stop responding to hormones. At menopause, the ovaries stop responding to FSH and so stop producing oestrogen (chapter 10.4).

- The **environment has an effect**. During normal metabolism, your cells produce small electrically charged molecules, called **free radicals**. These are very reactive and will react with proteins, DNA, minerals… they don't care! Free radicals can interfere with normal cell function, often causing irreversible damage which accumulates as we age.

  Free radicals are produced all the time, but in manageable quantities. The numbers produced increase with high levels of pollution and ultra violet (UVA) light.

- Many **personal factors are implicated**. It has been known for a long time that people on low calorie diets live longer. It has recently been confirmed that smoking and drinking alcohol can increase the number of free radicals produced. Experiments show that lack of exercise will result in loss of lean body mass. These are just a few of the personal choices we make (usually without thinking of the long term consequences).

Obviously the ageing process is very complex. One way of looking at it might be to think of these factors as contributing to the 'ticking clock'. One day the battery will run out and the clock will stop, but no one knows when or how quickly.

What are the signs of ageing?

There are many physical signs of ageing, such as wrinkles, grey hair, muscle loss and so on. And there are just as many symptoms that you cannot see, for example, stiff joints, feeling cold, brittle bones, mental confusion and so on. Some of these reasons are described in figure 1. Fortunately more and more people are living healthy and productive lives for longer.

How can we slow the rate of ageing?

Many of the changes associated with normal ageing can be delayed to some extent by:

- **Eating healthily**. A healthy balanced diet is essential for good health (chapters 2.3 and 12.4). As you get older the constituents of your diet may need to change, for example, after the menopause women will need more calcium.

- **Remaining physically active**. Activity helps your circulation, maintains muscle mass, increases metabolism, assists joint suppleness and stimulates your body's natural repair systems (chapter 12.5).

- **Getting enough rest**. Rest allows your body to remove wastes and repair damage (chapter 12.5).

- **Remaining mentally active**. The more you use your brain, the longer it will remain alert.

- **Remaining healthy**. Avoid smoking, drinking alcohol in excess or abusing drugs in order to stay healthy (chapters 12.7 and 12.8).

Death

It is often said that death is the only thing in life which you can be sure of. It comes to us all and yet it is still a big mystery as to what happens. The dictionary definition of death is '*the cessation of all physical and chemical processes that occur in the body or its cellular components*'. Clinical death is when there is no electrical activity in the brain stem.

Many people die after a long fulfilling life. Others die prematurely due to an accident or illness. The main causes of adult deaths in the UK are shown in chapter 12.1.

What do **you** know?

You should now be able to:

- Review the current theories as to why we age.
- Think ahead to your retirement age and describe some of the changes you would have expected to have happened to your body.
- Explain as many of these changes as you can.
- Suggest why the average life expectancy is different in different areas of the world.
- Explain why it is important for older people to remain physically and mentally active.
- Suggest how a person's lifestyle can contribute to premature death from such diseases as coronary heart disease, respiratory diseases and cancer.

Nervous and sensory systems

Brain – as cells die they are not replaced and short term memory may fail
– reactions slow
Eyes – lens loses its elasticity resulting in old sight
Ears – hearing deteriorates as sensory cells die
– unable to select sounds

Depression, confusion, Parkinsons, Alzheimer's, glaucoma, cataracts and insomnia

Skin

Skin – loses its elasticity and suppleness
– proteins cross link to form wrinkles
Hair – less grows
– becomes thinner and brittle loses pigment

Baldness

Muscular skeletal system

Bone – become thin and brittle as calcium is lost
Joints – become worn
– ligaments shrink and intervertebral discs flatten
Muscles – lose size, shape and strength
– loss of muscle tone results in posture problems

Osteoporosis, arthritis, backache

Excretory system

Kidneys – nephrons decline affecting ability to filter blood
Urethra – loss of muscle control

Kidney stones, incontinence

Respiratory and circulatory systems

Lungs – lose elastic tissue and become less effective so take up less oxygen
– respiratory infections more likely
Heart – heart valves thicken and heart pumps less blood
Blood vessels – hardening and narrowing of arteries increases blood pressure

Heart attack, hypertension, auto-immune diseases

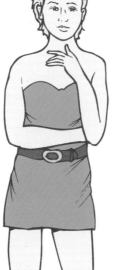
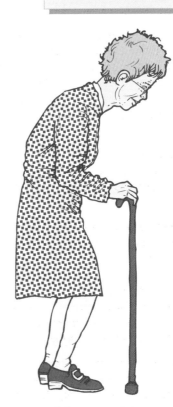

	1974	1984	1994	1997
% of population over 65	16.9	17.9	18.3	18.1
% of population over 75	4.9	6.3	6.8	7.2

18 to 80 years old

Digestive system

Guts – peristalsis slows as muscle tone is lost
Liver – ability to detoxify decreases
Pancreas – functions deteriorate

Constipation, IBS, haemorrhoids, gall stones and diabetes

Reproductive system

Female – organs deteriorate after menopause
– menstrual cycle stops
Male – prostate gland enlarges

Cancer of the breast and prostate glands

Figure 1 *Getting old happens to all of us. Fortunately not everyone will experience all of these.*

Chapter 10: Questions

1 The table shows how proportions of the parts of the human body change during growth.

| | Percentage of length of whole body | | | | |
	Birth	2½ Years	5 Years	15 Years	20 Years
Head and neck	27	27	22	17	15
Trunk	40	40	42	39	40
Legs	33	33	36	44	45

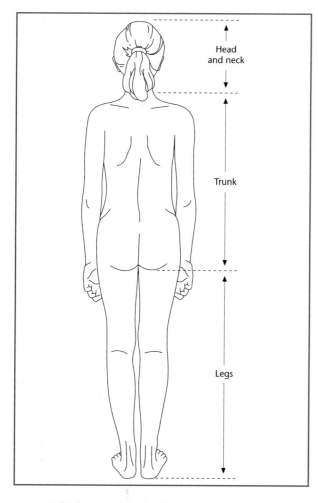

a Which part of the body
  i grows least?
  ii grows most? *(2 marks)*
b Growth hormone stimulates the growth of bones during childhood and adolescence. Suggest how a person who could not make enough hormone would differ in appearance from a normal person. *(2 marks)*
c In addition to an increase in size, other changes occur in the body during puberty. Give two of these changes which occur in the male. *(2 marks)*
(SEG June 1997)

2 The graph shows a typical pattern for the human growth curve. Use the graph to answer the questions that follow.

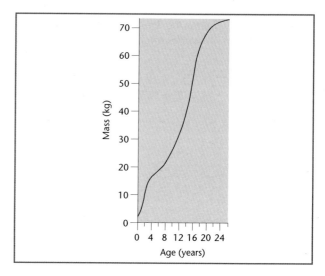

a During which 2 year period is growth the slowest? *(1 mark)*
b Describe the shape of the graph between the ages of 1 and 16. What are the causes of these changes in slope? *(4 marks)*
c For how long before the age of 0 (time of birth) does the graph begin? Explain why. *(2 marks)*
(SEG June 1992)

3 a State one function for each of the following parts of the reproductive system:
  i the scrotal sac,
  ii the oviduct,
  iii the urethra. *(3 marks)*
b Compare the development of secondary sexual characteristics in male and female by stating:
  i one visible change common to both male and female;
  ii one visible change that occurs in one sex only;
  iii the usual starting age of puberty in male and in female. *(3 marks)*
c The chart shows a female menstrual cycle:

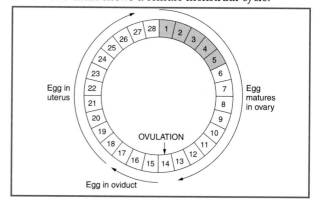

i Explain what happens between days 1 and 5 of the cycle. *(2 marks)*

ii Explain why days 11 to 16 are sometimes described as the 'fertile period'. *(4 marks)*

d What are the hormonal changes that occur if a woman becomes pregnant? *(3 marks)*

(SEG June 1992)

4 Sperm must travel through the female reproductive system in order to reach the egg.

a i Which organ produces eggs? *(1 mark)*

ii List the structures in order through which the sperm travels after it has entered the female body. *(3 marks)*

b What happens at fertilisation? *(1 mark)*

c In which organ of a female's body does a baby develop? *(1 mark)*

d What is the function of the placenta? *(2 marks)*

e The graph shows the growth curve for boys from birth to 18 years.

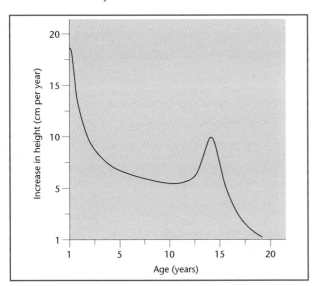

i Describe the shape of the curve from birth to age 5 years. *(1 mark)*

ii What causes the growth spurt, between ages 14–16? *(1 mark)*

iii Explain how the growth curve for girls would differ over the same period of time. *(1 mark)*

(NEAB June 1998)

5 Some students decided to investigate growth in humans by recording the heights of males and females at different ages. Their results are shown in Tables 1 and 2.

Heights of 12 year old students					
student	sex	height /cm	student	sex	height /cm
1	male	157	11	male	146
2	female	151	12	female	158
3	male	142	13	female	146
4	male	155	14	female	153
5	female	158	15	male	155
6	female	143	16	male	141
7	male	162	17	female	159
8	male	139	18	female	158
9	female	159	19	female	149
10	male	154	20	male	147

a i What was the height of the shortest student? *(1 mark)*

ii What was the sex of the tallest student? *(1 mark)*

iii Using data from Table 1, calculate the average (mean) height of the 12 year old girls. Use your answer to complete Table 2. *(4 marks)*

Age/years	Average heights of students/cm	
	males	females
12	149.8	....
14	166.7	163.1
16	176.4	167.4
18	181.1	170.2

b i Using the data in Table 2 draw line graphs, on a single set of axes to show the average heights of males and of females between the ages of 12 and 18 years old. Use the scales indicated. *(5 marks)*

ii At which age are males and females the same height? *(1 mark)*

iii Between which ages do females seem to be growing fastest? *(1 mark)*

c Suggest a reason why the average height of twelve year old females is greater than the average height of males of the same age. *(1 mark)*

(MEG June 1993)

11 Inheritance and variation

Your body is built to a blueprint. This blueprint is stored in the nucleus of every cell. It takes the form of genes. Each gene contains the information for the development of one particular characteristic of your body.

You inherited your genes from your parents, some from your mother and some from your father. They inherited theirs from their parents and if you have children, they will inherit some of your genes. In other words, they will have some of your characteristics, just as you have some of your parents' characteristics.

This chapter explains what genes are and how they are passed on from parents to children. It also explains why everyone is different.

After you have worked through this chapter, you should be able to:

- Explain what a gene is and the nature of the instructions it contains.

- Describe and explain the significance of the diploid and haploid conditions of a nucleus.

- Outline the structure of DNA and describe how it replicates to produce exact copies of itself.

- Outline the role of DNA in protein synthesis.

- Describe the behaviour of chromosomes during ordinary cell division (mitosis), and reduction division (meiosis).

- Discuss the significance of the two kinds of cell division.

- Explain the terminology of genetics and inheritance.

- Describe the basic laws of genetics.

- Do some genetic predicting using monohybrid inheritance.

- Explain how blood groups are inherited.

- Explain how sex is inherited and describe some sex-linked characteristics.

- Explain why people are all different.

- Describe the causes of genetic variation.

- Discuss how the environment may cause variation among characteristics.

- Explain what a mutation is and how they can be inherited.

Superbugs

Some people claim that the discovery of penicillin has added ten years to the average life span. Before antibiotics were discovered, people used to die from what are now considered minor ailments, like gum infections and infected cuts. Operations and even childbirth were impossibly dangerous. The discovery of antibiotics changed the outlook. There was now the means to kill bacteria and control infectious disease. Serious diseases like tuberculosis, gonorrhoea and pneumonia were at last brought under control and some virtually eliminated. Open heart surgery, hip replacements and kidney transplants became possible without the major worry of infection.

Antibiotic resistance

However, too much of a good thing has created a false sense of security. We are now faced with the prospect of returning to the days before antibiotics as more and more bacteria become resistant to them.

One strain of the bacterium *Staphylococcus aureus*, named **methicillin resistant *Staphylococcus aureus*** (MRSA) is normally harmless to healthy people, but if it gets into wounds after surgery, it can cause serious blood poisoning, often resulting in death. This bacterium has developed resistance to every type of antibiotic except one. It is now endemic in our hospitals and results in over 5000 hospital deaths per year.

These bacteria, or '**superbugs**' as they are known, have become the next major challenge for medicine in the 21st century. Just how serious is it? In 1941, penicillin annihilated 99% of all *Staphylococcus* strains and in 1999, it only killed 15% of them.

Most bacteria become resistant by the natural process of evolution. Take the 20 billion or so *Escherichia coli* (**E. coli**) living in the human intestine, it is possible that one million of these will contain mutated genes. If just one of these mutated genes offers the ability to resist penicillin, then when penicillin is used, all the other bacteria will be killed leaving the one resistant. This resistant bacterium will grow and reproduce to fill the available space it has been '**selected for**' and in a couple of days the intestine could contain millions of *E. coli*, all of which are resistant to penicillin.

The more antibiotics we use the more of these superbugs we are creating. In 1998, the government set up a select committee (SMAC) to look into this problem. From this came the CATNAP initiative, a two pronged campaign. The Campaign on Antibiotic Treatment is aimed at GP's urging them not to prescribe antibiotics unless it is absolutely necessary. The National Advice to the Public provides, through booklets in doctors waiting rooms etc, general information for patients about antibiotic use.

Antibiotics in foods

About half of the antibiotics used today are used to control infection in humans. The other half are used in animals for three reasons:

- to **treat disease**
- to **prevent disease**, especially in factory farming and other intensive rearing techniques
- as **growth promoters** – used this way antibiotics can increase the yield by as much as 8%.

Here again, the conditions are ideal for antibiotic resistant forms to survive while normal gut flora are killed. Some of these resistant forms can pass into humans through the food chain. For example, *Salmonella* is a common bacterium found in animal guts. In an outbreak of food poisoning in 1995, 87% of the *Salmonella* strain taken from the infected people was resistant to five major antibiotics.

What about genetically modified foods?

Genetically modified (GM) foods have been modified, through their genes, to give increased yields, resistance to disease, etc. One major concern is the use of antibiotic marker genes which are used to track the genetic modification (chapter 14.3). When, for example the gene conferring resistance to the European Corn Borer was spliced into maize, the gene conferring resistance to ampicillin went with it. This gene will therefore enter the food chain and may eventually find its way into humans.

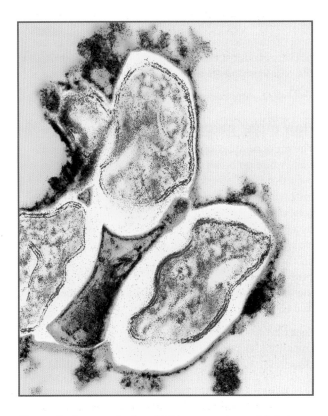

Figure 1 *A new strain of TB is emerging which is resistant to most antibiotics.*

11.1 Chromosomes and genes

What is a gene?

Do you ever wonder what makes you different from your friend? Why do you have blue eyes? Why does your friend have black hair? Characteristics like these depend upon the genes you inherit from your parents during the reproductive process. A **gene** contains instructions which the body can use to produce a particular characteristic. For example, a gene may contain the instructions to produce a certain eye colour. The usual way to describe this is to say that the gene **codes for** eye colour. Another gene might code for hair colour, and so on. Genes are often called the **units of inheritance** because they carry the characteristics from the parents to their children.

How are the instructions in genes used?

A simple way to look at this is to think of a gene as carrying the instructions for the manufacture of an enzyme. The presence or absence of an enzyme can be the difference between a characteristic being present or not. For example, if you have brown eyes, it is because you have the enzyme which helps in the production of the brown pigment. This enzyme can only be made if you have this gene.

The actual instructions of a gene are **encoded** into the molecule we call **DNA** (chapter 11.2). DNA is organised with proteins to form the **chromosomes** found in the nucleus of almost every living cell. Figure 1 illustrates the relationship between a gene, a chromosome and DNA.

How many chromosomes do cells have?

The more complex an organism is, the more genes it has. A human being is one of the most complex organisms and therefore has many genes (i.e. instructions for its assembly and functioning). These genes are carried on 23 chromosomes. All human cells, except the gametes (eggs and sperms), have these 23 chromosomes *plus* a copy of each. They therefore contain 46 chromosomes, more usually described as 23 **homologous pairs** of chromosomes. Homologous means 'the same'. Each pair consists of a chromosome and its identical copy.

Eggs and sperms only carry 23 chromosomes, one from each homologous pair. Cells which have two sets of chromosomes are described as being in the **diploid** state. The gametes with only one set of chromosomes, are in the **haploid** state. Sometimes diploid is simply represented by '**2n**' and haploid by '**n**'.

Why do gametes only have 23 chromosomes?

The gametes are produced by a special kind of cell division called **meiosis** (chapter 11.3). Meiosis separates the chromosomes of each homologous pair and directs them into different gametes. Each sperm produced will therefore contain half a man's chromosomes (the haploid state), and each egg will contain half a woman's chromosomes, one from each homologous pair. When these gametes fuse at fertilisation, the chromosomes are able to 'pair off again' (return to the diploid state), but now each homologous pair is made up of one chromosome from the father and one chromosome from the mother (see figure 2).

It is only possible to see the chromosomes in a nucleus when the nucleus is about to divide, and even then, they will need staining with a dye. When they are visible, they appear to be very tightly coiled, and consist of two parts joined at one point. These two parts are called **chromatids**. The chromosomes have replicated and the two parts are still joined together. Figure 3 shows the 23 homologous pairs of chromosomes (shown as chromatids) found in a human nucleus. This is called a **karyotype**.

The Human Genome Project

The Human Genome Project was established in 1990. It aims to discover what each of the 100 000 genes in the human genetic material codes for, exactly which chromosomes these are on, and where they are located on the chromosomes (called the **locus**). The task of 'gene mapping' is so enormous, that it is expected to take until the year 2005 to complete.

What do **you** know?

You should now be able to:

- Define the term gene.
- State where you got your genes from.
- Explain the relationship between a gene, chromosome and DNA.
- Explain the diploid and haploid states of a nucleus.
- Explain what homologous pairs of chromosomes are.
- Explain why gametes only contain 23 chromosomes, one from each homologous pair.
- Draw a labelled diagram of a chromatid and explain what it is.

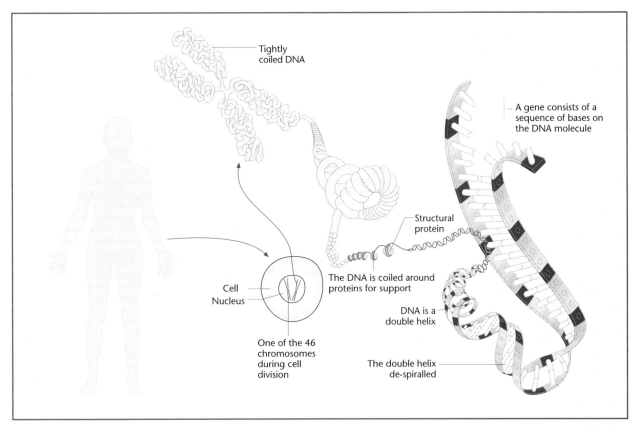

Figure 1 *Genes are part of the DNA molecule which forms the chromosomes in the nucleus of a cell.*

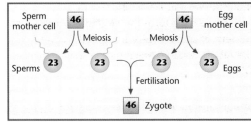

Figure 2 *Sexual reproduction restores the number of chromosomes to 46.*

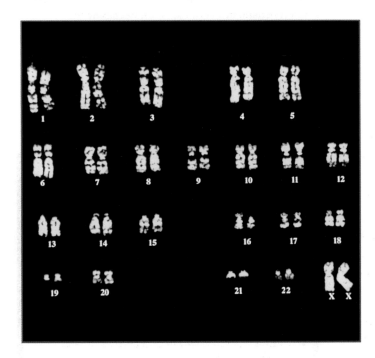

Figure 3 *The human karyotype consists of 23 homologous pairs of chromosomes.*

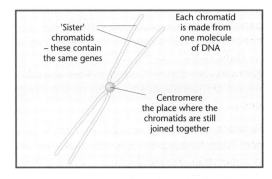

Figure 4 *Chromosomes are usually only visible when the cell is dividing and they have already replicated to form chromatids.*

INHERITANCE AND VARIATION 153

What is DNA?

DNA, which stands for **deoxyribonucleic acid,** is the very important molecule that contains our genes. The DNA forms part of a chromosome and is only found inside the nucleus of a cell (chapter 11.1).

Two more kinds of nucleic acid are **messenger ribonucleic acid** (mRNA), and **transfer ribonucleic acid** (tRNA). These are both found in the cytoplasm of a cell and are involved in protein synthesis (construction).

The structure of DNA

DNA is shaped like a ladder that has been twisted to form a helix, the so called **double helix**. The sides of the ladder are formed from alternate **sugar** (deoxyribose) and **phosphate** molecules. The rungs are formed from paired nitrogen **bases** (molecules containing nitrogen). These are joined by weak attractions called **hydrogen bonds**. There are four types of base, **adenine** (A) which always pairs with **thymine** (T), and **cytosine** (C) which always pairs with **guanine** (G). These are called **complimentary base pairs** (see figure 1b).

The sugar, phosphate and base combination is called a **nucleotide** (see figure 1a).

How DNA replicates

DNA is the only molecule that can replicate (copy) itself. With the help of enzymes, the DNA molecule unzips and new nucleotides are attached to each strand. Only complementary bases will bond, so an exact copy of the DNA is made every time (see figure 2). This is what happens when chromosomes replicate during cell division (chapter 11.3), and when a gene is copied for protein synthesis (see figure 3).

How can genes contain instructions?

A gene is part of a DNA molecule. The instructions are formed by the sequence of the bases in this part of the DNA. Every three bases, called a **triplet**, code for a particular amino acid. For example, the base sequence CCT codes for the amino acid proline, and TAT codes for the amino acid tyrosine.

There are 64 possible triplets, more than enough to code for the 20 amino acids found in proteins. This is how the genes contain instructions for the formation of proteins. It is called the **genetic code**.

Protein synthesis

Proteins are made from amino acids joined together to form a chain. The sequence of the amino acids is

important in determining the protein. This sequence is specified in the base sequence within a gene, i.e. the genetic code.

When a specific protein, which may be an enzyme is required by a cell, the gene for it is copied and used to produce the protein. The process of copying the gene is called **transcription**. The copy takes the form of (**mRNA**). Note that in RNA molecules, the base thymine is replaced by another base called **uracil**.

The mRNA leaves the nucleus and attaches to a **ribosome**. The code in the gene is then **translated** to produce the protein. This translation involves **tRNA**. Each tRNA carries the genetic code for a particular amino acid. It picks up the amino acid and delivers it to the ribosome. The full process is shown in figure 3.

Many of the proteins formed will be enzymes. The presence or absence of an enzyme can be the difference between developing a characteristic or not. This is how genes work.

Watson and Crick

The scientists James Watson and Francis Crick are generally credited with working out the double helix structure of DNA. They worked together at the University of Cambridge between 1951 and 1953 and based their work on observations made by the biophysicist Maurice Wilkins. The experimental proof of their model was later provided by the American biochemist Arthur Kornberg.

In 1962, Watson, Crick and Wilkins were awarded the Nobel Prize for their work on DNA.

What do **you** know?

You should now be able to:
- Name the different kinds of nucleic acids and state where they are located in a cell.
- Outline the structure of a DNA molecule.
- Describe a complementary base pair.
- Use diagrams to show how DNA can produce an exact copy of itself.
- Explain the genetic code.
- Use diagrams to show how the genetic code can be used to produce a protein.

Figure 1 *The DNA molecule forms a double helix.*

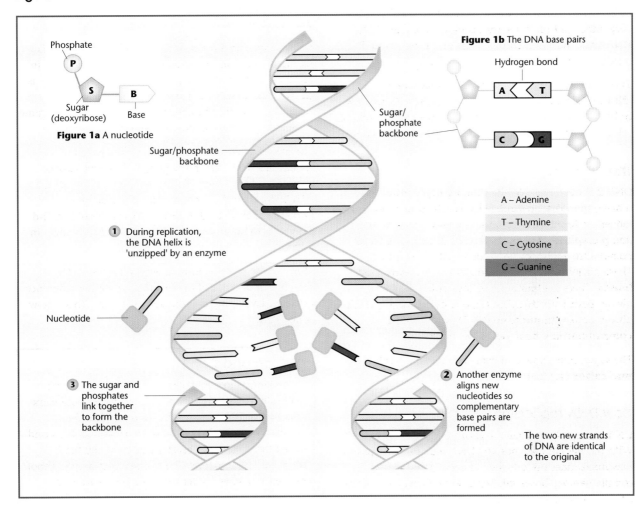

Figure 2 *DNA can replicate to produce identical copies of itself.*

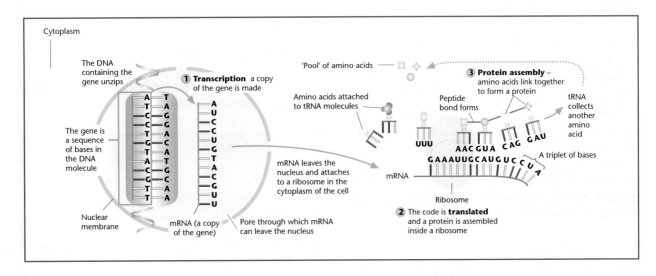

Figure 3 *Protein synthesis involves transcription, translation and assembly.*

11.3 Cell division

New cells are produced by the division of existing cells. During this cell division, the nucleus divides in one of two ways, by:

● **mitosis**, or

● **meiosis**.

Remember, it is the nucleus that contains the genetic instructions that will determine the structure and function of a cell in the human body. These instructions are in the genes on the chromosomes.

What happens in mitosis?

Mitosis is the type of cell division used to produce new cells for **growth**, and to replace worn out or damaged cells. The growth of a fertilised egg into a baby occurs through mitosis. The damaged cells of grazed skin are replaced by mitosis.

The most important thing about mitosis is that all the new cells produced have *exactly the same genes* in their nucleus. They are all **clones** in this respect, but the further development of the cells will depend upon which of these genes are 'switched on'. For example, the cells in an embryo are all produced from the original zygote by mitosis and thereforee contain the same genes. As the embryo grows into a foetus, some of these cells will develop into skin cells, others will develop into nerve cells and so on. This happens, not because they contain different genes, but because different genes in their genetic blueprint are 'switched on'.

The stages of mitosis are shown in figure 2.

Why is meiosis used?

Meiosis is *only* used to produce the gametes for sexual reproduction, i.e. eggs from the ovaries and sperms from the testes. It is often called reduction division because the gametes produced by meiosis contain half the genetic material (chromosomes) of the original cell. They are **haploid** cells produced from a **diploid** cell.

An outline of the process is shown in figure 3. There are two divisions of the nucleus resulting in four cells from each original cell. Each of these new cells will contain exactly half of the chromosomes, one from each **homologous pair**.

Random assortment of chromosomes

During meiosis, one chromosome from each homologous pair will go into each gamete. This means a cell with one homologous pair can produce two kinds of gamete, each containing one chromosome. A cell with two homologous pairs can produce four different gametes

(see figure 1). A cell with three pairs can produce eight different gametes and a human cell containing 23 pairs can produce 8 million different gametes! This is because it is pure chance as to which chromosome from each homologous pair goes into each gamete. We call this the **'random assortment** of chromosomes' and it is one reason why we are all different. Another reason is because of **crossing over**.

What is crossing over?

Before the homologous chromosomes pass into the gametes, they sometimes intertwine with one another and small parts often break off. These parts then join with the other chromosome thereby exchanging the genes on that part. This process, called **crossing over**, is described more fully in chapter 11.6.

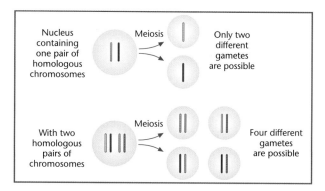

Figure 1 *How the chromosomes segregate into the gametes.*

What do **you** know?

You should now be able to:

● Name the 2 kinds of cell (nuclear) division and state when they are used.

● Show by means of diagrams why mitosis results in producing daughter cells with the same number of chromosomes.

● Explain why, although the new cells produced by mitosis have exactly the same genes, they may develop differently.

● State where meiosis takes place and what kind of cells are produced.

● Explain how a diploid cell produces haploid cells.

● Draw a diagrams to show how many gametes are produced by a cell containing 2 homologous pairs of chromosomes.

● Produce a table comparing mitosis with meiosis.

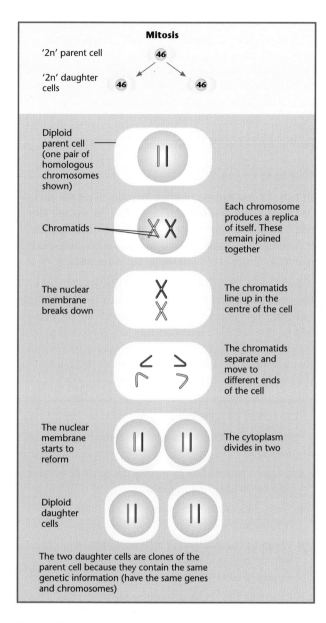

Figure 2 *Mitosis. The different stages can be seen in the photograph below.*

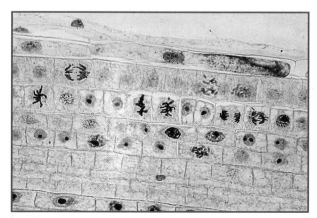

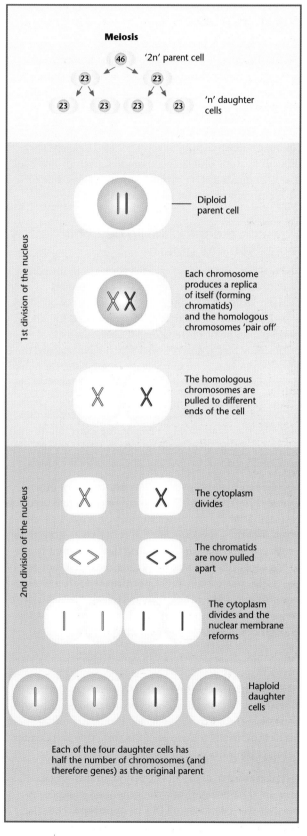

Figure 3 *Meiosis.*

Mendel and inheritance

Is each characteristic controlled by just one gene?

A characteristic is usually controlled by two genes which are on the different chromosomes of an homologous pair. When these chromosomes are separated during meiosis the two genes which control the characteristic are also separated.

Some of the more complex characteristics, such as skin colour, are controlled by several genes. These are very difficult to study and so the examples given in this book are all characteristics controlled by two genes, one on each chromosome of an homologous pair.

How can a characteristic be controlled by more than one gene?

Much of our knowledge of genetics comes from the early work of an Austrian monk called **Gregor Mendel**. Between 1856 and 1865 he carried out a series of breeding experiments with pea plants. Using **pure bred** tall and dwarf plants, he first investigated the characteristic of height. Pure bred plants are ones which have retained the same characteristics for many generations. From his results he concluded that the height of a plant was controlled by two genes. He further reasoned that these two genes were on the different chromosomes of a homologous pair, and although they both coded for height, the exact information contained within them could be different. For example, one gene could code for tallness and the other for dwarfness.

Mendel repeated his experiments using several other visible characteristics of pea plants and on each occasion he found that the characteristic was controlled by two genes, but the exact information contained within these genes could be different. He called these different forms of the gene, **alleles**. Mendel further reasoned that one of the alleles was usually more **dominant** than the other and this allele was always the one which the cell used as its instructions. The 'weaker' allele he referred to as the **recessive** allele. Details of one of Mendel's breeding experiments are shown in figure 1.

Genotype and phenotype

Normally when you describe a person, you describe their appearance; for example you say if they are tall or short, fat or thin. In the language of genetics, this is called the person's **phenotype**.

It is also possible to describe a person, or any organism, in terms of their genes, that is the genes that produce the phenotype. Geneticists call this its **genotype**. The genotype of a particular characteristic can be described as being **heterozygous** or **homozygous.**

Heterozygous means that the two genes coding for a particular character contain different information, i.e. are alleles. Homozygous means they contain the same information. **Homozygous dominant** means that they are both dominant genes and **homozygous recessive** means that they are both recessive.

The pure bred plants that Mendel used were homozygous for the characteristic he was studying (see figure 2).

The test cross

In figure 2 you can see that it is possible to get the same phenotype with two different genotypes, i.e. the tall plants could be either homozygous dominant or heterozygous. Sometimes it is useful to know which plants have which genotype and so a test cross may be performed.

A **test cross** involves crossing a tall plant with a pure breeding dwarf plant, i.e. a homozygous recessive. If the tall plant was homozygous dominant, all the offspring will be heterozygous and therefore tall. If the tall parent was heterozygous, 50% of the new offspring will be tall (heterozygous) and 50% will be dwarfs (homozygous recessive).

The laws of genetics

From his work Mendel established some basic laws of genetics:

- Characteristics of an organism are transferred from parents to offspring in genes.
- The genes are in pairs, one on each of the chromosomes forming an homologous pair.
- When the homologous pair of chromosomes are split up during gamete production (meiosis) the genes are also split up.
- One gene may be dominant to the other (the recessive). If both are present in an individual, the dominant one is used to produce the characteristic.

What do **you** know?

You should now be able to:
- Explain what alleles are and where they are found.
- Explain the terms dominant and recessive (for alleles).
- Using a cross between pure bred tall and pure bred dwarf pea plants, explain the terms homozygous, heterozygous and pure bred.
- Explain what you are describing by the terms phenotype and genotype.

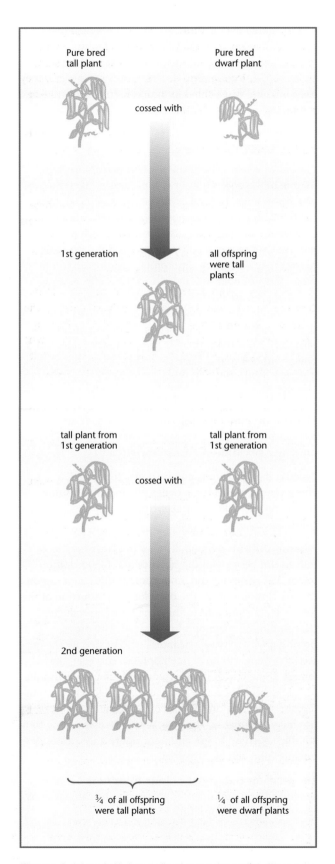

Figure 1 *Mendel's breeding experiments with peas.*

The gene (allele) for tallness is represented by **T**
The gene (allele) for dwarfness is represented by **t**
The two genes (alleles) are on seperate chromosomes

Parents:

Genes **T   T** Homologous chromosomes

t   t

Meiosis   Meiosis

Possible gametes

T   **T**   **t**   **t**

Possible fertilisations

1st generation

T   t   **T   t**   **T   t**   **T   t**

All heterozygous

4 tall plants –
because tall allele is dominant

New parents:

T   t   **T   t**

Meiosis   Meiosis

T   **t**   **T**   **t**

Possible fertilisations

2nd generation

T   T   **T   t**   **t   T**   **t   t**

Phenotypes   Genotypes

Homozygous dominant   Heterozygous   Homozygous recessive

3 tall plants   1 dwarf plant

Phenotypes   Genotypes

Figure 2 *The explanation of Mendel's observations.*

11.5 Genetic predicting

What will a baby look like?

For any characteristic which is controlled by one pair of alleles (i.e. **monohybrid inheritance**), it is possible to predict the genotypes and phenotypes of the offspring from two parents. All you need to know is which of the alleles is the dominant form of the characteristic. Taken to its extreme, it is even possible to select genotypes for breeding, so you can be certain that only good characteristics are passed on. This is common in plant breeding and some animal breeding, but there are laws against geneticists trying it with humans.

The rules of genetic predicting

The basic laws of inheritance were established by Gregor Mendel with his work on peas. And there are a few simple rules that should be followed when using these to make predictions:

1 Each allele is represented by a letter, the dominant allele having the capital form of the letter.

2 Although the alleles are on homologous chromosomes, the chromosomes are not actually drawn as this avoids confusion.

3 Two gametes from each parent are always shown. Each gamete will receive one of the genes/alleles. These can be different or the same.

4 Possible fertilisations are usually shown by a **Punnett square** which shows all the possible offspring from the gametes (see figure 1).

5 The first generation of offspring are referred to as the F_1 **generation** and the second as the F_2 **generation**.

Cystic fibrosis is a disease that affects about 1 in 1600 people. The symptoms are described on page 223. It is an inherited disease and an example of monohybrid inheritance.

The inheritance of blood groups – an example of multiple alleles

A person's blood group is determined by the presence or absence of **antigens** on the surface of the red blood cells. There are two antigens, **antigen A** and **antigen B**. The presence or absence of these is determined by your genes.

There are three possible alleles in this case, I^A, I^B and I^0. The 'I' stands for the type of protein molecule that the antigen is made from. Alleles I^A and I^B are both dominant forms and allele I^0 is the recessive form. You can have any two of these. Figure 2 shows how this works in the genotype. Notice that blood group AB is determined by two dominant alleles and in this case both antigens are produced. This is an example of **co-dominance**, when the dominant and recessive rule does not apply.

What determines sex?

The genes which control the sex of a person are found on one homologous pair of chromosomes called the **sex chromosomes**. In the karyotype (chapter 11.1), these are the 23rd pair of chromosomes. The sex chromosomes in a female are identical just like any other homologous pair and are represented by the letters **XX**. In a male, however, one of the chromosomes is smaller than the other. It is just over half the size of the X chromosome and is represented by the letter Y. A male's sex chromosomes are therefore **XY**. Figure 3 shows how these chromosomes are passed on from parents to offspring. Notice that there is always a 50% chance of a boy or girl being produced.

Sex linked characteristics

The sex chromosomes also carry genes which are responsible for determining other characteristics. These are called **sex-linked characteristics**.

Because the Y chromosome is shorter than the X chromosome, it has some genes missing. The result is that some sex-linked characteristics in men are controlled by only one gene.

Haemophilia is a blood disorder in which the blood fails to clot because of the absence of a blood clotting factor. The genes for the production of this factor are on the sex chromosomes. The gene for the production of the factor (**H**) is dominant to the gene for non-production (**h**) resulting in haemophilia. Females who are homozygous recessive – or males who have only the one recessive gene will have haemophilia. However, the female gamete with homozygous recessive genes usually fails to develop beyond the zygote stage. A heterozygous female is called a **carrier** because although she does not have the disease, she does have a recessive gene that can be passed on to her children. Figure 4 illustrates how haemophilia can be inherited.

The genes for **red-green colour blindness** are also sex-linked and are inherited in exactly the same way as the genes for haemophilia.

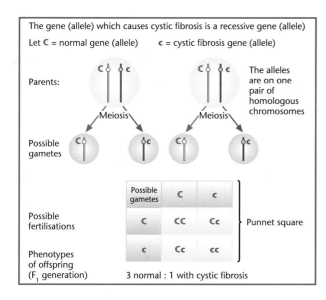

Figure 1 *Cystic fibrosis is inherited.*

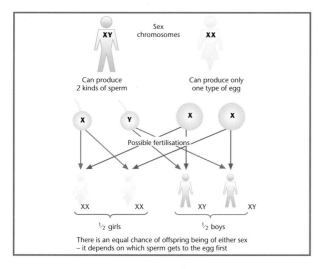

Figure 3 *How the sex of a child is determined.*

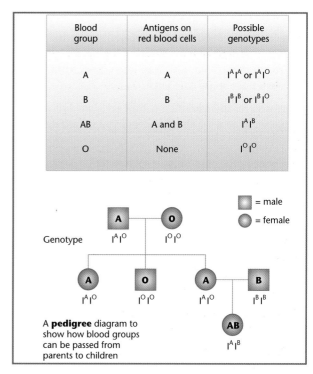

Figure 2 *The inheritance of blood groups.*

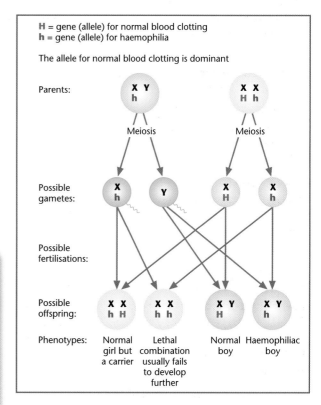

Figure 4 *The inheritance of haemophilia is linked to the inheritance of gender because the genes are on the sex chromosomes.*

What do **you** know?

You should now be able to:

- Explain the term monohybrid inheritance.
- Using the rules of genetic predicting, show how cystic fibrosis is inherited.
- Draw a genetic inheritance diagram to show how ABO blood groups are inherited.
- Explain what a pedigree diagram shows.
- Explain how the sex of a child is determined.
- Draw a genetic inheritance diagram to show how the sex-linked disorder haemophilia is inherited.

INHERITANCE AND VARIATION

11.6 Variation

Why do people vary so much?

There are about 6000 million people on Earth and every one is different. They have different heights, weights, skin colour, eye colour, IQ's, and so on. Even identical twins will have some differences.

The reason for this variation is that everyone has a unique set of genes. The set of genes you inherit depends on:

- the genes your parents have to pass on

- the **random assortment of chromosomes** during meiosis which results in every gamete getting a different set (chapter 11.3).

- the way small portions of the chromosomes and the genes they contain are exchanged during the production of the gametes – called **crossing over** (see figure 1).

The processes above can produce over eight million different sperms and eight million potential eggs with respect to the genes in one nucleus. It is entirely random which single egg and single sperm take part in fertilisation.

The odds against the same two people producing identical children by separate fertilisations is 64 billion to 1! This is one reason why we are all different.

How can identical twins be different?

Identical twins will contain the same genes, but if they are raised in different environments and given different stimuli, they can develop some major differences. For example, they will contain the genotype for a particular weight and height, but will only achieve these if they eat enough food. They will have the same potential IQ, but will only achieve it with the right kind of stimulus and education.

Variation within human beings is therefore the result of two things:

- the genes inherited from your parents

- the environment you live in.

Discontinuous and continuous variation

Variation within a population of organisms falls into two categories.

- **Discontinuous variation** is the kind where there is a small number of distinct types within a range. It is due entirely to the genes present in the individual. The characteristics displaying this kind of variation are usually coded for by one pair of genes, e.g. you can either roll your tongue or you cannot, you are either

haemophilic or you are not, your blood group is A, B, AB or O (chapter 11.4).

- **Continuous variation** is the kind where there is a range of intermediate types between two extremes. For example, if you measure the height of the individuals in a population, and plot these, it would look like the graph in figure 2. This is described as a 'bell-shaped' graph and shows what is called a **normal distribution**. This type of distribution is typical of characteristics that show continuous variation. Most people are in the mid-range.

Characteristics which show continuous variation are often **polygenic**, that is controlled by more than one pair of genes. For example, skin colour is controlled by several pairs of genes and each pair has a dominant and recessive version (alleles). Each dominant allele present in the genotype contributes to the skin colour of the individual. Figure 4 shows how this works.

The influence of the environment

The changes caused by the environment only alter the phenotype of a person. For example sun bathing will change the colour of your skin, but this new colour cannot be passed on to your children. The main environmental influences which can cause these sort of changes are:

- the food you eat

- how much you exercise

- the diseases/illnesses you catch

- how much alcohol you drink

- whether you smoke or abuse drugs

- your education.

These are all covered in other chapters.

What do **you** know?

You should now be able to:

- List 3 causes of genetic variation.
- Suggest how the environment can create differences between people.
- Show, by means of diagrams, why so many different kinds of eggs and sperms can be produced.
- Draw some diagrams to show how genes can be exchanged during meiosis.
- Explain what discontinuous and continuous variation are and state two examples of each.

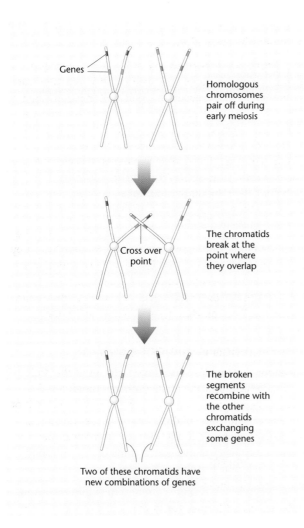

Genes

Homologous chromosomes pair off during early meiosis

Cross over point

The chromatids break at the point where they overlap

The broken segments recombine with the other chromatids exchanging some genes

Two of these chromatids have new combinations of genes

Figure 1 *Crossing over can move genes about.*

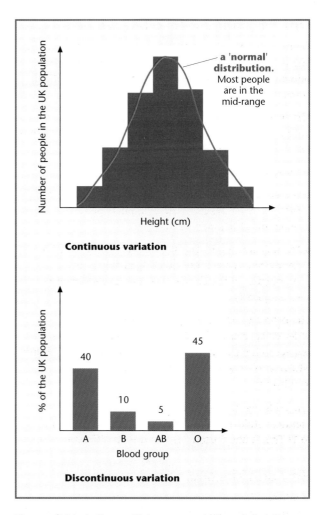

a 'normal' distribution. Most people are in the mid-range

Number of people in the UK population

Height (cm)

Continuous variation

% of the UK population

40

10

5

45

A   B   AB   O

Blood group

Discontinuous variation

Figure 2 *Variation within a population falls into two categories.*

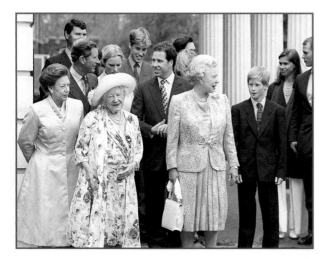

Figure 3 *It is easy to tell these are all members of the same family even though they are not identical.*

AABBCC Six dominant alleles	– very dark brown skin
AABBCc	– dark brown skin
AABbCc	
AaBbCC Three dominant alleles	– medium brown skin
AaBbcc	
Aabbcc	– pale brown skin
aabbcc No dominant alleles	– very pale skin

Figure 4 *Skin colour is determined by three pairs of alleles. Each dominant allele contributes to colour.*

11.7 Mutations

Can the environment alter your genotype?

It is possible for the environment to alter your genotype. This can be studied by events during pregnancy. It is known that the phenotype of a child is very dependent upon aspects of the mother's environment and in particular, the drugs that she takes during pregnancy. Many of these drugs can pass through the placental membranes and enter the embryo/foetus, often with disastrous consequences. Some of the effects are described in chapter 12.7. Many of the developmental changes are the result of alterations to the genes within individual cells. These alterations are called **mutations**.

What are mutations?

A mutation is a change in the genetic material of a cell. This alters the instructions. The change can be to a single gene or a whole chromosome. This can lead to a structural change or a change in the amount of protein produced. The most important changes are those which can be passed on to the offspring. In humans, this means the mutation must occur to the genetic material in the cells which produce the gametes, i.e. in the ovaries and testes.

Mutations usually occur spontaneously, but can also be caused by **mutagens**.

What are mutagens?

Mutagens are environmental factors that can cause mutations. They include:

- Ionising radiations such as X-rays, alpha, beta and gamma rays
- ultra violet (UV) light
- chemicals, such as benzene in cigarette smoke.

Chemicals which turn cells into cancer cells are called **carcinogens**. These work by inducing mutations. Chemicals which can cause genetic changes in a developing embryo or foetus are called **teratogens**.

Gene mutations

A gene mutation is a change in the structure of the DNA that forms the gene, such as a base sequence change. This, in turn, will result in a change in the characteristic.

Most gene mutations produce recessive alleles as in the disease, **sickle cell anaemia**. An individual who is homozygous for the normal dominant allele (N) will produce normal haemoglobin. An individual who is homozygous for the mutated recessive allele (n) will produce abnormal haemoglobin. The cells containing abnormal haemoglobin become sickle shaped (see figure 3). This haemoglobin cannot carry as much oxygen as normal haemoglobin and the condition can result in death.

Carriers of the recessive allele (Nn), produce a mixture of normal and abnormal haemoglobin. At high oxygen concentrations they are healthy, but if the oxygen concentration falls, their red blood cells revert to the sickle shape and they cannot carry enough oxygen. They are said to have the **sickle cell trait**. Strangely, carriers are more resistant to malaria, which helps them survive in certain parts of the world.

Changes of a dominant allele to a recessive allele have also caused **cystic fibrosis**, **haemophilia**, **albinism** and **polydactyly**. **Huntington's chorea** is a degenerative disease of the nervous system caused by the change of a recessive allele to a dominant allele (see figure 2).

A gene mutation may be responsible for a new strain of influenza virus (see chapter 13.8).

Chromosome mutations

Chromosome mutations result in whole blocks of genes becoming altered, exchanged, duplicated or deleted. They produce conditions called **syndromes**.

For example, **Down's syndrome** is the result of a fault in meiosis, which results in female gametes containing an extra copy of the 21st chromosome (see figure 4). This extra chromosome has enormous effects on the phenotype. A Down's syndrome child will have characteristic physical features including a flattish face, small hands with short fingers and some learning difficulties.

Down's syndrome is more common in children born to older women. It is possible to detect this condition in a foetus using amniocentesis (chapter 9.7).

Can we predict the results of mutated genes?

Genetic screening does just this. Parents who may be at risk of producing a disabled child can attend **Genetic Counselling Units** where an in depth investigation will be undertaken and the appropriate advice given. If high risk parents do decide to have a child, the counsellors will then spend time on preparing the parents for raising a physically challenged child and help with schooling arrangements.

In the near future, gene therapy may eliminate these kinds of problem (chapter 14.7).

Are mutations ever beneficial?

Occasionally, mutations may improve on a characteristic. Occurrences are very rare but extremely important because they form the basis of **evolution**. Nature **selects** these improved variants and they go on to breed and produce future offspring. This process, over a period of millions of years, has resulted in all the different life forms on Earth.

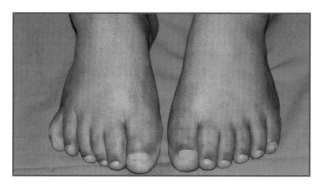

Figure 1 *This child has polydactyl (an extra digit) due to a gene mutation.*

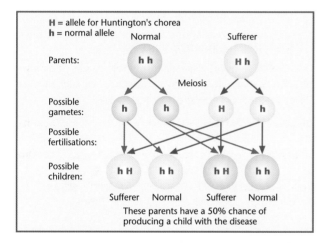

Figure 2 *Huntington's chorea is caused by change of a recessive allele to a dominant allele.*

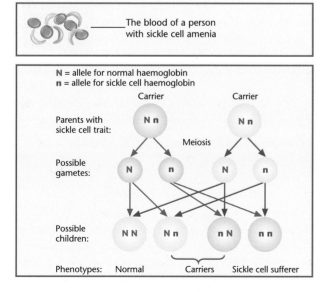

Figure 3 *A gene mutation causes sickle cell anaemia.*

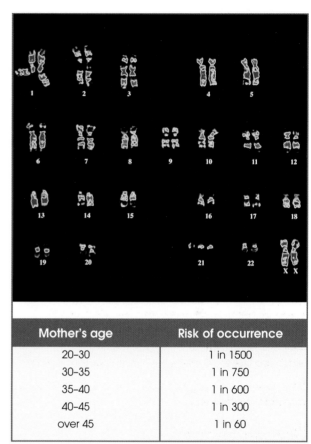

Mother's age	Risk of occurrence
20–30	1 in 1500
30–35	1 in 750
35–40	1 in 600
40–45	1 in 300
over 45	1 in 60

Figure 4 *A chromosome mutation can cause Down's syndrome. The risk of mutation increases with the mother's age.*

What do **you** know?

You should now be able to:

- Explain what mutations are.
- Name 4 substances that can cause mutations.
- Explain what a gene mutation is and list 4 examples.
- Describe the cause and effects of sickle cell anaemia.
- Explain why sickle cell anaemia will never die out in certain parts of the world.
- Explain what Huntington's chorea is and why it is different.
- Using diagrams explain how a Down's child might be produced.
- Discuss how mutations may have helped in the development of all the different life forms.

Chapter 11: Questions

1 There is a serious human disease called thalassaemia. It causes the haemoglobin in the red blood cells to be abnormal and less able to carry out their normal function.

  a What is the normal function of haemoglobin?

    (1 mark)

  b What would you expect to be one major effect of thalassaemia on people with the disease? *(1 mark)*

  c The diagram below shows the members of a family in which one of the children has thalassaemia.

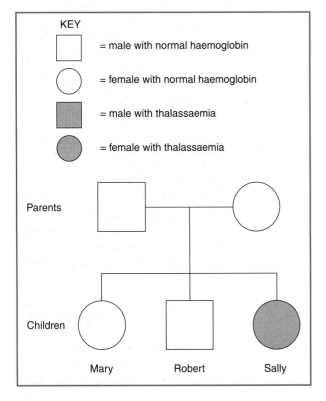

    KEY

    ☐ = male with normal haemoglobin

    ○ = female with normal haemoglobin

    ■ = male with thalassaemia

    ● = female with thalassaemia

Thalassaemia is inherited, and the allele of the gene which causes it is recessive.
(H = gene for normal haemoglobin,
h = gene for thalassaemia.)
Copy and complete the following diagram to show why Sally has thalassaemia.

		Mother	Father
Parent's genes		Hh	_____
Gene in:	egg which produced Sally _____	sperm which produced Sally _____
Genes in:		Sally _____	*(3 marks)*

  d Explain how Mary and Robert can have normal haemoglobin. *(1 mark)*

  e If the parents decided to have a fourth child, what would be the chance of this child having thalassaemia? *(1 mark)*

    (NEAB Sample Assessment)

2 The diagram shows a simplified animal cell just before division.

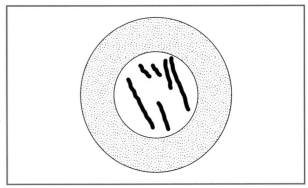

  a Give one important difference you would show if you drew a similar human cell. *(1 mark)*

  b The diagrams below show the result of the division of the cell shown above.

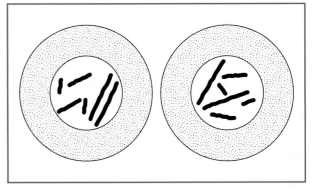

The cell has divided by mitosis. Give two features present in these diagrams which show this.

    (2 marks)

    (SEG June 1990)

3 The diagram shows part of a DNA molecule.

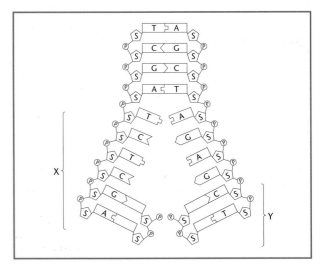

a What general name is given to the structures labelled A, C, G and T? *(1 mark)*

b What is happening to the DNA molecule in region X? *(1 mark)*

c Suggest the correct letters (A, C, G or T) for the spaces on the diagram in region Y. *(1 mark)*

d In what way is the structure of a DNA molecule related to the structure of a protein molecule? *(2 marks)*

(SEG June 1999)

4 Cystic fibrosis is an inherited condition which affects the lungs. It is caused by a recessive allele. People who are homozygous for the unaffected allele and people who are heterozygous, do not suffer from cystic fibrosis.
N = the unaffected allele
n = the allele for cystic fibrosis
A person could have one of the following genotypes.
          NN   Nn   nn

a **i** Give two possible genotypes of an unaffected person.

ii Give the genotype of a person who has cystic fibrosis. *(3 marks)*

b A man and his wife are both unaffected but their first child suffers from cystic fibrosis. Copy and complete the diagram below to show the genotypes and phenotypes of the offspring. *(4 marks)*

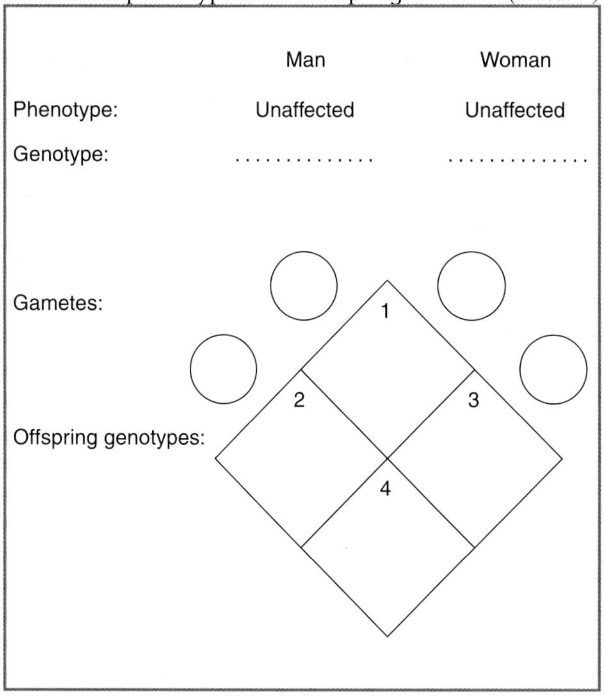

	Man	Woman
Phenotype:	Unaffected	Unaffected
Genotype:	. . . .	. . . .

Gametes:

Offspring genotypes:
(diagram with circles numbered 1, 3 at top; circles at left; boxes numbered 2, 4)

c What is the probability that this couple's next child will have cystic fibrosis?
    none   1 in 3   1 in 4   2 in 4   3 in 4
(1 mark)
(SEG June 1998)

5 Phenylketonuria (PKU) is an inherited condition. It is an example of **discontinuous variation** and was originally caused by a **mutation** which produced a **recessive** allele of a certain **gene**.

a What is meant by each of the following biological terms?
  i Discontinuous variation *(2 marks)*
  ii Mutation *(1 mark)*
  iii Recessive *(1 mark)*
  iv Gene. *(2 marks)*

b A man and his wife are both heterozygous for PKU. They do not suffer from the disease.
  i This couple has so far had two children, both girls. Neither of these has PKU. Draw a suitable genetic diagram to show how it is possible for the man and his wife to produce some children who suffer from PKU and some that do not. Use the following symbols:
    N = allele for not suffering from PKU
    n = allele for PKU *(4 marks)*
  ii The wife is pregnant again. What is the probability that her new child
    1 will suffer from PKU?
    2 will be a boy? *(2 marks)*

c The effects of PKU are due to accumulation of large amounts of the amino acid phenylalanine in the tissues of the body. Normally the following reactions occur in the body cells to break down the phenylalanine:

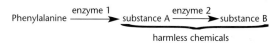

Phenylalanine $\xrightarrow{\text{enzyme 1}}$ substance A $\xrightarrow{\text{enzyme 2}}$ substance B
harmless chemicals

  i Explain why a mutation in the gene for enzyme 1 would cause a rise in the concentration of phenylalanine in the tissues. *(2 marks)*

  ii Why must a baby with PKU be fed a low-protein diet or be fed with a diet containing artificial proteins? *(1 mark)*
(SEG June 1999)

12 Health

How much are you responsible for your own health? If a member of your family gets asthma, will you also get it? How can you improve your health? This chapter answers these questions and explains what *good health* is.

After you have worked through this chapter, you should be able to:

- Discuss the meaning of health.
- Outline the inbuilt factors which can affect your health.
- Describe the environmental influences on health.
- Discuss the importance of health behaviour.
- Describe the causes and prevention of gum disease and tooth rot.

- Describe the results of neglecting your feet.
- Outline the importance of eating healthily.
- Assess the importance of regular exercise and rest.
- Define and explain the causes of mental illness.
- Discuss the problems associated with abusing drugs.
- Describe the effects on the body of the main groups of drugs.

Health and social class

What is social class?

Social class is a classification of people based on their occupation. This arranges them into divisions often just called I, II, III, IV, and V (table 1).

Social class	Examples of occupation
I Professional	Doctor, solicitor
II Managerial	Teacher, policeman
III Skilled (a) non-manual (b) manual	Secretary, draughtsman Bricklayer, cook
IV Partly skilled	Barperson, postman
V Unskilled	Labourer, window cleaner

Table 1 *Social classification of people by occupation.*

How is health linked to social class?

In the United Kingdom health has always been linked to social class. Statistics can be used to show this link very clearly. Widely used indicators of health are the life expectancy at birth and the infant mortality rate (table 2).

Social class	Life expectancy	Infant mortality rate (1995)
I Professional	74.9	4.5
II Managerial	74.9	4.8
III Skilled		
(a) non-manual	73.5	5.5
(b) manual	72.4	5.9
IV Partly skilled	69.7	6.6
V Unskilled	69.7	6.7

Table 2 *Infant mortality.*

Statistics also show that:

- People in social class V are more than twice as likely to die before they reach retirement age.
- Men in social class V are four times more likely to suffer from mental illness.
- More people in social class IV and V suffer from long standing illness. This is called chronic illness (see figure 1).

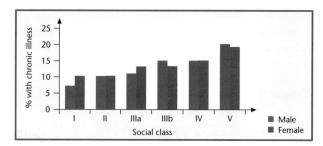

Figure 1 *Chronic illness. (1994)*

- In nearly all cases the highest mortality from diseases is in the lower social classes.

- The incidence of high blood pressure is higher in social class V (table 3).

| Social class | Percentage with high blood pressure | |
---	Male	Female
I Professional	16	22
II Managerial	19	20
III Skilled		
(a) non-manual	21	23
(b) manual	20	24
IV Partly skilled	20	25
V Unskilled	24	26

Table 3 *Percentage with high blood pressure.*

Why do these differences exist?

We can only guess at the reason for the differences, although there is evidence that:

- Classes IV and V do not make as much use of the preventative medical services, such as dentists (see figure 2).

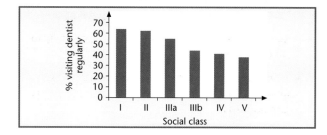

Figure 2 *Dentists. (1995)*

- Classes IV and V usually have lower incomes and as such cannot afford some of the necessities for a healthy life such as good food and housing.

- More people in classes IV and V smoke thereby increasing their chances of suffering certain diseases and creating an unpleasant environment for their children (see table 4).

- Women in social class V are nearly twice as likely to be obese.

| Social class | Percentage who smoke | |
---	Male	Female
I Professional	15	14
II Managerial	21	20
III Skilled		
(a) non-manual	21	21
(b) manual	36	31
IV Partly skilled	38	33
V Unskilled	45	33

Table 4 *Smokers. (1998)*

- Children in social class V are five times more likely to suffer accidental death than those in social class I.

What is the solution to these problems?

In 1948 the Government introduced the National Health Service (NHS) as a solution to these problems. The NHS made good medical treatment available to every member of a community whether rich or poor. Its success, to some extent, can be judged on statistics which show:

- A higher percentage of the population now make use of the health services.

- Generally, the health of the population is improving. The life expectancy is increasing and infant mortality rates are falling. Less people are dying from disease.

- The biggest improvement has been in the health of social classes I and II.

Health inequalities like these have been the focus of a recent independent enquiry commissioned by the government. The findings have been taken very seriously and tackling these inequalities is one of the twin aims in the government's new public health strategy, *Saving Lives: Our Healthier Nation.*

How healthy are you?

Everybody at some time experiences poor health, but just how healthy are we the rest of the time? If you are in perfect health this usually means your body is working at peak efficiency both physically and mentally. According to the **World Health Organisation** (WHO), good health is '*a state of complete physical, mental and social well being, and not just the absence of disease or infirmity*'. Anything less than this and you are unhealthy in some way or another. So not many of us can say we have perfect health! But clearly there are degrees of unhealthiness: a person could just be a bit unfit; or they could be seriously ill with cancer.

Figure 2 shows one way of looking at health. Your position on the line depends, to a large extent, on your environment and lifestyle. These can either promote good health or lead to sickness.

Health and homeostasis

Good health is about your body maintaining homeostasis regardless of changes in your environment or behaviour. Homeostasis will be affected by the food you eat, the air you breathe, the alcohol you drink, even the thoughts you think (stress), but it must overcome all of these to preserve good health. If it fails, you become diseased and sick. You may even die. We can all help our body by adopting good health behaviour.

Figure 3 shows some of the ways your environment and behaviour can affect your health. Some examples are explored in the rest of this chapter.

Are there things that affect our health that we have no control over?

Your health is not only affected by almost everything you do, but also by what you are – inbuilt factors that we a cannot change.

- **Genotype**. Every child inherits from its parents a 'blueprint' for its future growth and development. Unfortunately, this set of instructions will also include any inheritable disorders, such as haemophilia, cystic fibrosis and Huntingdon's chorea. Figure 1 shows how haemophilia has been passed through the generations of the royal family.

- **Age**. Many diseases and disorders take time to develop and are therefore associated with old age. Alzheimer's (a progressive disease of the brain, resulting in dementia), and Parkinson's diseases are rare before the age of 60. Many types of cancer and heart disease also seem to come later in life, probably partly due to a genetic disposition and partly due to the accumulative

effects of wear and tear from living life. Figure 5 shows the main causes of death at different ages for women and men.

- **Sex**. Many illnesses seem to affect one sex more than the other. Pre-menstrual tension (PMT) clearly only affects women and prostate cancer only affects men. Some disorders are sex-linked and are therefore more common in males, e.g. haemophilia and red-green colour blindness. Many diseases, which are not sex-linked, also seem to affect one sex more than the other. For example, three times more men than women suffer from lung cancer, but it is not clear why.

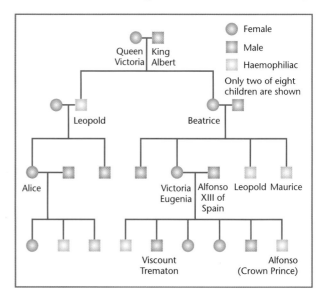

Figure 1 *Haemophilia in the Royal family.*

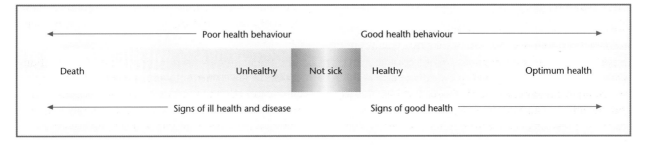

Figure 2 *Where do you fall on the health line?*

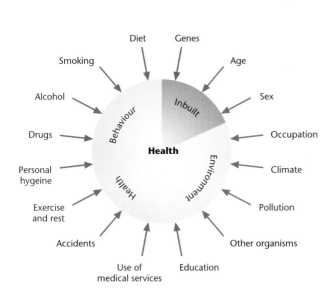

Figure 3 *Your health is affected by almost everything.*

Table 1 *UK adults' views of what is bad for their health (1996).*

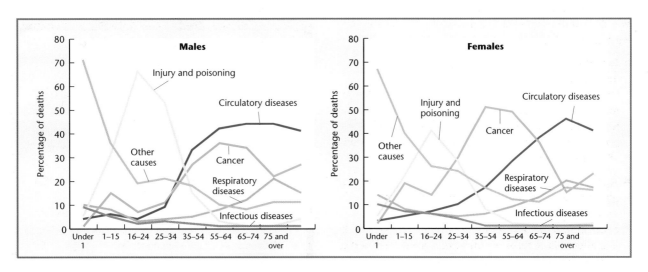

Figure 5 *The major causes of death for people in the UK in 1997.*

The 'blueprint' you are born with affects your health, as does your environment, for instance:

- **Where you live**. For example, the country you live in can have a large effect on your health. Its climate alone can contribute to good and poor health. Sunlight is required to make vitamin D in your skin, yet too much of it can damage your skin and even cause cancer.

- Your **occupation**. A person's occupation exposes them to many potentially harmful situations and substances. Some of these hazards are described below.

- Your **social class**. In the UK, social class is linked to occupation. There is a lot of evidence to suggest that there are large health differences within the social classes (page 168).

- The **health education** you receive. To live a healthy life you must be aware of what is considered good and bad for you. In the UK there is now a carefully planned programme of health education in schools and the community.

- **Pollution**. In an industrialised society such as ours, pollution is inevitable (see chapter 16).

- **Other organisms**. Many organisms obtain their food from others and in doing so cause or spread disease. (see chapter 13).

It is difficult to separate these factors, because they are dependent upon each other. For example, if you live in an industrial town, you are more likely to be affected by pollution which may reduce the efficiency of your immune system. Clearly, some people are disadvantaged more than others.

How can occupation affect health?

Hazards to health at work include a variety of **occupational diseases** and accidents. The resulting ill health can include: headaches, backache, **repetitive strain injury** (RSI), deafness, cancer, dermatitis, infectious diseases, depression, loss of limbs and even death. These account for the loss of millions of working days and many premature deaths every year. However, work-related illness is almost always avoidable, with a bit of foresight. For example:

- **Occupational factors** (the nature of the job). If the job requires a lot of lifting, then an employer should offer a 'lifting and handling course' to its employees so they know how to lift correctly.

- **Environmental factors** (the workplace). In noisy environments, it is advisable to wear ear protection.

- **Human factors**. Carelessness, haste and short cuts can result in accidents. These can be avoided by

careful action planning, with realistic timing for tasks and adequate breaks.

The 'Health and Safety at Work Act'

In 1974, the government published a set of legal requirements relating to the health and safety of employees at work. It is a set of rules for employers and employees to follow to encourage good practice. An important part of it relates to **Risk Assessment** which sets out guidelines for employers on how to identify potential hazards and how to minimise risk (see figure 2).

Another important set of regulations, the **Control of Substances Hazardous to Health** (COSHH) was introduced in 1988. These regulations require an employer to identify hazardous substances in the workplace, identify who is at risk and take measures to minimise this risk. This, for example, may mean correctly labelling and storing substances, or putting in place procedures for handling them.

Health and safety laws are enforced by the **Health and Safety Inspectorate** and **Environmental Health Officers**.

What about 'special needs'?

Special needs is a term used to describe people who need a bit of extra help to perform tasks that most able-bodied people can manage. It includes people with chronic illnesses, broken bones, hearing problems, dyslexia, other learning disabilities, mental retardation and even heavily pregnant women. The help covers mobility, extra time for learning, special therapy, and so on. Meeting special needs is about providing access to situations and environments that would normally be out of reach, thereby improving quality of life and position on the health line.

What do **you** know?

You should now be able to:

- Outline how your environment could be affecting your health.
- Explain why it is often difficult to assign a cause.
- Describe some of the health risks in different occupations.
- Describe three ways health related illness could be avoided.
- Explain what a risk assessment is and draw a flow diagram to show how you would carry this out.
- Explain what COSHH stands for.
- Explain how noise pollution can damage your health.

Health Risk	Ill Health Effects
Handling heavy loads	Back ache, strains and sprains
Repetitive movements e.g. typing	Repetitive strain injury (RSI)
Breathing or handling hazardous chemicals	Cancer, asthma, dermatitis. poisoning
Noisy surrounds	Deafness, tinnitus
Continuous vibrations	White finger, backache
Exposure to radiations e.g. UV, X-rays	Cancer, eye damage, burns
Exposure to micro-organisms	Infectious diseases
Stressors e.g. excessive workload	Stress, hypertension, burn out

Figure 1 *Some occupational hazards.*

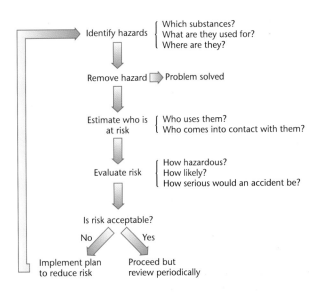

Identify hazards — Which substances? What are they used for? Where are they?

Remove hazard ⇨ Problem solved

Estimate who is at risk — Who uses them? Who comes into contact with them?

Evaluate risk — How hazardous? How likely? How serious would an accident be?

Is risk acceptable?

No — Implement plan to reduce risk

Yes — Proceed but review periodically

Figure 2 *A risk assessment should be carried out for all dangerous activities.*

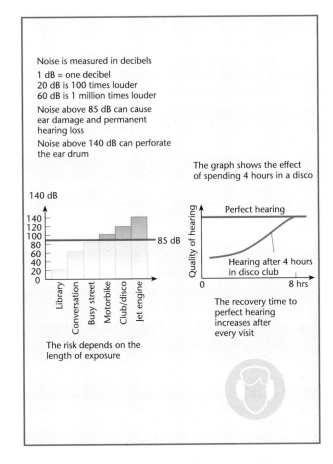

Noise is measured in decibels

1 dB = one decibel
20 dB is 100 times louder
60 dB is 1 million times louder

Noise above 85 dB can cause ear damage and permanent hearing loss

Noise above 140 dB can perforate the ear drum

140 dB

85 dB

Library, Conversation, Busy street, Motorbike, Club/disco, Jet engine

The risk depends on the length of exposure

The graph shows the effect of spending 4 hours in a disco

Perfect hearing

Quality of hearing

Hearing after 4 hours in disco club

0 — 8 hrs

The recovery time to perfect hearing increases after every visit

Figure 4 *Noise pollution is a serious problem.*

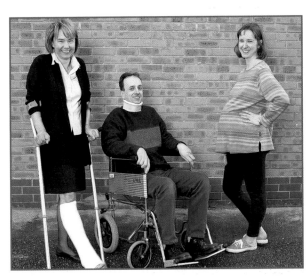

Figure 3 *Photograph of some people with special needs.*

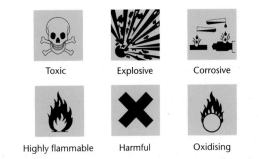

Toxic · Explosive · Corrosive

Highly flammable · Harmful · Oxidising

Figure 5 *Some hazard warning symbols used for chemicals.*

Personal hygiene

Good health behaviour can be described as a lifestyle which promotes good health, and maximises our potential for physical, mental and social well being. This means:

- maintaining good personal hygiene
- eating a good healthy balanced diet
- taking regular exercise and getting plenty of rest
- staying free from stress
- not smoking
- not drinking alcohol in excess
- using the preventive medical services.

A clean body is obviously essential to good health. It is something that everybody can achieve and only requires a little time. For example, washing daily will prevent **body odour** (BO) and possible infections. Your skin contains two kinds of gland, **sweat** and **sebaceous** (oil) **glands**. Sweat which is mainly salt and water, is used to cool your body. If it is not washed away, bacteria will feed on it producing unpleasant odours. Most of your sweat glands are on your forehead, armpits, groin and soles of your feet, so these places, in particular, need frequent washing.

Sebaceous glands produce an oil called **sebum**, which is used to keep your skin and hair supple and prevent drying out. They are mainly found in the hairy parts of your body. During adolescence, sebaceous glands produce more sebum which can block the pores, resulting in spots. Thorough cleansing can help prevent these becoming infected and developing into **acne**. A balanced diet combined with outdoor exercise can also prevent overproduction of sebum.

Why should I clean my teeth?

We all have natural bacteria in our mouths. These bacteria feed on the sugar in food and produce acid, which can dissolve the enamel of your teeth and irritate the gums, causing **dental caries** and **gum disease**. This can result in bad breath, and eventually loss of teeth.

Dental caries is the main cause of tooth loss in children and teenagers. If your teeth are not cleaned properly, the acid produced by the bacteria dissolves a hole in the enamel and then the dentine. If the hole reaches the pulp, the nerve is exposed and this causes the pain of toothache. Infection can develop and quickly spread through the pulp causing inflammation, more pain and, eventually, an **abscess**.

Gum disease is more common in older people. If bacteria build up in the mouth they irritate the gums. The gums become sore, swell up and bleed easily, especially when brushed. At this early stage the disease is called **gingivitis**. If it is not treated, the inflammation will reach the root of the tooth and the jaw bone, destroying the cement and fibres holding the tooth in place (see figure 4).

The bacteria and sugary food can build up on the surface of teeth forming **plaque**. You can see this more clearly by chewing a **disclosing tablet**, which contains a harmless vegetable dye (see figure 3). Plaque can react with saliva to produce a hard yellow deposit called **calculus**. Once this has formed, you will need a dentist or hygienist to remove it.

Can you prevent caries and gum disease?

The way to do this is to prevent excess acid being produced in your mouth. This can be achieved in two ways:

- by avoiding sugary foods, or at least cleaning your teeth and mouth after eating them
- by preventing the build up of plaque by thorough cleaning, every morning and night
- by visiting the dentist for regular check-ups.

Why do teeth become sensitive?

Receding gums, due to ageing or gum disease, will leave the root of the tooth exposed. As the root does not have a hard coating of enamel the dentine is exposed. Tiny pores in the dentine allow hot, cold or sweet substances to enter and trigger the nerve in the pulp cavity, causing pain. Some toothpastes temporarily block these pores, reducing tooth sensitivity.

What do **you** know?

You should now be able to:

- Write a list of things you would consider to be poor health behaviour.
- Explain why washing daily is good health behaviour.
- Describe the causes of tooth rot and gum disease and explain how these can be avoided.
- Explain why teeth sometimes become sensitive.
- Outline the potential problems of neglecting your feet.

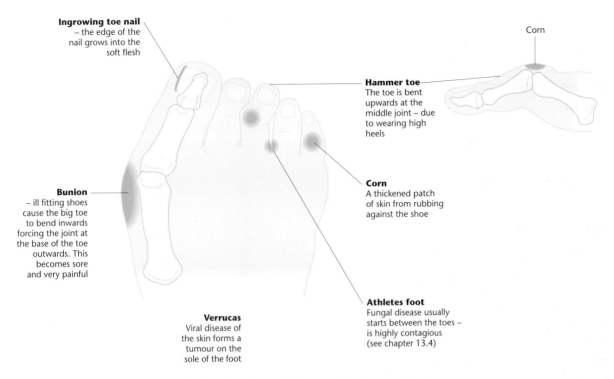

Ingrowing toe nail – the edge of the nail grows into the soft flesh

Corn

Hammer toe The toe is bent upwards at the middle joint – due to wearing high heels

Bunion – ill fitting shoes cause the big toe to bend inwards forcing the joint at the base of the toe outwards. This becomes sore and very painful

Corn A thickened patch of skin from rubbing against the shoe

Verrucas Viral disease of the skin forms a tumour on the sole of the foot

Athletes foot Fungal disease usually starts between the toes – is highly contagious (see chapter 13.4)

Figure 1 *The feet need frequent attention to avoid unwanted complaints.*

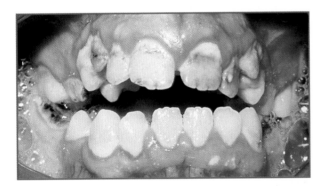

Figure 2 *Neglected teeth and gums.*

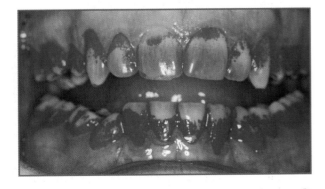

Figure 3 *Neglected teeth and gums after using a disclosing tablet.*

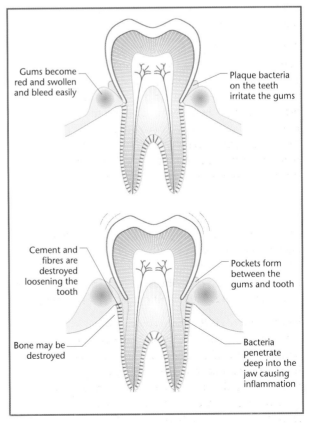

Gums become red and swollen and bleed easily

Plaque bacteria on the teeth irritate the gums

Cement and fibres are destroyed loosening the tooth

Pockets form between the gums and tooth

Bone may be destroyed

Bacteria penetrate deep into the jaw causing inflammation

Figure 4 *The process of gum disease.*

12.4 Diet and weight control

What is a healthy balanced diet?

In an ideal world we would all:

● eat a healthy balanced diet

● eat just enough to maintain a good body weight.

In reality this rarely happens, creating many health problems. Figure 1 shows some of the consequences.

The components of a healthy balanced diet are described in chapter 2.3. Surveys consistently show that in the UK we are eating:

● **too much fat**. We need some fat in our diet to provide energy, make cell membranes, some hormones and vitamin D. Too much fat causes **obesity** and all its associated problems (see figure 2). Research suggests that too much saturated animal fat can also increase blood cholesterol levels increasing your chances of heart disease (chapter 3.5), having a stroke and getting gall stones.

● **too much refined sugar**. Most processed foods now contain added refined sugar. Too much sugar can result in obesity and tooth decay (chapter 12.3).

● **too much salt**. Salt is essential for the normal functioning of nerves and muscles. Too little will result in cramp and too much will increase blood pressure, increasing your chances of heart disease and a stroke.

Salt is often added to canned or processed foods to improve flavour. It is important to realise that infants cannot tolerate high salt levels because their kidneys cannot excrete the excess.

● **too little fibre**. Increasing your fibre intake can help you reduce the amount of food you eat and help protect against colon cancer and other digestive problems such as constipation and irritable bowel syndrome (IBS).

How much food do you need to eat?

Your food must supply the materials your body requires for growth and repair, to stay healthy, and your energy needs. We require different amounts at different times of our lives. Even day to day we need different amounts depending on the outside temperature and how active we are. To obtain the right amount of food you need to balance energy intake with the energy used. The **Department of Health** has suggested that no more than 35% of your daily energy intake should come from fat, with less than 11% from saturated fat. A further 15% should come from protein and the rest from carbohydrates, mainly natural sugars and starch. For the average adult female using 8100 kJ of energy per day,

this is equal to 74 g fat, 71 g protein and 238 g of carbohydrates. Figure 1 in chapter 2.3 shows the **recommended nutrient intakes** (RNI) for different age groups.

What will happen if you eat too much food?

If you eat more food than your body requires, that is your energy intake exceeds your energy output, the excess food is turned into fat and stored. You will put on weight and may even become **obese**. Obesity is defined by means of the **body mass index** (BMI). An obese person has a BMI of more than 30. Table 1 shows how obesity in the UK is on the increase.

Obesity carries health risks, some of these are shown in figure 2. Another way of assessing your health risk is to compare your **waist-hip ratio** (WHR). A WHR of less than 1 for men and 0.8 for women is considered healthy.

Fat should make up between 12–18% of a man's body and 18–25% of a woman's body weight, depending on age. This fat is stored in special cells under your skin and around some of your vital organs. For every 38 kJ of excess food eaten, a further 1 g of fat will be stored.

What will happen if you eat too little?

Eating too little food will result in poor health and deficiency diseases (see figure 1). Eating too few energy foods will lead to **starvation**. Your body will use its carbohydrate and fat reserves to produce energy but when these are exhausted your body uses proteins. This can quickly lead to death.

Many people starve themselves on purpose, in an attempt to lose weight. This is the idea behind slimming diets, i.e. reduce your consumption of the energy foods slightly so that your fat reserves are used. If this is to work without causing serious illness, it is important that the rest of the diet remains the same so that you still get enough of the other nutrients. It is also important to exercise whilst slimming, to maintain muscle mass. Dieting is a very complex business and should always be approved by a health professional. For some, it can lead to serious illness.

People suffering from **anorexia nervosa** develop a morbid fear of fatness and strive for thinness by starving themselves. They can become so thin that it starts to affect their health and can often result in death.

A person with **bulimia nervosa** will eat exceptionally large amounts of food, and then expel it by vomiting or using laxatives. The effect on health is just as worrying as anorexia. Both conditions need urgent and sensitive medical support.

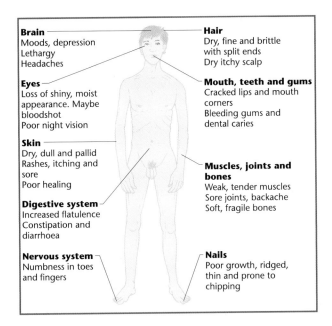

Brain
Moods, depression
Lethargy
Headaches

Eyes
Loss of shiny, moist
appearance. Maybe
bloodshot
Poor night vision

Skin
Dry, dull and pallid
Rashes, itching and
sore
Poor healing

Digestive system
Increased flatulence
Constipation and
diarrhoea

Nervous system
Numbness in toes
and fingers

Hair
Dry, fine and brittle
with split ends
Dry itchy scalp

Mouth, teeth and gums
Cracked lips and mouth
corners
Bleeding gums and
dental caries

**Muscles, joints and
bones**
Weak, tender muscles
Sore joints, backache
Soft, fragile bones

Nails
Poor growth, ridged,
thin and prone to
chipping

Figure 1 *Some of the effects of malnutrition.*

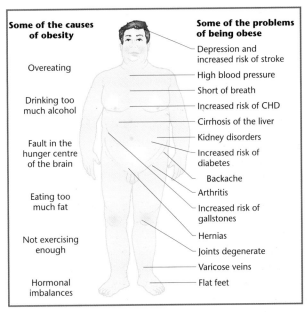

**Some of the causes
of obesity**

Overeating

Drinking too
much alcohol

Fault in the
hunger centre
of the brain

Eating too
much fat

Not exercising
enough

Hormonal
imbalances

**Some of the problems
of being obese**

Depression and
increased risk of stroke

High blood pressure

Short of breath

Increased risk of CHD

Cirrhosis of the liver

Kidney disorders

Increased risk of
diabetes

Backache

Arthritis

Increased risk of
gallstones

Hernias

Joints degenerate

Varicose veins

Flat feet

Figure 2 *Some of the causes and problems
created by obesity.*

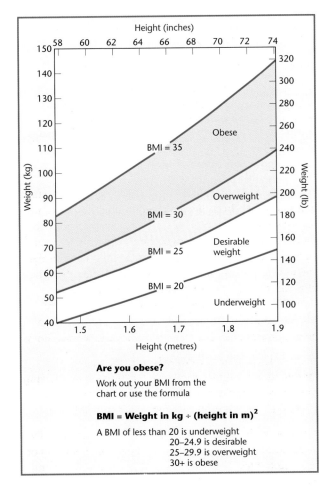

Are you obese?

Work out your BMI from the
chart or use the formula

BMI = Weight in kg ÷ (height in m)²

A BMI of less than 20 is underweight
 20–24.9 is desirable
 25–29.9 is overweight
 30+ is obese

Figure 3 *Work out your body mass index (BMI).*

	1986		1996	
	Men	Women	Men	Women
% overweight	38	24	45	34
% obese	8	12	16	17

Table 1 *Obesity in the UK is increasing.*

What do **you** know?

You should now be able to:

- Review the components of a healthy balanced diet.
- Outline what is generally considered to be wrong
with the average UK diet.
- Work out how much fat, protein and carbohydrate
you should be eating every day.
- Work out your BMI and waist-hip ratio and
assess your health risk.
- Describe some of the health risks associated
with obesity.
- Give some examples of how malnutrition can
affect your health.
- Explain the difference between anorexia and
bulimia nervosa.

12.5 Exercise and rest

Why should I exercise regularly?

Regular exercise will keep your body working at its maximum efficiency. It does this by:

- improving your general **fitness**

- stimulating natural maintenance and repair systems such as the **immune system** so that, for example, wounds heal more quickly

- improving the circulation of the blood by strengthening your heart muscle (making it more powerful) and so reducing your resting pulse rate and blood pressure

- reducing the amount of fatty substances in the blood thereby helping prevent heart disease

- improving lung capacity by strengthening the diaphragm and increasing the expansion of the alveoli, which increases the amount of oxygen intake

- increasing **lean body mass** (muscle), which leads to an increase in metabolic rate so that food is used up more quickly

- improving the strength of ligaments and tendons

- improving muscle tone and posture (chapter 5.4).

Exercise can be used to reduce weight, but you need to do a lot of exercise regularly to really make a difference. For instance, it takes over half an hour of jogging to work off the energy provided by a 60 g portion of cheese. Table 1 shows the amount of energy various activities require.

Too much exercise can sometimes be harmful. For example, many athletes suffer joint problems later in life.

What is fitness?

Physical fitness is a measure of your ability to cope with the physical demands of everyday life. It can be divided into three parts:

- **Stamina**. This is your ability to keep going without becoming short of breath or collapsing from exhaustion. It will be largely determined by the efficiency of your **cardiovascular** and **respiratory** systems.

- **Suppleness**. Every joint in your body is capable of a range of movements brought about by the muscles near it. Your suppleness is a measure of how well they can achieve these. The more a joint is used, the more flexible it tends to become. A top gymnast will have more flexible joints because he or she will use the full range of movements more often.

- **Strength**. Your strength is determined by the size of your muscles relative to your body size. Each muscle is capable of generating a force. The bigger the muscle, the bigger the force. A fit person tends to have bigger muscles. Figure 1 shows which muscles are developed by participating in different sports.

How can fitness be improved?

Surveys regularly show that two thirds of adults in the UK do not take enough exercise to keep themselves healthy. Table 1 opposite shows some of the exercises you could do and gives an indication of how effective they are for improving fitness.

How important is rest?

No matter how fit you are, there always comes a time when your body is exhausted and needs to rest. The best kind of rest is sleep. This allows your body to remove the waste which has accumulated during the day and to make any necessary repairs. It is a time when your brain can sort itself out and posture muscles can relax. In young people it is the time when most of the growth hormone is released.

The amount of sleep a person needs alters with age. Newborn babies need up to 18 hours a day whereas most adults can manage on 6–8 hours. Research suggests that the quantity is not as important as the quality of your sleep.

Sleep tends to follow a cycle of 30–40 minutes of **quiet sleep** followed by 30–40 minutes of **deep sleep**. Dreaming occurs after you have come out of deep sleep. This period is called **REM sleep** because it is accompanied by rapid eye movements. Figure 2 illustrates the stages of sleep.

What do **you** know?

You should now be able to:

- Describe the health benefits of regular exercise.
- Explain the term fitness.
- Assess the effectiveness in improving stamina, strength and suppleness of the exercises you do.
- List some of the muscles your exercises target.
- Explain why exercising will never be an effective way of losing weight, yet must form part of a weight-loss diet.
- Describe the benefits of a good night's sleep.

Exercise	Average energy expenditure (kJ per min)	Stamina	Suppleness	Strength	Risk of injury
Golf	10--20	poor	fair	poor	moderate
Walking slowly		fair	poor	poor	low
Tennis		fair	good	fair	moderate
Gymnastics		fair	excellent	good	high
Jogging	21--30	excellent	fair	fair	moderate
Cycling slowly		good	fair	good	low
Walking quickly		good	poor	poor	low
Football/rugby		good	good	good	high
Swimming		excellent	excellent	excellent	low
Squash	31--40	excellent	good	fair	high
Cycling fast		excellent	fair	good	low
Disco dancing		good	excellent	poor	low

Table 1 *Which exercise is best?*

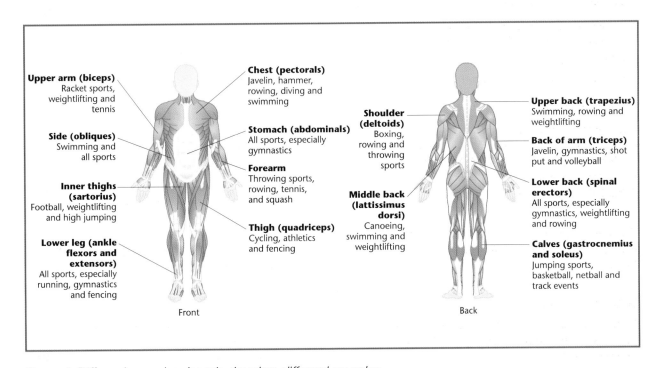

Figure 1 *Different exercises/sports develop different muscles.*

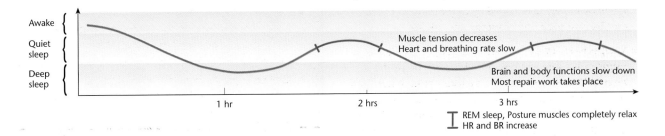

Figure 2 *Sleep follows a regular cycle.*

12.6 Mental health

What can affect mental health?

Your brain controls your body. For good health this must be functioning properly. The functioning of the brain can be affected by mental illness, disease, accidental damage, and stress.

What is mental illness?

Mental illness is an illness of the mind which results in abnormal behaviour. About one in ten of the UK population will be affected by such an illness – it may last a few weeks or a lifetime. Most sufferers however, make a full recovery.

There are two main groups of mental illness (see figure 2):

- **Neuroses** are illnesses which usually have an emotional or social cause, such as the death of a loved one. People with neuroses are fully *aware* of their problem

- **Psychoses** can also result from emotional stress, but not always. Often there is a loss of brain function due to some form of damage or ageing. A psychotic person loses touch with reality and his or her behaviour often becomes anti-social. People with psychoses are usually *unaware* of their problem.

Diseases of the nervous system

The damage caused to the nervous system by disease is often irreparable and can result in the loss of some mental functions. Some of the more serious diseases of the nervous system are shown in table 2.

Accidents to the head can also result in brain damage and loss of mental functions.

What is mental handicap?

Mental illness should not be confused with mental handicap. A **mentally handicapped** person has a particular condition present from birth, which usually can not be cured, but often can be overcome with special help. Mental handicap can result from failure of the brain to develop fully during pregnancy or through toxic shock from the mother smoking or drinking alcohol during pregnancy. In a few cases it is caused by oxygen deprivation at birth.

What is stress?

Stress is very difficult to define, yet most people will have experienced it at some time. It is the feeling of being overburdened, under pressure and so anxious that you cannot cope with everything in your life. The outside pressures on you start to interfere with the delicate balance within your body resulting in illness, abnormal behaviour and even death.

What causes stress?

Factors that cause stress are called **stressors**. Figure 1 lists some of the main stressors identified in the last census. Many of them are major changes or conflicts, but some are everyday activities. For many people, everyday life is stressful.

When you face a stressor, your body will release more adrenaline which initiates the 'fight or flight' reaction. This prepares your body to deal with the stressor before returning to normal. Put another way, normal homeostatic mechanisms have countered the stress to maintain a balanced internal environment.

If stress occurs regularly, your body maintains its state of arousal instead of returning to normal, so you have permanent high blood pressure and blood sugar levels, increased muscle tension and slower digestion. This **exhaustion stage** is also characterised by abnormal behaviour sometimes called 'burn-out'.

Eventually body systems start to fail. The immune response becomes less efficient and disease follows. Death usually comes from stress induced diseases like cancer or heart disease.

How can you avoid or reduce stress?

There is no easy answer to this. Everyone will have their own way of coping with stress. For some it might simply be a good cry. What is generally recognised is that you should always treat the cause not the symptoms. Work out what your individual stressors are and when they are most likely to cause you stress. For example, doing your homework on a Saturday afternoon might be more stressful than doing it on a Friday night, so change your habits. If you can do this with most of your stressors, the ones you cannot do anything about will be more bearable. Remember stress can kill so do something about it sooner rather than later.

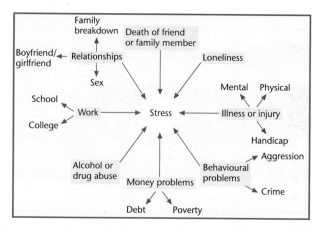

Figure 1 *Some of the main stressors.*

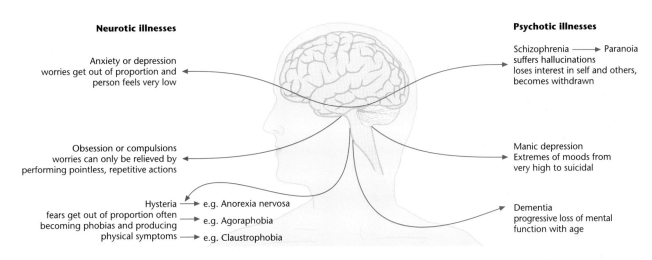

Figure 2 *Mental illness can be grouped into two types, neurotic and psychotic illness.*

Disease or disorder	Effects on the nervous system
Alzheimer's	Degeneration of brain tissue and changes in brain chemistry resulting in loss of memory and personality changes.
Epilepsy	Abnormal electrical activity in the brain causing seizures, blackouts and convulsions.
Migraine	Reduction in blood flow to parts of the brain resulting in a throbbing headache and sensitivity to bright light.
Meningitis	Inflammation of the meninges resulting in headaches, skin rash and flu like symptoms.
Parkinson's	Degeneration of nerve cells resulting in loss of voluntary movements.
Stroke	Reduction in blood supply to parts of the brain resulting in loss of function of that area.
Multiple sclerosis	Destruction of myelin resulting in tremors, loss of speech and paralysis.

Table 2 *Diseases and disorders of the nervous system.*

Physical	Emotional
headache	depression
sweating	irritable
insomnia/constant tiredness	loss of self esteem
indigestion	anxiety
diarrhoea	short temper
constipation	feeling alone
muscular aches and pains	feeling unable to cope suicidal
excessive sweating	tearful
breathlessness	inability to show feelings
itchy skin	
Behavioural	**Organisational**
increased smoking or drinking	difficulty in making decisions
loss of interest in things/life	lateness
binge eating	low productivity
loss of appetite	inability to complete tasks
withdrawal	

Table 1 *Symptoms of stress.*

What do **you** know?

You should now be able to:

- Describe the 2 main groups of mental illnesses.
- Describe 3 neurotic and three psychotic illnesses.
- Explain what stress is and how you would recognise someone who is stressed.
- Write a list of your own stressors.
- Explain how you cope with stress.
- Outline how long term stress can cause death.

12.7 Drug use and abuse

What is a drug?

A **drug** is a chemical substance that can alter the way your mind or body works. This includes substances like alcohol, nicotine, medicines and solvents. **Medicines** are usually preparations which contain drugs, but not all drugs are medicines.

Why take drugs?

Drugs are usually taken for medical reasons, to fight an infection or illness, or to help control pain. Some of these have to be **prescribed** (see chapter 13) by a doctor, but others can be bought from chemist shops.

Drugs are also used for non-medical reasons, for the affects which they have on the body. This kind of drug use is called **drug abuse**. There are three main kinds of drug abuse:

- to improve sporting performance, for example **steroids** can help build muscle and thereby increase strength: **amphetamines** improve alertness.

- to create a feeling of well being. Unfortunately, this initial 'high' soon disappears, and is replaced by a 'low' feeling. This can create a craving for the drug, which can lead to **dependence**.

- to create or enhance mood, for example drugs such as alcohol, nicotine (in tobacco) are used socially. Although these are legal in this country, they can still cause many problems for the user, including dependence.

Drug abuse can be defined as the use of drugs leading to physical, economic and social harm.

What is drug addiction?

When we refer to an 'addict', we usually mean someone whose whole life is devoted to obtaining and taking drugs. The term 'drug addiction' has been replaced by '**drug dependence**'. This describes the compulsion to continue taking a drug as a result of taking it in the past. Drugs can induce two kinds of dependence:

- **Physical dependence** results from regular use of drugs like heroin and barbiturates. These drugs become part of the body chemistry or make changes to it, so that when you stop taking them, you suffer physical withdrawal symptoms, such as sweating, shaking and vomiting. Your body will often become tolerant to drugs which cause physical dependence. This means to get the same effect, you need to increase the amount taken. This is shown by smokers who go from 5 to 40 cigarettes a day.

- **Psychological dependence** is simply a craving for the substance. You feel you cannot do without it, but in fact if you stopped taking it, you would not have any physical withdrawal effects. Nearly all drugs are capable of inducing this kind of dependence.

Table 1 shows the level of physical and psychological dependence created by some drugs.

What are the other risks of taking drugs?

- **Side effects**. All drugs have side effects, even medicines and social drugs. The seriousness of the side effects will often depend upon the size of the dose.

- **Cutting agents**. Many illegal drugs are mixed, or cut, with other substances, such as caffeine, quinine, talcum powder and flour. These can cause serious damage to blood vessels and the mucous membranes of the lungs.

- **Sharing needles**. There are real risks of transmitting serious diseases, such as hepatitis and AIDS, by sharing unclean needles. Injection sites can also become infected and develop abscesses.

- **Mixing drugs**. Many drugs interact with one another causing more powerful effects, especially side effects. For example, mixing moderate amounts of two depressants such as barbiturates and alcohol can result in a fatal coma.

- **Taking drugs when pregnant**. Any drugs taken during pregnancy should always be under medical supervision. The effects on the foetus will depend on the stage of the pregnancy and the length of use.

How drugs pass through the body

Most drugs need to pass into the blood to reach their site of action. How quickly a drug gets to the blood and by which route will depend on how it is taken and in what form (pill, liquid or spray). Figure 1 shows the main routes through which drugs can enter a body. Most drugs are eventually processed by the liver and excreted by the kidneys. If the drug is present in excessive amounts, the organs may not be able to cope and will become diseased.

For example, when alcohol enters your body, a little of it is excreted, but most passes to the liver where it is used as a source of energy. The poison acetaldehyde and fat are produced during metabolism. The poison causes inflammation of the liver, called **hepatitis** (jaundice is often the first sign of hepatitis as the liver fails to deal with the breakdown products of red blood cells); the excess fat is deposited making the liver swell, often called **fatty liver**; the blood supply is reduced and eventually, as liver cells die they are replaced by fibrous tissue resulting in the condition called **cirrhosis**.

Figure 1 *The speed with which a drug gets into the blood stream depends on the method of delivery.*

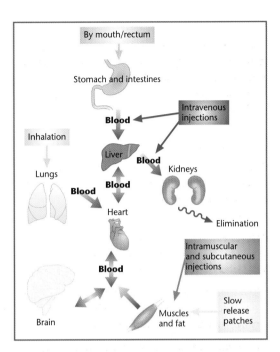

Drug	Physical dependence	Psychological dependence	Tolerance
Alcohol	*	***	✓
Amphetamines	*	***	✓
Barbiturates	***	*	
Cannabis	*	**	
Cocaine		***	
Crack	***	***	✓
Ecstasy			
Heroin	***	***	✓
LSD		*	
Nicotine	*	**	✓
Solvents		*	
Tranquillisers	*	*	✓

Table 1 *Drugs vary in their ability to cause dependence.*

Drug	Possible effects on embryo/foetus
Alcohol	Abnormalities, poor physical and mental development, foetal alcohol syndrome, low birth weight
Amphetamines	Heart defects, low birth weight
Antibiotics	Deafness, jaundice, deformities (depends on type)
Barbiturates	Abnormalities, withdrawal symptoms after birth
Caffeine	Stimulates foetal nervous system causing foetal distress
Cannabis	Premature birth
Cocaine	Stimulates nervous system, renal and brain abnormalities
Heroin	Foetal dependence, low birth weight
LSD	Increased risk of miscarriage, possible DNA damage
Nicotine	Low birth weight

Table 2 *Taking drugs during pregnancy should always be under medical supervision.*

Drugs and the law

The Misuse of Drugs Act divides drugs into three classes:

- *CLASS A* cocaine, crack, ecstacy, heroin, LSD, magic mushrooms, some amphetamikes
- *CLASS B* cannabis, some amphetamines
- *CLASS C* steroids, tranquillisers

There are penalties for breaking the Misuse of Drugs Act:

Possession 2–7 years prison/ and/or fine

Supply 5 years to life imprisonment and/or fine depending on the class.

Table 3 *Some drugs are also covered by the Medicine Act.*

What do **you** know?

You should now be able to:

- Explain what a drug is and the difference between a drug and a medicine.
- Define drug abuse and describe the 3 main kinds.
- Outline the difference between psychological and physical drug dependence.
- Explain what a cutting agent is.
- Discuss why it is unwise to share needles.
- Explain why it is unwise to take any drugs other than those prescribed during pregnancy.
- Describe how alcohol is metabolised by your body and how over consumption can lead to cirrhosis of the liver.

12.8 Drugs of abuse

Amphetamines, methedrine and cocaine

These are all **stimulants** and speed up the actions of the central nervous system. In the short term they make you feel more alert, energetic and confident, but the side effects include disturbed sleep, loss of appetite and an increased heart rate and blood pressure.

When taken for long periods they all cause physical dependence. A tolerance to amphetamines and methedrine can quickly develop. Amphetamines and methedrine produce serious depression and regular cocaine use can result in paranoia.

Caffeine and **nicotine** are mild stimulants. The main effects of these are shown in figures 1 and 2.

Barbiturates and tranquillisers

These are **depressants** and slow down the actions of your central nervous system. In the short term they can relieve anxiety and tension, remove inhibitions and make you feel more relaxed. But they also make you feel drowsy and affect co-ordination and judgement.

Long term use can result in physical dependency. You can also rapidly build up a tolerance to tranquillisers and easily overdose on any depressants.

Heroin and morphine

These are sometimes called **analgesics** because they are pain killers. Their action is similar to depressants except that they work mainly on the part of your brain which registers pain.

Heroin is an excellent painkiller, but unfortunately is also one of the most abused drugs bringing misery and great distress to many people. When first taken, it produces a feeling of great happiness, warmth and contentment, but also rapidly leads to dependency. Such dependency often leads to early death through an accidental overdose, infection or suicide.

Aspirin and **paracetamol** are mild painkillers used for headaches and fever. Aspirin also reduces inflammation.

Ecstasy, LSD and cannabis

These drugs alter your senses, often producing mental illusions, and are therefore called **hallucinogens**.

LSD is made from a fungus called ergot. People who take it often have vivid hallucinations. They talk of the experience as 'tripping'. The nature of the 'trip' depends upon the person's mood or frame of mind. It can be terrifying, or sometimes very joyous and mystical. There is evidence that long term use of LSD can cause serious depression.

Ecstasy is a 'stimulant hallucinogen'. It gives the user a heightened awareness of the surroundings and feelings of great love and energy. Most of the side effects are caused by dehydration and salt loss. These include stiffness of joints, sweating, loss of appetite, anxiety and panic attacks. People have died form taking ecstasy.

Cannabis is a 'depressant hallucinogen'. It produces a relaxed feeling in which the user becomes very talkative and the importance of everyday objects is sometimes exaggerated. Regular use can result in mental problems such as paranoia for people who already have problems. The biggest risk with cannabis is in the method of taking the drug.

Solvents

The fumes or vapours from glues, lighter fluid, nail varnish removers and cleaning chemicals act as depressants of the central nervous system. In the short term they may remove inhibitions and cause a euphoric feeling, but they will also create headaches, dizziness, confusion, drowsiness, nausea and vomiting.

Longer term effects will depend on the solvent used, but these may include brain, liver and kidney damage. Although users have a low risk of physical dependence, many die from the toxic effects.

Alcohol

Alcohol is a depressant drug. You can develop a tolerance to it and it can lead to dependence, yet over 90% of the adult population regularly drink it. It is particularly easy to become dependent on alcohol given the lifestyle and attitudes in the UK. Most men and women who drink moderate amounts are probably not harming their health. Recent studies have even suggested that small amounts can be good for health. Problems arise with alcohol when it is regularly taken in excess. One in 20 people in the UK drink alcohol in excessive amounts and become **alcoholics**.

The effects of alcohol depend on the quantities consumed. In small quantities, it produces a feeling of well being because it reduces anxiety and inhibitions, and increases the blood flow to the skin making you feel warm. This in itself can cause serious loss of body heat. Larger quantities can result in a lowering of blood glucose levels, thereby reducing the energy supply to the brain. This causes the mental confusion we call drunkenness. Regularly drinking excessive quantities can cause many problems (see figure 3), at worst alcoholism, which can kill.

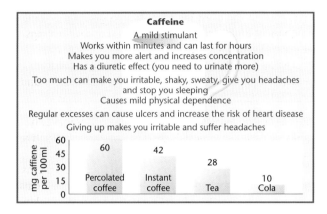

Figure 1 *Caffeine is a stimulant drug.*

Figure 2 *Nicotine is a stimulant drug.*

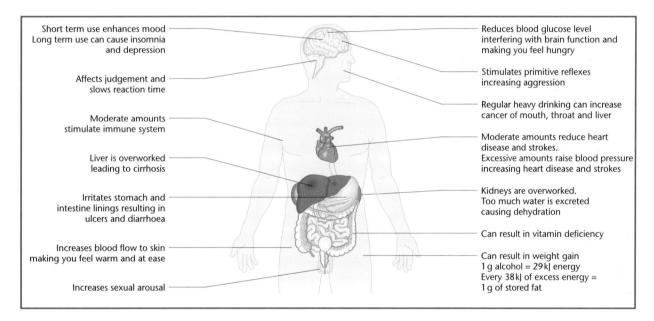

Figure 3 *Alcohol is a depressent drug. It can affect your health in many ways.*

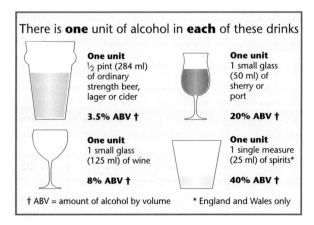

Figure 4 *How much alcohol does a drink contain?*

What do **you** know?

You should now be able to:

- Describe how drugs are classified into 4 main groups.
- For each group state some of the short term and long term effects of taking them.
- Produce a table showing the relative ability of each group to produce dependence and tolerance.
- List some examples of each group.
- List some of the problems associated with the long term use of alcohol.

Chapter 12: Questions

1 a The graph shows the relationship between body weight and body height.

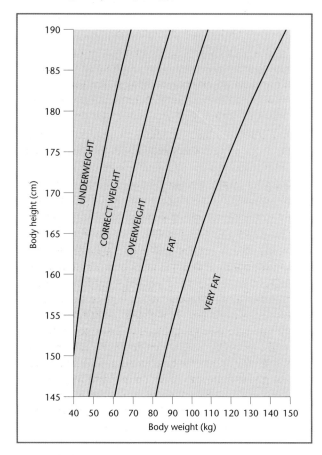

i A person has a body height of 165 cm and a body weight of 100 kg. *(1 mark)* Which description from the graph fits this person? *(1 mark)*

ii What is the maximum correct weight for a person with a body height of 175 cm?

iii Two persons have the same body height, 180 cm. Person A has a body weight of 140 kg. Person B has a body weight of 55 kg. Each person wishes to reach their correct weight. Give one suitable change in diet for each person. *(2 marks)*

iv Give one health problem for a person who is very fat for many years. *(1 mark)*

b Several years ago it was thought that for a person to be healthy a diet should be rich in eggs, milk, cheese and red meat but low in bread and potatoes. Now it is thought that less eggs, milk, cheese and red meat should be eaten but more bread and potatoes should be included in the diet. Suggest two reasons why the diet now recommended is thought to be healthier. *(2 marks)*
(SEG June 1994)

2 A student did an experiment to investigate a possible cause of tooth decay. Loose material and debris was carefully scraped from between the teeth.
The apparatus was set up as shown in the diagram and left in an incubator at 37 °C for 24 hours.

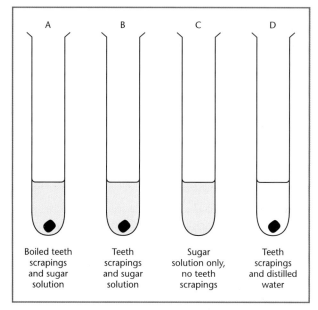

After this time the test tubes were removed from the incubator and the same amount of universal indicator was added to each of them. This indicator is green when neutral, blue in alkaline conditions and orange when acidic. The table shows the results of testing with universal indicator.

Test tube	Colour produced
A	Green
B	Orange
C	Green
D	Green

a Suggest why the student decided to incubate the test tubes at 37 °C. *(1 mark)*

b Name another indicator which could have been used to find the pH conditions in the test tubes. *(2 marks)*

c Suggest an explanation for the results obtained. *(6 marks)*

d Suggest how your explanation shows the possible connection between the material around the teeth and tooth decay. *(2 marks)*
(SEG June 1994)

3 The graph shows the effect of different amounts of alcohol on the average reaction time of a group of people.

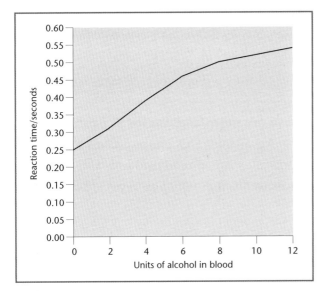

Reaction time/seconds (y-axis, 0.00 to 0.60)
Units of alcohol in blood (x-axis, 0 to 12)

a Calculate the change in the reaction time when the level of alcohol increases from 0 to 4 units.

(2 marks)

b Explain why it is dangerous to drink and drive.

(3 marks)

c Read the following passage and answer the questions which follow.

DRUG ABUSE AND DRUG DEPENDENCE

Drug abuse is defined as the use of drugs leading to physical, economic, mental or social harm. The term is commonly associated with taking illegal drugs such as heroin and LSD but also applies to drugs such as alcohol, nicotine, prescription drugs and solvents.

Drug dependence is of two types:

i psychological – i.e. an emotional state of craving for a drug.

ii physical – i.e. a condition where the body undergoes chemical changes as a result of taking the drug. If it is withdrawn severe physical disturbances, called withdrawal symptoms, occur. These symptoms range from sweating, vomiting and mental confusion to uncontrolled muscular spasms and coma. These symptoms can be fatal.

---

   i Explain why the body becomes physically dependent upon a drug. *(1 mark)*

   ii Name one withdrawal symptom. *(1 mark)*

d i Explain why drug addicts have a higher risk of developing AIDS. *(2 marks)*

   ii Suggest two examples of physical harm which may result from long term drug abuse.

(2 marks)
(NEAB June 1997)

4 Read the following passage about alcohol.

Alcohol is a small molecule which can dissolve in water and fat. This means that alcohol can easily pass through fatty cell membranes.

Men have an enzyme in the stomach which can break down some of the alcohol. Women have much less or none of this enzyme. Women are usually smaller than men. As a result the same quantity of alcohol has more effect on women than men.

Once it is in the blood alcohol spreads quickly around the body. About 2–4% is excreted. In the liver alcohol is oxidised and used for energy release and the formation of fats. This leads to a build up of fats in the liver which interferes with its function. It also causes high fat and low glucose in the blood which interferes with the functions of the brain, liver and blood vessels.

Regular, heavy drinkers become tolerant to alcohol because the liver produces more enzymes to remove it. This means that more alcohol is needed to keep the blood alcohol concentration high enough for any mood-altering effects. Nerve cells become less responsive to alcohol. Substances produced in the breakdown of alcohol are produced in much higher quantities and react with proteins in liver cells. These changed proteins can cause an immune response which damages the liver. This can lead to jaundice (yellow eyes and skin) as the damaged liver cannot remove broken down blood pigments.

Eventually the build up of fats causes the liver to swell and cirrhosis develops. Damaged cells are replaced by fibrous material which becomes hard and receives little blood. As blood flow into the liver becomes more and more blocked it is diverted into blood vessels around the gullet causing internal bleeding and vomiting of blood.

a Explain why alcohol can enter body cells so quickly. *(1 mark)*

b Give two reasons why the same quantity of alcohol has more effect on women than men. *(2 marks)*

c Suggest why the quantity of alcohol in the blood can be measured using

   i a breathalyzer (breath test); *(1 mark)*

   ii a urine sample. *(1 mark)*

d The same amount of alcohol does not have the same mood-altering effect on men who are regular, heavy drinkers as it does on men who are only occasional drinkers. Explain why. *(2 marks)*

e Describe three ways in which regular, heavy drinking damages the liver. *(3 marks)*

f Explain why alcohol has 'mood-altering' effects.

(2 marks)
(NEAB June 1999)

CHAPTER

13 Disease

Most people are ill at some time in their lives. There are many reasons for ill health, but most of the diseases we suffer are caused by micro-organisms. This chapter is all about these micro-organisms; how they cause disease, how they are spread and how this can be prevented. It also describes how your body responds to disease, why you recover and what help is available.

After you have worked through this chapter, you should be able to:

- Outline the main cause of disease.
- Describe the main cause of infectious disease.
- Describe the causative organism, symptoms, methods of transmission and control of influenza, cholera, tuberculosis, athlete's foot, thrush and malaria.
- Outline how infectious diseases can be spread.
- Describe the main sexually transmitted diseases.
- Outline the causes, symptoms and transmission routes for HIV.
- Explain what cancer is, what can cause it and the current methods of treatment.
- Describe your body's natural barriers to infection.
- Explain the role of your blood in preventing the development of disease.

- Explain how you can develop immunity to diseases.
- Outline some of the problems this can cause for blood transfusions and transplants.
- Describe the course of an infectious disease.
- Describe the use of antibiotics to control disease.
- Explain how the fight against disease is taking place at the personal, community and worldwide levels.
- Outline the processes involved in supplying clean safe water.
- Explain what happens to domestic refuse.
- Explain how sewage is disposed of safely.
- Describe the causes and prevention of food poisoning.
- Explain the principles of hygienic food handling and food preservation.

Allergic responses

What is an allergy?

An allergy is an over-reaction by your body's defence system to a normally harmless foreign substance. This results in symptoms from a runny nose, itchy eyes and tight chest to, in extreme cases, death.

The allergic response

Any substance which causes an allergic response is called an **allergen**. The most common allergens are pollen, dust mites, mould spores, insects, industrial chemicals, medicines, foods and pets. The first time your body comes in contact with an allergen, it is **sensitised** to it. It produces **antibodies** which attach

to special white blood cells (called **mast cells**) in the tissues. The next contact with the allergen results in the release of **histamine** and other chemicals (see figure 1). This reaction is called the '**shocking**' response. The size of the shocking response is determined by the amount of allergen. It can result in mild discomfort or an **anaphylactic** response resulting in death.

The histamine and other chemicals cause a general **inflammation response** and other effects depending on location. In the nose it increases the secretion of mucus, hence the runny nose. In the skin it can cause little 'weals' or red 'flares'. Some food allergies result in eczema, especially in babies and toddlers (see page 16).

Types of allergic response

An allergic response can be immediate or delayed. Both types can be caused by the same allergen.

Immediate responses are seen with hay fever, perennial rhinitis, asthma and many food allergies. A visible reaction occurs within seconds or minutes of contact with the allergen. This is mostly due to the histamine released.

A delayed response can take hours or days to develop. It involves a different kind of immune response in which no histamine is released. The allergen is isolated at the point of contact by a localised cellular reaction. The test for tuberculosis (TB) sensitivity is based on this. TB bacterial proteins are introduced into the skin. If you are already sensitised to these, red spots appear after a few days.

Anaphylactic shock

An anaphylactic shock is a severe reaction to a large amount of allergen after having been sensitised to a small amount. It is an immediate reaction and can be caused by almost any allergen, but usually it is food or drugs. Blood pressure drops dramatically and airways usually narrow. The skin becomes pallid, the chest tightens and there may be swelling and a rash. It can result in death, but if not, recovery is often just as rapid.

The management of allergies

The best way to prevent allergies is to avoid the allergens or, at least, minimise your contact with them, by for example, not stroking cats or eating certain foods. If this is not possible, there are various medical treatments available:

- **Desensitisation** is useful for hay fever and house mites. This involves being injected with progressively larger amounts of the allergen so your body builds up antibodies to fight it.

- **Anti-histamine** drugs can be taken to stop the production of histamine. People with asthma are usually given inhalers containing **bronchodilators** to relax the smooth muscle in the walls of the bronchioles and **steroids** to reduce the inflammation.

- **Adrenaline** is given to reverse anaphylactic shock.

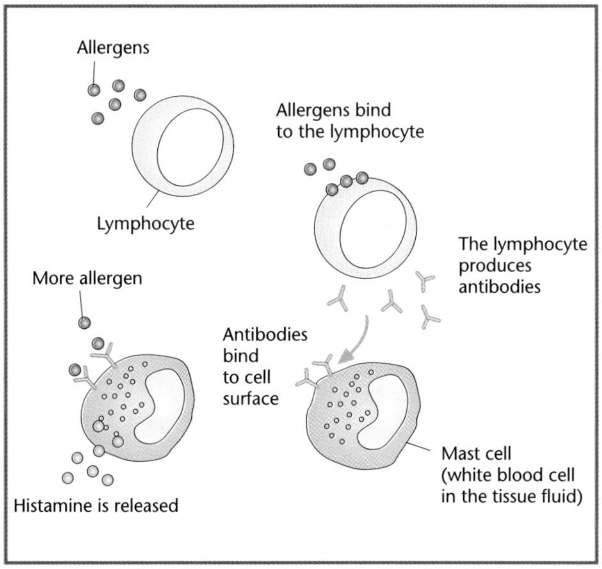

Figure 1 *The allergic reaction.*

Allergy	Allergen	Symptoms	Site affected
Hay fever	pollen grains	runny nose, itchy eyes, sneezing, facial swelling	nose, eyes
Perennial rhinitis	dust mites, mould spores	runny nose, sneezing, itchy eyes	nose, eyes
Asthma	pollen, dust mites, foods feathers	wheezing	bronchial tubes
Utricaria	foods, medicines	itchy red bumps	skin

Table 1 *The most common types of allergy.*

13.1 Disease

What is disease?

A disease is a condition that prevents your body, or part of it, working properly. There are many different kinds of disease, each having its own specific cause (see table 1). Diseases are classed as infectious or non-infectious.

- **infectious diseases** are caused by other organisms and can be caught. Organisms which cause disease are called **pathogens**.

- **non-infectious diseases** cannot be caught because they are not caused by other organisms. They are either inherited, the result of ageing, or due to poor health behaviour.

How can you identify a disease?

Every disease will have it's own collection of signs and **symptoms**. Your doctor recognizes a disease by assessing your symptoms, but he or she will also want to do some tests to confirm the cause before giving you treatment. These tests may be to:

- Look for the causative organism by taking samples of body fluids (e.g. blood) and sending these samples to a microbiology laboratory for culturing (chapter 14.1).

- Look for more **clinical signs** which are very specific to a particular disease. For example, a high blood sugar level indicates diabetes mellitus.

- Look for physical signs, lumps in the breasts for example might be a sign of breast cancer.

- Use X-rays and other **imaging techniques** to look inside your body for damage. For example, MRI scanning is used to locate damage to bones, especially the backbone (see page 2).

Which organisms cause disease?

Many diseases are caused by organisms entering your body and then feeding and reproducing in it. In doing so, they may interfere with the functioning of the body by causing physical damage, or poison it by excreting poisonous waste substances called **toxins**. Many of these organisms are very small, such as **viruses**, **bacteria**, **protozoa** and **fungi**. They are often called **micro-organisms**. Others, such as **insects** and **worms**, can be quite large.

What are viruses?

Viruses are very simple organisms consisting of two parts only, a protein coat and a strand of genetic material which can be either DNA or RNA (see figure 1). They are the smallest of all living things and can only be seen by using an electron microscope. All viruses are parasites and can cause disease. They can only reproduce inside the cells of other living organisms, such as plants, animals or bacteria.

How do viruses cause disease?

How a virus causes disease can be illustrated by the **influenza** virus. Influenza is an infection of the respiratory passages. The virus infects the lining cells, enters the nucleus and takes over the control of the cell. The cell is made to stop all its normal work and start making more influenza viruses. Eventually the cell bursts, releasing the new viruses, or sometimes new viruses are budded out (see figure 1). Each of these new viruses will enter another body cell and reproduce itself. In a matter of hours, tens of thousands of cells can be destroyed. It is this destruction of cells which usually results in the symptoms of disease, in this case a sore throat, fever, nausea and general weakness. Sometimes bacteria may invade the area and cause a **secondary infection** such as **pneumonia**. The influenza virus is spread from person to person in tiny droplets of moisture released when you breathe out.

Viral diseases can often be very serious because there are no drugs which a doctor can give you to fight them. It is up to your own body to initiate making antibodies, and if you are incapable of doing this as many older people and young children are, you may die.

Figure 2 shows some of the main human viral diseases. Viral diseases also do a lot of damage to our crops and domestic animals.

Are there any useful viruses?

Viruses have no natural uses, but as we learn more about them we are able to use them to our advantage. For example, the control of insect pests such as caterpillars can now be achieved using viruses which infect the caterpillars. A virus used in this way is called a **biological control agent**.

Viruses which infect bacteria are also used to transfer genes into the bacteria so that they can make products for us (chapter 14.3).

Cause of disease	Example of disease
Infection by other organisms	Food poisoning, influenza, malaria, thrush
Nutritional deficiencies	Malnutrition, starvation, obesity
Inherited in the genes	Haemophilia, colour blindness, cystic fibrosis
Occupation (as one factor)	Asbestosis, stress, cancer
Social behaviour	Alcoholism, drug addiction
Ageing (as one factor)	Arthritis, dementia, cancer
Metabolic disorders	Diabetes, phenylketonuria, cancer
Pollution (as one factor)	Bronchitis, asthma

Table 1 *There are many different causes of disease.*

Disease		Some symptoms
AIDS	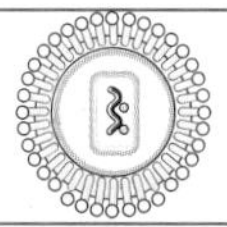	Prolonged tiredness, fever, diarrhoea and excessive weight loss
Common cold	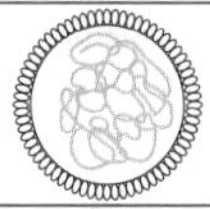	Sneezing bouts, runny nose, shivering, streaming eyes
German measles	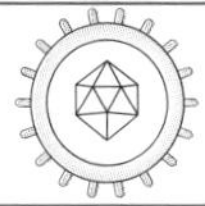	Small pink spots covering the skin, swollen glands, mild fever
Hepatitis	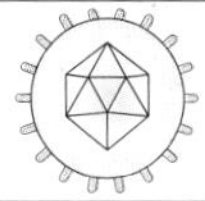	Headache, muscle pain, nausea, vomiting, jaundice
Influenza	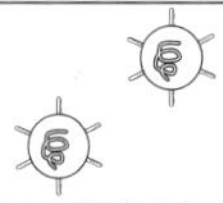	Same symptoms as the common cold plus aching muscles, fever and a cough
Measles	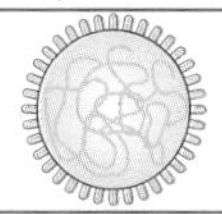	Runny nose, streaming eyes, followed by spots on the back and arms, white spots in mouth
Mumps	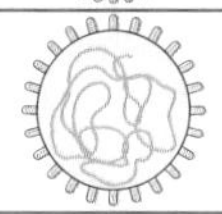	Fever, sore throat, shivering and swollen glands
Polio	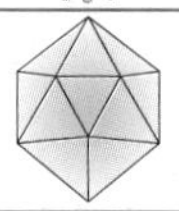	Mild fever, stiffness of muscles and eventually paralysis
Rabies	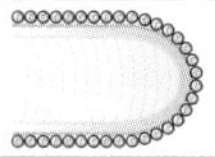	Headaches, muscular spasms and breathing difficulties

Figure 2 *Some common viral diseases and their symptoms.*

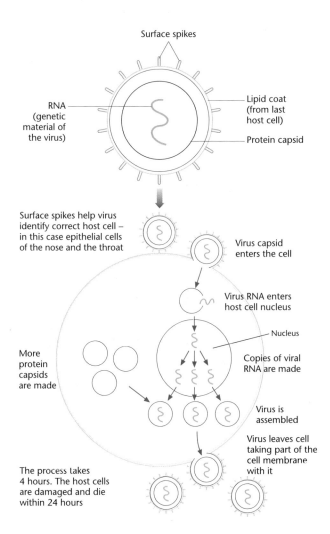

Figure 1 *The infection cycle of the influenza virus.*

What do **you** know?

You should now be able to:

- Define disease and list some of the main causes of disease.
- Describe 4 ways you can identify a disease.
- Explain what infectious diseases are.
- List the main types of organisms which cause infectious diseases.
- Draw and label a diagram of an influenza virus.
- Explain with sketches, the life cycle of an influenza virus.
- State 2 reasons why an influenza infection can cause illness.
- Explain why you usually recover from a viral infection.

What is AIDS?

AIDS stands for **aquired immune deficiency syndrome**. It is a condition which develops because an infected body's defences are not working properly. The condition is characterised by a particular pattern of illnesses, two of the most serious being a rare form of skin cancer (Kaposi's sarcoma) and a form of pneumonia. People who die from AIDS usually die from one of these illnesses or a combination of factors which their body cannot fight.

AIDS is caused by a virus called **human immuno-deficiency virus** (HIV: see figure 1). This infects the **T lymphocytes** and **macrophages** in your blood preventing them defending your body against attack by other agents.

What are the symptoms of AIDS?

AIDS has a variety of symptoms, many of which are very common symptoms of other diseases and disorders. When diagnosing AIDS, a doctor will look for a pattern to the symptoms. Some of the symptoms which may suggest AIDS are:

- profound sweating which my last for weeks
- swollen lymph nodes
- rapid and excessive weight loss
- persistent fever and night sweats
- persistent shortness of breath
- a persistent dry cough
- diarrhoea which lasts for more than a week
- pink or purple patches on the skin
- lethargy and depression.

People with HIV are particularly susceptible to other infections, especially thrush, warts, eczema and pneumonia.

Does it take long for the symptoms to show?

After the initial infection, minor symptoms such as fever, sweats, headaches, sore throats and swollen glands may develop, but these will soon disappear as your immune system produces **antibodies** to fight the infection. These antibodies can be present from three weeks and a person with them is described as **HIV positive**.

This initial period is usually followed by a symptom free period of many years (average 10 years). The virus remains dormant inside the lymphocytes: the cells which should be destroying it. During this time the person is infectious and can spread the disease. Eventually, the symptoms return as viruses are released from the

lymphocytes into the blood. As the immune system becomes overloaded, minor infections such as thrush take hold. This second stage, often called **ARC** (Aids Related Complex) will develop into the full syndrome as the immune system starts to fail allowing more serious infections and cancers to develop. The HIV may also infect the brain causing personality changes.

How is HIV passed on?

HIV can only be transmitted from person to person in body fluids, such as blood and seminal fluid. Surprisingly, the virus is remarkably fragile when outside an organism and can be killed by heat and simple chemicals such as alcohol and bleach.

Over 90% of the transmissions in the UK are during sexual intercourse, both heterosexual and homosexual (see figure 3). In theory, this is preventable by practising safe sex, such as using a condom. HIV also crosses the placental membranes and can, therefore, be passed onto a foetus in the womb. Infants can be infected during birth or whilst breastfeeding.

When little was known about AIDS, some people were infected through blood transfusions, but now all blood in the UK is heat treated to destroy the virus. Similarly, haemophiliacs caught it from contaminated blood clotting factors, but again these are now safe.

Can AIDS be treated or cured?

There are no cures for AIDS yet, but work on a vaccine is progressing. There are drugs available which can prolong life and delay the onset of AIDS. These do, however, have some serious side effects. In the meantime, a massive health education campaign has been taking place in the developed world to educate people about the need for safe sex and the risks of sharing needles. But AIDS is a worldwide disease and needs to be treated as such.

What do **you** know?

You should now be able to:

- Explain what AIDS stands for, what causes it and the symptoms.
- Explain what HIV positive means.
- Describe the main methods of transmission of HIV and suggest how these can be minimised.
- Describe the pattern of infection leading to full AIDS.
- Explain why people with HIV have a greater risk of developing other diseases.

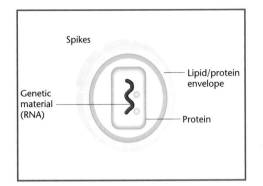

Figure 1 *The human immunodeficiency virus.*

Transmission group	Up to 1994	1995	1996	1997	Cumulative total
Heterosexuals	1258	307	438	410	2413
Homo/bisexuals	7427	969	1128	741	10265
Injecting drug users	770	143	175	123	1211
Blood recipient	564	109	60	34	767
Perinatal	149	33	33	48	263
Unknown	98	11	22	31	162
All	10266	1572	1856	1387	15081

Table 1 *Reported AIDS cases by means of transmission (UK).*

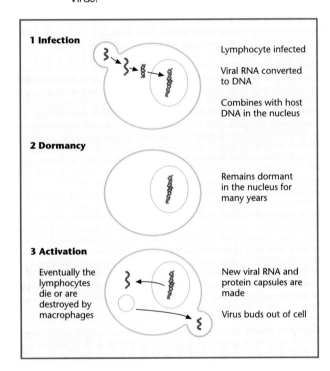

Figure 2 *The life cycle of a HIV particle.*

Figure 3 *Diagnosed HIV infections by age in UK (1997).*

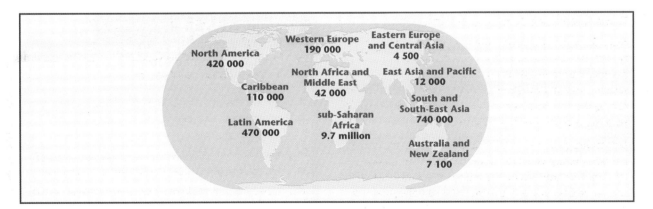

Figure 4 *Estimated deaths from AIDS from the beginning of the epidemic (to the end of 1997).*

Bacteria

What are bacteria?

Bacteria are very small and primitive single-celled organisms (see figure 1). They were first seen by a Dutchman called Van Leeuwenhoek when he examined scrapings from his teeth through a microscope. We now know that bacteria are found almost everywhere. Most are very useful and have an important role in nature but a few also cause serious diseases in humans, in the animals we breed and in the plants we use for food.

How are bacteria useful?

Bacteria have many uses, some of which are:

- the recycling of nutrients e.g. nitrogen (chapter 15.4)
- the treatment of sewage (chapter 13.13)
- the production of vitamin K in our intestines
- the digestion of cellulose in the stomachs of herbivores
- the production of cheese, yoghurt and vinegar (chapter 14.5)
- the production of drugs (chapter 14.7)
- the production of silage
- as a high protein food source (chapter 14.5).

Many of these are described further in the relevant chapters.

How are bacteria harmful?

Bacteria are harmful to us in two ways:

- Some of them cause diseases (see figure 2). These are referred to as **pathogenic** bacteria.
- Some of them feed on our food, making it go bad. Organisms that feed on dead plants and animals causing it to decay are called **saprophytes** (chapter 13.4). The main saprophytes are bacteria and fungi. More effects of bacteria on our food are described in chapters 13.14 and 13.15.

How do bacteria cause disease?

Most bacteria cause disease by releasing poisonous substances called **toxins**. These are usually released to help the bacteria penetrate the host cells or alter the cell chemistry. The toxins produced by *Salmonella* bacteria for example, cause ulceration of the gut lining and result in dehydration and fever.

The link between bacteria and disease was first discovered by Louis Pasteur when he was working with diseased silk moths. Twenty years later, Robert Koch managed to show that a killer disease of cattle (anthrax) was also caused by bacteria. The technique he used to do this is still used today in pathology laboratories. We now know of hundreds of diseases caused by bacteria some of which are shown in figure 2.

Some types of bacteria, including many which live and feed on our food are capable of producing resistant stages called **spores**. These can withstand extreme conditions, including for short periods, high temperatures. This is of particular concern in food. Cooking and re-heating food must be done for long enough at a high temperature to destroy these spores, otherwise they could still spoil the food and even cause food poisoning.

Tuberculosis (TB)

TB is a serious bacterial infection of the organs of the body, usually the lungs. The bacteria invade the lung tissue causing cell death and scarring. These scars can be seen on X-rays and this is the one form of diagnosis. The symptoms include weight loss, fever, persistent coughing and blood stained sputum. Transmission is by droplets of moisture and direct contact with body fluids. The disease will usually only develop if the immune system is weakened for some reason. Treatment is by use of antibiotics.

Until recently, all school children were vaccinated against TB using the BCG vaccine and there were very few cases of TB in the UK. It is now on the increase.

Cholera

Cholera is found in areas with poor sanitation. The bacteria which cause it are transmitted in water. They infect the large intestine causing severe diarrhoea and abdominal pain. The dehydration resulting from fluid loss can cause death within 24 hours. The death rate during an epidemic can be as high as 50%. Treatment involves replacing the fluids by a saline drip and taking antibiotics to kill the bacteria.

What do **you** know?

You should now be able to:

- List 6 ways bacteria are useful.
- Explain why bacteria spoil food.
- Explain what spores are and why they can be dangerous in food.
- Explain how bacteria cause disease.
- List 6 diseases caused by bacteria.
- Outline the cause, method of transmission, symptoms and treatments for TB and cholera.

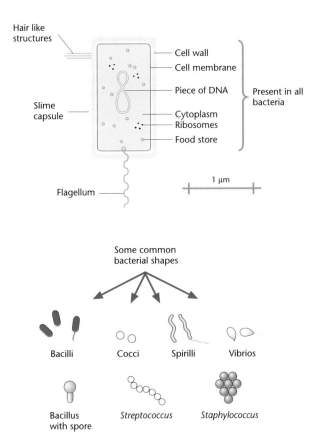

Figure 1 labels:
Hair like structures
Cell wall
Cell membrane
Piece of DNA
Present in all bacteria
Slime capsule
Cytoplasm
Ribosomes
Food store
Flagellum
1 μm

Some common bacterial shapes
Bacilli
Cocci
Spirilli
Vibrios
Bacillus with spore
Streptococcus
Staphylococcus

Figure 1 *The structure of a typical bacterium and some comon bacterial shapes.*

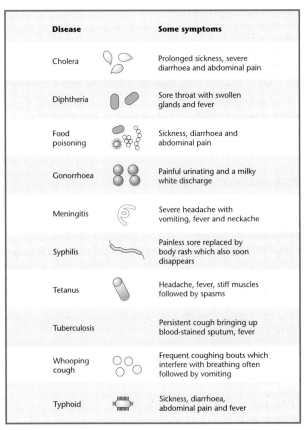

Disease		Some symptoms
Cholera		Prolonged sickness, severe diarrhoea and abdominal pain
Diphtheria		Sore throat with swollen glands and fever
Food poisoning		Sickness, diarrhoea and abdominal pain
Gonorrhoea		Painful urinating and a milky white discharge
Meningitis		Severe headache with vomiting, fever and neckache
Syphilis		Painless sore replaced by body rash which also soon disappears
Tetanus		Headache, fever, stiff muscles followed by spasms
Tuberculosis		Persistent cough bringing up blood-stained sputum, fever
Whooping cough		Frequent coughing bouts which interfere with breathing often followed by vomiting
Typhoid		Sickness, diarrhoea, abdominal pain and fever

Figure 2 *Some common bacterial diseases and their symptoms.*

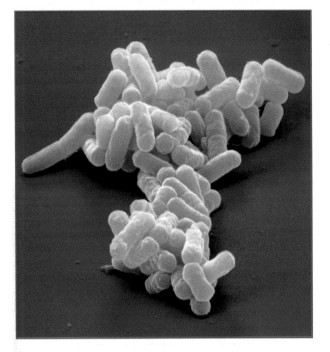

Figure 3 E. coli *is a rod-shaped form of bacteria.*

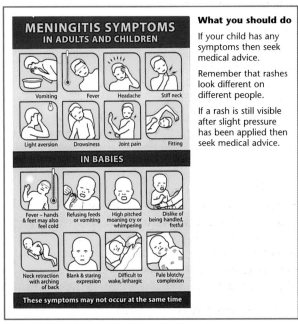

MENINGITIS SYMPTOMS
IN ADULTS AND CHILDREN

Vomiting | Fever | Headache | Stiff neck
Light aversion | Drowsiness | Joint pain | Fitting

IN BABIES

Fever – hands & feet may also feel cold | Refusing feeds or vomiting | High pitched moaning cry or whimpering | Dislike of being handled, fretful
Neck retraction with arching of back | Blank & staring expression | Difficult to wake, lethargic | Pale blotchy complexion

These symptoms may not occur at the same time

What you should do

If your child has any symptoms then seek medical advice.

Remember that rashes look different on different people.

If a rash is still visible after slight pressure has been applied then seek medical advice.

Figure 4 *Meningitis can be caused by bacteria and viruses.*

13.4 Fungi

What are fungi?

Fungi are the **yeasts**, **moulds** and **mushrooms**. They are neither plants nor animals, but form their own group. Most feed as **saprophytes**, and live in or on their food. Some are **parasites**. The body of a fungus is called a **mycelium** (see figure 1). It consists of fine tubular threads called **hyphae**, which penetrate the food. These hyphae secrete digestive enzymes into the food which digest proteins, fats and carbohydrates. They then absorb these products of digestion and use them to grow. Just before the food runs out, the fungus produces lots of microscopic **spores** which are liberated into the surrounding air.

Yeasts are the exception to this. They are single-celled organisms which reproduce by a process called budding (see figure 2).

How are fungi useful?

The Chinese were using yeast for bread making and a mould to produce soy sauce over 2000 years ago. These processes have changed very little. Some present day uses of fungi include the following:

- Yeast is used by the **baking industry** to produce carbon dioxide to make dough rise.

- Yeast is used by the **brewing industry** to produce alcohol from sugars.

- Moulds are used to **produce antibiotics**, e.g. *Penicillium* is used to produce **penicillin** (chapter 14.7).

- Moulds are used by the cheese manufacturers to **ripen cheeses** and give them their individual flavours, e.g. one kind of *Penicillium* is used in Camembert cheese. Blue cheeses actually contain moulds.

- Mushrooms and truffles are **used as food**.

- Various fungi are used to produce **protein concentrates** (single cell protein – chapter 14.5).

- Various fungi are used for the large scale production of **enzymes**, e.g. *Aspergillus* is used to produce amylase which is used by the brewing industry (chapter 14.4).

How are fungi harmful?

Fungi are harmful to us in four ways:

- Some of them **spoil our food**.

- Some **destroy our crops**, e.g. potato blight, powdery mildew of cereals, black stem rust of wheat.

- Some **destroy our houses** and furniture, e.g. dry rot.

- Some **cause diseases**, e.g. athletes foot, thrush.

How do fungi cause disease?

A small number of fungi cause diseases in humans. They live on dead or living cells causing irritation and cellular damage. Some produce spores which can cause allergic reactions e.g *Aspergillus* spores cause farmer's lung. Two of the more common fungal infections are:

- **Athlete's foot**. This disease is caused by a mould type of fungus called *Tinea*. It lives and feeds on the dead, sweaty skin between your toes. This feeding damages the living skin underneath, causing soreness and inflammation. Athlete's foot is extremely contagious and is usually passed on in public places such as swimming pools and communal changing rooms. It can be cured by a **fungicide** lotion spread on the infected area. Avoid sharing towels or socks and dry your feet thoroughly, especially after swimming, to keep the bacteria at bay.

- **Thrush**. This is caused by a yeast-like fungus called *Candida*. It lives and feeds in the delicate mucous membranes lining your body's natural openings, such as the mouth and vagina. Most poeple have *Candida* present in their body, but not in sufficient quantities to cause a problem. When you are 'run down' and unwell, or have been taking a course of drugs which have altered the normal balance of micro-organisms in your body, it can grow rapidly and produce itching, soreness and inflammation. Thrush can be cured by **anti-fungal** preparations.

Women often suffer from mild thrush during menstruation. Normally the *Candida* is held in check by the acid pH in the vagina, but during menstruation, the pH becomes less acid allowing it to grow.

What do **you** know?

You should now be able to:

- Name the 3 kinds of fungi.
- Draw a diagram to explain the structure of a typical mould fungus.
- Explain how a typical mould fungus feeds.
- Explain how the feeding activity of *Tinea* fungus causes athletes foot.
- Suggest how the spread of athlete's foot can be controlled.
- Explain what thrush is and why it can be classed as an opportunistic infection.
- List 3 more ways fungi are harmful to us.
- List 6 ways we make use of fungi.

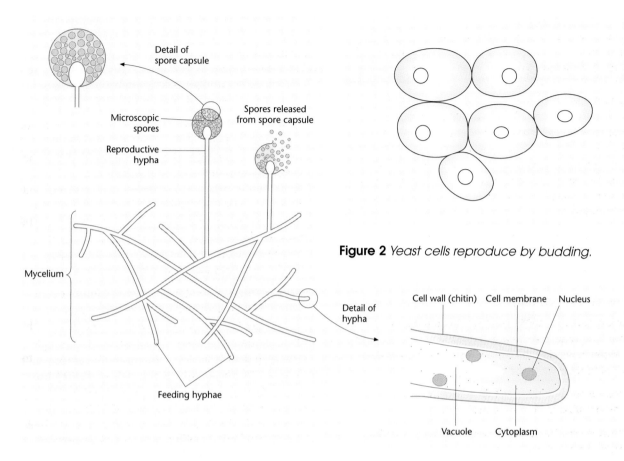

Figure 2 *Yeast cells reproduce by budding.*

Figure 1 *The structure of a typical mould.*

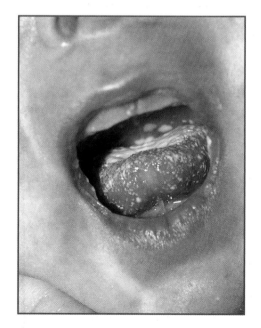

Figure 3 *Oral thrush shows up as white patches on the tongue and roof of the mouth.*

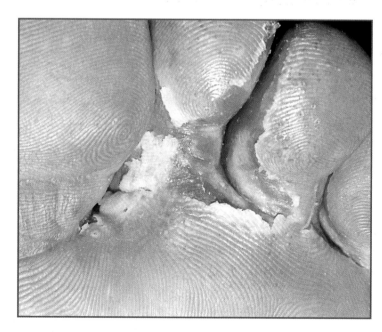

Figure 4 *Athlete's foot is caused by the fungus* Tinea. *The spread of it can be reduced by using disinfectants in communal bathing facilities.*

13.5　Parasites

What are parasites?

Parasites are organisms that live on or in another living organism, the **host**. They obtain their food from the host, often causing illness, disease and even death.

There are many human parasites. Three groups particularly worth mentioning are the **insects**, **protozoa** and **worms**.

Do insects cause disease?

Insects are the most abundant of all animals, but surprisingly, very few are directly responsible for human diseases. Many, however, are **vectors** of disease and are harmful in other ways:

- as vectors for diseases of our crops, e.g. greenfly carry plant viruses
- as vectors of the diseases that affect our domestic animals, e.g. fleas transmit myxomatosis
- by destroying our crops, e.g. locusts and cabbage white butterfly caterpillars eat the leaves
- by spoiling our food, e.g. weevils taint flour
- by damaging our buildings and furniture, e.g. termites damage wood; clothes moths damage clothing
- by causing disease by removing blood, e.g. bedbugs can cause anaemia in humans.

Some of the insects that can cause illness and spread disease are shown in figure 1.

What are protozoa?

Protozoa are single-celled animals, slightly larger than bacteria but still microscopic. Most are harmless and some are even useful. For example, some protozoa live in the alimentary canal of animals and help them digest cellulose. In return they get food and shelter. This kind of relationship where both organisms benefit is called a **symbiotic relationship**. Others are used to digest the organic matter and destroy pathogens in sewage.

A few protozoa cause very serious diseases, the most widespread being:

- **Malaria**. About 500 million people a year catch malaria and about three million die as a result. Many of the rest continue to suffer from the illness for the rest of their lives.

The protozoan that causes malaria is called *Plasmodium*. This has a complex life cycle involving both mammals (including humans) and the mosquito (see figure 2). The mosquito transmits the protozoan from one mammal to another. We call it the **vector**.

- **Dysentery**. Dysentery is particularly common in countries where there is poor sanitation. It has many different causes, one of which is the protozoan *Entamoeba* (figure 4). This lives in your intestine, feeding on bacteria and occasionally on the lining cells. The symptoms of dysentery are severe diarrhoea, sickness and ulcers. People die from dysentery.

The vector is often the housefly, but it is sometimes passed on by humans. The parasites are passed out in human faeces. If they get into drinking water, because of bad sanitation, or food, because of poor personal cleanliness, the disease can rapidly spread to many more people.

Are there worms which cause disease?

The two groups of worm that cause disease are the **roundworms** and the **flatworms**. The names of these worms describe the shape of their bodies.

Tapeworms are flatworms. They are the largest of all disease-causing organisms, sometimes reaching lengths of several metres. They have two hosts: the one in which they reach sexual maturity is called the **primary host** and the other is called the **secondary host**. The fish, beef (see figure 3), and pork tapeworms all have humans as their primary host. All tapeworm infestations can be prevented by cooking food properly and disposing of sewage effectively.

Roundworm infestations are rare in the UK, but in other parts of the world, particularly the underdeveloped regions, infestation levels can be as high as 75%.

What do **you** know?

You should now be able to:

- Explain what a parasite is and name 3 groups of parasites.
- List 6 ways insects are harmful to us.
- Explain what a vector of disease is.
- Name 3 diseases spread by insect vectors.
- Name 2 serious diseases caused by protozoa.
- Explain, with an example, a symbiotic relationship.
- Name 2 groups of worms which are responsible for human diseases.
- Using a diagram explain how the tapeworm anchors itself in the gut.
- Explain how tapeworm infestations could come about.

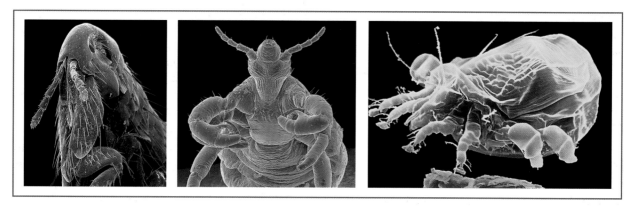

Figure 1 *Some insects spread disease: the human flea transmits typhus; the body louse transmits typhus and impetigo; and the scabies mite transmits impetigo, eczema and scabies.*

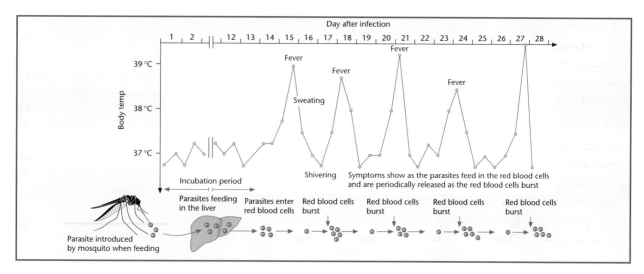

Figure 2 *Many people catch malaria whilst holidaying in tropical countries, but only show symptoms when they return to the UK.*

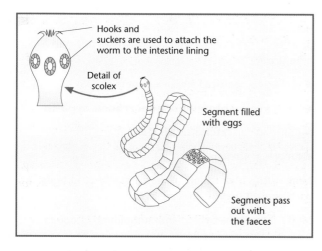

Figure 3 *A pork tapeworm can live in a human intestine.*

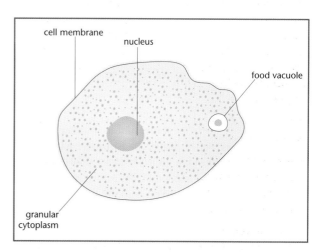

Figure 4 *Entamoeba is a parasitic protozoan which lives in your intestine and can cause dysentery.*

13.6 Infectious disease

Diseases that a person can catch from someone else or somewhere else, are called **infectious diseases**. The organisms that cause these diseases are called **pathogens**.

How are pathogens spread?

Pathogenic organisms can be spread in five ways:

- **In the air**. Coughing, sneezing, breathing and even talking release tiny droplets of moisture into the air. Microbes cling to these droplets and may enter a person's body when he or she breathes in. Diseases such as the **common cold** and **influenza** are spread in this way, particularly in crowded, stuffy places like buses, trains, pubs and lifts. **Diphtheria** and **tetanus** bacteria cling to dust particles in the air and many fungi release spores which we can breathe in.

- **By infected food and water**. Food can be contaminated in many ways. For example it may have been handled with dirty hands or carved up with a dirty knife. The guts of many animals contain *Salmonella* bacteria and if cooked meat is stored alongside fresh meat, this may result in contamination and lead to food poisoning (chapter 13.14). Water is often contaminated by discharging raw sewage into it. This can help to spread serious diseases like **dysentery** and **cholera**.

- **By objects**. Diseases like **impetigo** can be caught from sharing hairbrushes or sleeping in the same sheets. **Athlete's foot** can be caught from sharing towels, socks and shoes, and even the floor in showers.

- **By direct contact**. Some pathogens can only be passed on by direct contact with an infected person. These diseases are said to be **contagious**. The organisms involved can only live inside a body. Many of the sexually transmitted diseases are spread in this way (see figure 2). Some people have the pathogens in their body but do not become ill. These people are called **carriers** and present a real problem for the prevention of infection.

- **By insects and other animals**. Organisms that spread disease from one individual to another are called **vectors**. For example, the **bubonic plague** which wiped out a large number of the population in England in 1665, was spread from rats to humans by fleas. Impetigo can be spread by body lice.

Figure 1 shows how flies spread disease.

Which vectors spread which diseases?

A lot of the world's most serious diseases (in terms of number of people affected), are spread by insects.

Mosquitoes spread **malaria** and tsetse flies spread **sleeping sickness**. These two alone account for over four million deaths per year.

By far the worst insect vector is the **housefly**. It is responsible for the spread of over one hundred different diseases, including **cholera**, **polio** and **dysentery** (see figure 1).

Rats and mice are not only vectors of disease but also do serious damage to property. The diseases they have been known to spread are **food poisoning**, **bubonic plague** and **infective jaundice**.

Dogs, cats and foxes are vectors of the disease called **rabies**. Rabies is a very serious disease, **endemic** (ever present) in most countries of the world, but so far it has not entered the UK, mainly due to a history of strict **quarantine** regulations. Quarantine is a period of isolation which, until recently, all animals had to go through before they could enter the UK and many other countries. The animals are kept in isolation for a period, which exceeds the **incubation period** of any diseases it could be carrying.

What are epidemics?

An **epidemic** is an outbreak of a disease which spreads rapidly infecting a lot of people in a population. We often get epidemics of influenza in the UK. Some particularly virulent strains of influenza virus can spread from other countries. When a disease is epidemic in several countries it is described as being **pandemic**.

Sexually transmitted diseases (STDs)

Sexually transmitted diseases, as the name suggests, are infectious diseases which are transferred from person to person during sexual intercourse or other sexual practices. They are caused by a variety of different organisms:

- viruses e.g. **genital herpes**, **warts**, **AIDS**

- bacteria e.g. **chlamydia**, **gonorrhoea**, **syphilis**

- protozoa e.g. **trichomoniasis**

- fungi e.g. **thrush**

More details about some of these are shown in figure 2. AIDS is dealt with in chapter 13.2.

Most STDs can be treated with antibiotics, although penicillin resistant varieties of gonorrhoea have recently been reported. Prevention in this case is much better. By practising safe sex, many of these diseases can be avoided.

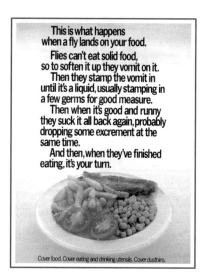

Figure 1 *Would you eat this food now?*

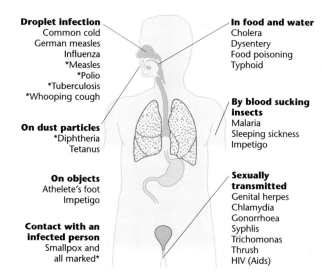

Figure 2 *How some common diseases may be spread.*

Disease	Infective agent	Time for first symptoms to show	Symptoms	Estimated cases in the UK 1997* male	female
Chlamydia	Bacterium	Up to 4 weeks	Green discharge from penis Blockage of penis by pus Painful urination Swollen lymph nodes Pelvic inflammatory disease	13694	18163
Gonorrhoea	Bacterium	2–10 days	Painful urination May be a yellow discharge	7749	3902
Syphilis	Bacterium	Average 21 days	Painfully sore on sex organs (inside vagina in women) Skin rash	84	33
Trichomoniasis	Protozoan	Up to 1 month	Men: rare Women: yellowish green discharge from vagina, soreness and itching	231	5302

Table 1 *These sexually transmitted diseases can easily be prevented.*

What do **you** know?

You should now be able to:

- Explain what an infectious disease is.
- List the main ways by which infectious diseases can be spread.
- State how influenza, tuberculosis, typhoid, cholera, salmonella food poisoning, gonorrhoea, syphilis, athlete's foot and rabies are spread.
- Name 3 insect vectors and the diseases they spread.

- Describe how the housefly transmits diseases.
- Explain why rabies has, so far, not entered the UK.
- Explain what epidemics and pandemics are.
- Name a disease that is endemic in the UK.
- Describe the causative agent, the main symptoms and the incubation period for chlamydia.
- Suggest how sexually transmitted diseases could be avoided.

13.7 Cancer

What is a cancer?

Your body is constantly producing new cells to grow and to repair damaged tissues. The new cells are produced by cell division which normally takes place in a very controlled way. Sometimes the control signals go wrong and a cell divides for no apparent reason, i.e. when no growth is taking place or when repair is not necessary. The new cells accumulate to form a ball of cells called a **tumour**. The tumour can often be felt as a hard lump because the cells forming it are packed more closely together than normal cells. There are two kinds of tumour:

Benign tumours are slow growing and often stop after a while. The tumour does not invade the surrounding tissue or spread throughout the body. Most warts are benign tumours.

Malignant tumours are cancers. They are irregular balls of cells formed from rapidly dividing cells. Malignant tumours never stop growing and often take over important organs, preventing them from working properly. The cancerous cells break away and spread to other parts of the body, where they produce new tumours called **secondary tumours**. The cancer is said to have **metastasised**.

What are the causes of cancer?

There are over 200 different types of cancer. We think we know what causes some of these. For example, research suggests that smoking causes lung cancer. However, some people develop lung cancer having never smoked. Others who have smoked heavily throughout their lives may never develop lung cancer. Clearly some people are more likely to develop cancer than others. This may be due to their lifestyle or having inherited characteristics which make the cells of certain organs more likely to turn cancerous.

Substances, which are capable of causing cancer, are called **carcinogens**. There are some well documented ones:

- **Chemical carcinogens,** such as benzene, found in many fuels cause cancers of the bladder and scrotum. Benzopyrene and other chemicals found in cigarette smoke cause, amongst others, lung, mouth and bladder cancers. Heavy use of alcohol is associated with cancers of the mouth, throat, oesophagus and liver.

- **Ionising radiations** such as X-rays may cause cancer of the bone marrow resulting in leukaemia.

- **UV radiation** in sunlight causes skin cancers.

- **Chemical irritants** such as asbestos dust and particles in smoke increase the risk of cancers of the mucous membranes and lungs.

- Some **viruses** such as the human papilloma virus (warts) are associated with an increased risk of cancer. People with HIV often develop Kaposi's sarcoma.

Can cancer be cured?

One in three people will be affected by cancer at some stage of their life but not all will die because of it. Some cancers, if discovered early enough, can be cured. The success of the treatment depends partly on the type of cancer and how soon the cancerous cells are discovered. Treatments for cancer are improving and deaths from cancer have been falling (see table 2).

What are the treatments for cancer?

Treatment usually begins soon after the cancer is diagnosed. The main types of treatment are:

- **surgery** to remove all or as much as possible of the cancerous growth

- **radiotherapy** which uses radiation to destroy the cancer cells. Most cancer cells are more sensitive to radiations such as X-rays so these are targeted at them. The treatment is usually painless, but can have some side effcts such as red itchy skin – like a mild sunburn.

- **chemotherapy** uses strong drugs called **cytotoxic drugs** because they destroy rapidly dividing cells. They work on the basis that cancer cells divide more rapidly than normal cells and so more will be killed more readily. Because the drugs do kill some normal cells, chemotherapy is given in stages with rests in between to allow normal cells to recover. Unfortunately, there are almost always side effects such as nausea, tiredness and sometimes hair loss.

There are also many new treatments becoming available. These include **bone marrow transplants, peripheral blood stem cell transplants, monoclonal antibodies** (chapter 14.7) and **hormone therapy**.

And just as many complementary therapies such as herbalism, homeopathy, reflexology, and so on.

What do **you** know?

You should now be able to:

- Explain what a cancer is and explain the difference between malignant and benign tumours.
- Describe how a cancer can spread from one part of the body into another.
- Describe 5 types of carcinogen.
- Describe the 3 main treatments for cancer and explain how they work.
- List the cancers which are increasing and those which are decreasing.

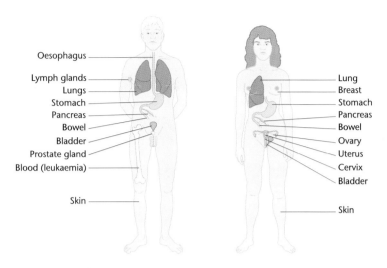

Oesophagus
Lymph glands
Lungs
Stomach
Pancreas
Bowel
Bladder
Prostate gland
Blood (leukaemia)
Skin

Lung
Breast
Stomach
Pancreas
Bowel
Ovary
Uterus
Cervix
Bladder
Skin

Figure 1 *The ten most common cancers in men and women (UK, 1997).*

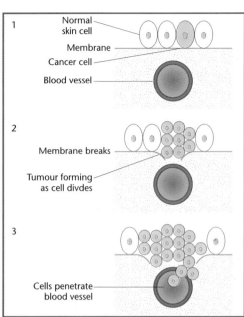

1 Normal
skin cell
Membrane
Cancer cell
Blood vessel

2 Membrane breaks
Tumour forming
as cell divdes

3 Cells penetrate
blood vessel

Figure 3 *How cancer can spread throughout the body.*

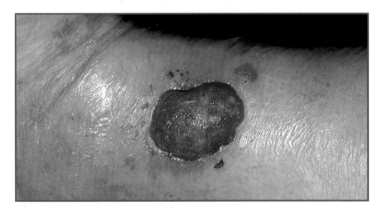

Figure 2 *Skin cancer is on the increase yet is one of the most preventable cancers.*

Type	Organ/tissue affected
Carcinoma	Skin, glands and lining tissues of organs
Sarcoma	Muscles, bones and fibrous tissues blood vessel lining
Leukaemia	White blood cells
Lymphoma	Lymphatic tissue

Table 1 *Cancers can be classified by the tissues they invade.*

	Cancer	Rates per 100,000 population		
		1991	1994	1997
Male	Stomach	20.1	17.9	15.5
	Colon, rectum, rectosigmoid junction and anus	33.7	30.7	30.1
	Pancreas	11.8	10.9	10.8
	Lung	92.9	82.7	74.0
	Prostate	34.1	34.1	32.9
Female	Stomach	12.4	10.9	9.6
	Colon, rectum, rectosigmoid junction and anus	32.7	30.0	27.6
	Pancreas	11.7	11.4	11.2
	Lung	41.7	41.5	40.8
	Breast	52.7	48.2	45.0
	Uterus	11.8	9.8	9.4

Table 2 *Death rates for selected cancers 1991–97 (UK).*

Preventing infection

To cause disease most pathogens have to enter the body. Your body has many natural ways of preventing invasion (see figure 2):

- Your skin provides a **physical barrier** to infection.

- Cavities such as your mouth, nose, vagina, and anus, together with your bronchial tubes, are lined by **mucous membranes**. These provide a physical barrier to pathogens and also produce **mucus**, which can trap them. Pathogens which are trapped in the mucus lining the bronchial tubes are then moved by **cilia** to the throat and swallowed.

- Many of your body secretions contain chemicals which make conditions very harsh for most micro-organisms. For example, sweat, tears, and nasal secretions all contain acid which slows down the growth of bacteria. They also contain an enzyme called **lysosyme** which destroys many pathogens. Vaginal secretions are also acidic.

- Pathogens in food are firstly attacked by lysosyme in saliva. This also washes them off the teeth. If they reach the stomach, the **hydrochloric acid** there makes the pH a low level, which kills them.

- Pathogens are **washed out** of the urethra by urine.

You may think that these defence mechanisms will make you safe from disease, but many pathogens do get into your body – where the blood responds.

How does your blood react to pathogens?

When your natural defences are breached, for example, your skin is damaged allowing pathogens into your body, your blood continues the defence against disease in two ways:

- **Non specific responses**. These are localised responses in the area where the tissues have been damaged. They include **inflammation** and **phagocytosis,** which are described in chapter 3.2.

- **Specific responses**, called this because the type of response depends on the type of pathogen. These responses involve the **immune system** and in particular the **lymphocytes**.

What is the role of the lymphocytes?

There are two kinds of lymphocytes. These have different roles in the defence against pathogens. **T lymphocytes** destroy virus-infected cells, parasites and fungi. They also destroy your own cells that have become cancerous.

B lymphocytes produce **antibodies** to destroy pathogens or the toxins they produce (see figure 1).

What are antibodies?

Antibodies are special proteins which can destroy or lead to the destruction of any foreign substances which enter the body. Their production is triggered by another type of chemical called an **antigen**. Antigens are attached to the cell surface of all cells, including pathogens. Each type of antigen will result in a specific antibody being produced to destroy it (see figure 3).

When a pathogen invades your body, its antigens activate a specific type of B lymphocyte. There are only a few of these in the blood, so this takes time, several weeks in some cases. The B lymphocyte now produces clones of itself which start producing lots of antibodies. These antibodies spread quickly throughout the body destroying any of the antigens they come across and thereby the pathogen.

Why don't we attack our own antigens?

Your immune system is programmed not to destroy your own antigens. In technical terms, it can recognise 'self ' from 'non-self'. Occasionally this does breakdown, and your body starts to attack itself, especially as you enter old age. When this happens you develop an **auto-immune disease** such as **multiple sclerosis (MS)**, **rheumatoid arthritis** and **insulin-dependent diabetes mellitus**. For example, in diabetes, you produce antibodies which destroy the insulin producing cells, and in MS, your own T lymphocytes start to destroy the myelin sheath around nerve cells.

Cancer cells are destroyed because they change their surface antigens and are treated as 'non-self'.

What do **you** know?

You should now be able to:

- Describe your body's first line of defences against infection.
- Review the non-specific responses of your blood to infection.
- Outline the role of the T lymphocytes in preventing a disease developing.
- Define the terms antigen and antibody.
- Draw a diagram to show the relationship between antigens, B lymphocytes and antibodies.
- Explain why some people develop autoimmune diseases.

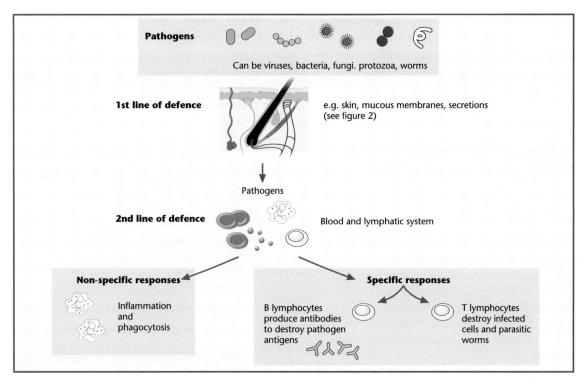

Figure 1 *The body's main defences against disease.*

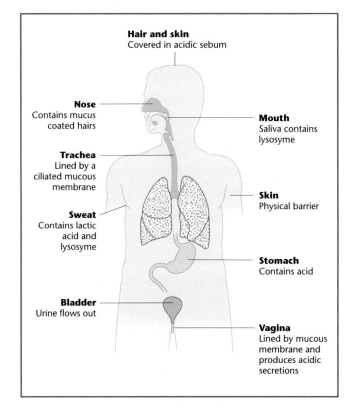

Figure 2 *The body has many barriers to infection.*

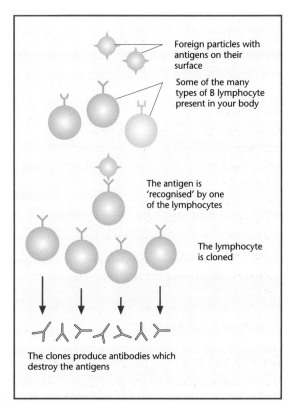

Figure 3 *Antibodies are produced in response to an antigen.*

Why do you develop immunity to a disease?

Once you have recovered from a disease, most of the cloned B lymphocytes die, but not all. The B lymphocytes which remain in the blood become **memory cells**. The next time the same pathogen invades your body, its antigens are quickly recognised by these extra memory cells (much more quickly than before) and antibodies are again produced to destroy the pathogen before it can cause disease. You are said to be **immune** to the disease as it has no chance to develop.

Can you be given immunity to a disease?

To become immune to a disease, you need to have had the initial infection so that you have memory cells and are therefore primed for a quick response. This is often called **active immunity** because you produce your own antibodies. Active immunity can be acquired naturally or artificially by being injected with a **vaccine**. The vaccine needs to cause the production of antibodies and memory cells, but without resulting in the disease. It can take several forms, as:

- **Dead organisms** which still have antigens on their surfaces yet cannot grow and reproduce. The antigens cause the production of antibodies and memory cells without disease, e.g. diphtheria and whooping cough vaccines.

- **Attenuated organisms** which are less virulent forms of the organisms. They are still living, but have lost the ability to reproduce, e.g. measles and TB vaccines.

- **Toxoids** are modified forms of the toxins produced by some bacteria. They are not poisonous, yet contain antigens which can stimulate the production of antibodies, e.g. tetanus vaccine.

Once acquired, active immunity can last a lifetime, but not always. For example, you must be re-vaccinated against diphtheria every five years to maintain immunity. This re-vaccination is called a **booster** because it boosts the level of memory cells in your blood. Table 1 shows the type of vaccine used for some common diseases and how long the immunity can last.

In England there is a programme of vaccinations which starts when you are two months old and continues into adulthood (see figure 2). Some parents choose not to have their children vaccinated because not all vaccines are one hundred per cent safe. Parents have to weigh up the risks of suffering from a disease against the risk of the vaccine. The ability of mass vaccination to reduce the death rate from a disease is clearly shown in figure 1.

Can you be given antibodies?

It is possible to get temporary immunity to a disease by acquiring antibodies made somewhere else. This **passive immunity** only lasts as long as the antibodies remain active. Breast fed babies receive antibodies from their mother, particularly in the first few days. Some of the smaller antibodies also cross the placenta during pregnancy. These help babies resist disease over the initial period when their immune system may not be fully functional.

Passive immunity can be given to people who are going to parts of the world where certain diseases are endemic. It only lasts for short periods, usually a maximum of six weeks. Nowadays most antibodies are usually produced in culture vessels by genetically modified micro-organisms (chapter 14.7)

Can the immune response cause problems?

The problem of **autoimmune** diseases has already been mentioned. In addition, the immune response can cause problems with blood transfusions, organ transplants and tissue grafts.

- **Blood transfusions**. When giving blood transfusions, the blood groups have to be matched very carefully, because different blood groups contain different antibodies. It is very dangerous to give someone unmatched blood (chapter 3.2).

- **Organ transplants and tissue grafts**. If cells with surface antigens which your immune system does not recognise as 'self' are put into your body, they will be destroyed by the T lymphocytes. This will lead to rejection.

  Before using an organ for transplantation, its cells will be **tissue-typed** to find out its cell surface antigens. The ideal organ would have the same antigens on its cells as the recipient cells. If this is not possible (and it rarely is), rejection can be avoided after the transplant by taking **immunosuppressant** drugs, such as cyclosporin. This inhibits the action of the T lymphocytes. Unfortunately, it also reduces the efficiency of the immune system to fight off other infections.

Do antigens ever change?

Some pathogens regularly change their cell surface antigens (they mutate) giving rise to new strains. The immunity you develop to one strain of pathogen will not be effective against any new strain, leaving you open to the disease. Influenza does just this and, whilst it is possible to be vaccinated against it, the vaccine will not always be effective against all the strains.

Disease	Nature of vaccine	Recommended vaccination time (UK)
Diphtheria	Dead organisms ⎫	Usually given as a combined vaccine (DTP vaccine)
Tetanus	Toxoids ⎬	at 2, 3 and 4 months
Whooping cough	Dead organisms ⎭	Boosters for tetanus and diphtheria at 5, 15 and 19 years, then tetanus every 7 years
Haemophilus influenzae B (meningitis)	Bacterial capsule (HIB vaccine)	Three doses at 2, 3 and 4 months Booster at 5 years
Polio	Attenuated organisms	Given at 2, 3 and 4 months. Booster after 5 years
Measles	Attenuated organisms ⎫	Usually given as a combined vaccine
Mumps	Attenuated organisms ⎬	(MMR vaccine) at 15 months
German measles (rubella)	Attenuated organisms ⎭	Girls have a rubella booster at 13 years
Tuberculosis	Attenuated organisms	Recommended at 13 years
Hepatitis B	Genetically engineered antigens	Recommended for health workers and when travelling to some countries

Table 1 *Some vaccinations are recommended in the UK.*

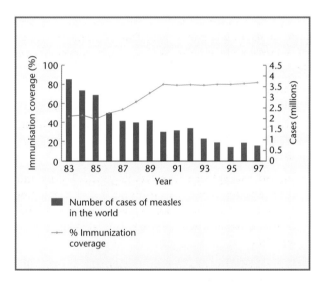

Figure 1 *Mass immunisation is an effective way of reducing the spread of measles.*

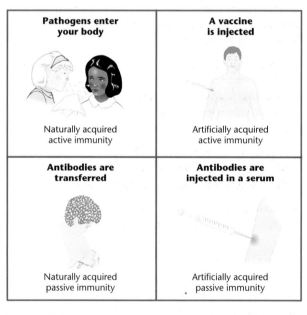

Figure 2 *There are several ways of becoming immune.*

What do **you** know?

You should now be able to:

- Explain what must happen for you to develop immunity to a disease.
- Explain how you can develop the different kinds of immunity.
- Outline the vaccination programme for tetanus and explain why 3 separate injections are required.
- State what kind of vaccine is used and why.

- Describe the other 2 kinds of vaccine.
- Suggest why mothers are encouraged to breast feed their babies.
- Review the problem the immune response causes for blood transfusions.
- Outline the problems of transplanting organs and suggest how these could be minimised.

The course of an infectious disease

After infection with pathogens, except for massive doses, there follows a period of no symptoms. This is the **incubation period** (see table 2), during which time the microbes are reproducing and building up in number. Cell damage may be immediate, but the **symptoms** of illness only start to appear when sufficient damage has occurred.

Soon after infection your body starts to mobilise its defences. Sometimes the defences may destroy the pathogens before they can do enough damage to cause ill health, in which case you will never know you have been infected. As part of the defence mechanism, the pathogen will be '**typed**' and eventually **antibodies** will be produced which generally result in your recovery. The full course of an infectious disease is described in figure 1.

Why does body temperature go up?

Some bacterial and viral pathogens release **toxins**. These stimulate the white blood cells to produce substances called **pyrogens** which reset the body thermostat so body temperature goes up a few degrees. As your body temperature rises, you may start to shiver and feel cold. This is called a **chill** and is the result of your body's response to its core temperature being below that set by the thermostat (chapter 8.5). Once reached, the new higher temperature interferes with the pathogen's reproduction and toxin production. It also stimulates and mobilises your body's defences so that you can deal more quickly with the pathogens. As the amount of toxin falls, less pyrogens are released and the thermostat resets to normal body temperature. The return to normal is accompanied by heavy sweating to lose excess heat.

Are there any drugs to help fight infections?

There are many drugs to help fight infections. Most of these are **antibacterial** although there are substantial **antifungal** and **antiprotozoan** drugs. Unfortunately there are very few **antiviral** drugs. Drugs are used when the immune system is not coping and needs some extra help. They usually work by killing the pathogens or stopping them from reproducing.

One of the first drugs to be discovered was the antibiotic **penicillin**. Penicillin, produced by the mould *Penicillium* was discovered almost by accident in 1928 by Alexander Fleming. It soon became one of the most useful drugs against bacterial infections. Since then many more have been discovered or developed, each effective against a particular range of bacteria.

Antibiotics

Antibiotics are chemicals produced by living organisms (bacteria and fungi) which can be used to kill bacteria inside the human body. They are possibly the most prescribed drugs today. There are antibiotics which are effective against almost all bacterial infections and they are able to kill these bacteria inside the human body without harming the host. A few may have minor side effects and some can cause serious allergic reactions (see page 188), but generally if taken as intended they are relatively safe.

The biggest problem has come from the overuse of antibiotics. Antibiotics are often used unnecessarily and this has resulted in strains of resistant bacteria (see page 150). The overuse can also upset the balance of the normal micro-organisms which live in the human body. The lack of competition allows some of the more pathogenic ones to flourish, such as *Candida*, which causes thrush.

What do painkillers do?

Painkillers, more properly called **analgesics**, cannot help your body fight infection. They simply relieve the symptom of pain, thereby making you feel better. There are two main kinds of analgesics.

Morphine is a **narcotic** and a very strong pain killer only used for intense pain in a hospital setting.

Aspirin and **paracetamol** are non-narcotic drugs use to treat things like headaches and the discomfort of a sore throat. Aspirin also reduces inflammation.

What do **you** know?

You should now be able to:

- Describe the course of a typical infectious disease form infection to complete recovery.
- Describe why your temperature usually rises and explain the usefulness of this.
- Suggest why your pulse rate goes up when you have an infection.
- Explain why antibiotics are so useful against bacterial infections.
- Use a diagram to explain how you could test the effectiveness of an antibiotic against a particular bacterium.
- Explain what the analgesics morphine, aspirin and paracetamol are used for.

Group & examples	Isolated from	Good for
Penicillins e.g. Benzylpenicillin Ampicillin	Fungus (mould)	Blood poisoning Throat infections Gonorrhoea and syphilis Bronchitis Pneumonia
Cephalosporins e.g. Cephalexin	Fungus (mould)	Food poisoning Urinary infections
Macrolides e.g. Erythromycin	Bacteria (streptomycetes)	Used instead of penicillin if person is allergic to it
Aminoglycosides e.g. Streptomycin Gentamycin	Bacteria (streptomycetes)	Used in conjunction with penicillin to kill bacteria in the gut and urinary tract
Tetracyclines e.g. Tetracycline	Bacteria (streptomycetes)	A broad spectrum drug especially good for fevers and diarrhoea
Antifungals e.g. Nystatin Griseofulvin	Bacteria (streptomycetes)	Thrush Ringworm Fungal disease of skin
Antivirals e.g. Acyclovir	Mostly synthetic	Cold sores Genital herpes
Antiprotozoans e.g. Chloroquine Pyrimethamine	Plants or synthetic	Malaria Toxoplasmosis

Table 1 *Different kinds of drugs are used for fighting different infections.*

Disease	Incubation period
AIDS	6 months to 8 years
Chicken pox	17 days
Cholera	1–5 days
Common cold	average 4 days
Diphtheria	2–5 days
Dysentery	average 3 days
Food poisoning	average 1 day
Gonorrhoea	5 to 10 days
Influenza	2–4 days
Malaria	12–30 days
Measles	10–15 days
Mumps	18 days
Rabies	1–6 months
Rubella	10–21 days
Tuberculosis	4–6 weeks
Whooping cough	7–14 days

Table 2 *The incubation periods of some common diseases.*

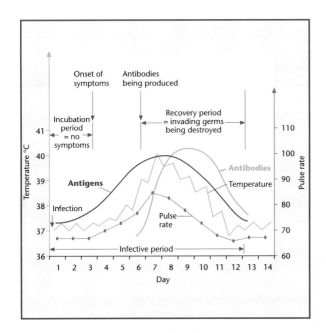

Figure 1 *The normal course of an infectious disease.*

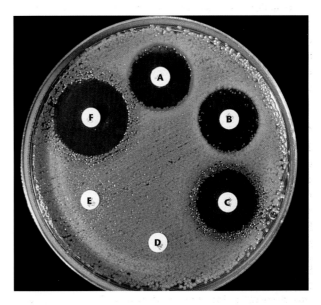

Figure 2 *To test the effectiveness of an antibiotic it is placed on a small disc which is then put onto the surface of an agar plate inoculated with the bacterium. In this case, antibiotic F is the most effective.*

The fight against disease

The fight against disease involves prevention and management. It is being fought at three levels, the **personal level**, the **community level** and the **worldwide level**.

On the personal level it involves maintaining good health behaviour. This is described more fully in chapter 12.3.

The role of the community in fighting disease

Most of us live in cities, towns or villages. We share a lot of facilities and services with our neighbours, many of which can affect our health. Providing these facilities and services in England is the responsibility of local government. Each local authority has to provide, by law, certain services for the community. They must:

- **provide safe water** for drinking, washing, etc. (chapter 13.12)

- **deal with the sewage and refuse** made by the community (chapter 13.13)

- **provide medical care** for those who require it. Community health care in the UK is provided by the **National Health Service** (NHS). This was set up in 1948, with the intention of making good medical treatment and facilities available to every member of a community, whether rich or poor. In attempting to achieve its goals, the NHS has gone through many re-organisations. The latest model is outlined in figure 1.

- **monitor standards of health and hygiene** within the community and implement amongst others, the Food Safety Act (1990), the Health and Safety at Work Act (1974) and the Factories Act (1961).

This is largely carried out by the **Environmental Health Services** who employ Environmental Health Officers and Public Health Inspectors to keep checks on standards, investigate complaints and if necessary, take legal action. However, much of their work is giving advice and making sure people are equipped with the knowledge to do things correctly.

Most local governments also provide many additional services.

What is health education?

Any long term strategy aimed at preventing diseases and improving health must include **health education**. If people know why they become ill, they will take precautions to prevent it. Health education is all about improving your awareness of health issues and related factors so that you can make informed decisions about anything that might affect your health, now or in the future. It is also about developing good positive attitudes to health so that the health of the community will improve.

Health education in England forms part of the government's wider public health strategy called *Saving Lives: Our Healthier Nation*. The two aims of this are (i) to improve the health of the population and (ii) to reduce the health gap (health inequalities). Figure 2 outlines some recent health education campaigns.

Fighting disease on a worldwide level

There are many organisations concerned with world health, but the largest and most influential is the **World Health Organisation** (WHO). This was set up by the United Nations Assembly in Geneva in 1948 and still retains its headquarters there. The objective of the WHO is '*the attainment, by all peoples, of the highest possible levels of health*'. At present there are 191 Member States involved and with their co-operation the WHO is active in the following areas:

- setting global standards for health

- the planning, promotion and development of comprehensive health services and programmes

- the monitoring of health and disease

- the prevention and control of disease

- the improvement of environmental conditions

- establishing standards for drugs, pesticides, etc.

- the co-ordination of research programmes, the training and provision of health personnel.

There have already been some successes in some of these areas. For example, the **infant mortality rate** in many countries has fallen dramatically due to work done on behalf of the health of mothers and babies – in particular, education and diet. The promotion of **mass immunisation** has wiped out smallpox all over the world. This was officially declared **eradicated** in 1980. Malaria, polio and leprosy have been eradicated from many areas of the world and safe water is now available to millions more people.

The WHO also works in conjunction with other agencies such as the **Federal Agricultural Organisations** (FAO) and United Nations Educational, Scientific and Cultural Organisation (**UNESCO**) to tackle problems like starvation and malnutrition in developing countries. A successful partnership has been forged with United Nations Children's Fund (**UNICEF**), UNESCO and the **World Bank** to tackle the growing problem of AIDS. There are many more organisations such as the **International Red Cross**, **Christian Aid** and **Oxfam**, which are also deeply involved in all aspects of world health, and nearly 1200 other health related institutions currently collaborating with the WHO.

Priority and target (by 2010)	Some strategies
Cancer To reduce the death rate (DR) from cancer in people under 75 by one-fifth	• raising awareness of the risk factors • raising awareness of and access to screening • investment in cancer services
Coronary heart disease and stroke To reduce the DR from CHD and stroke for people under 75 by two-fifths	• raising awareness of the risk factors • providing high quality services for prevention and treatment • funding more cardiac surgery
Accidents To reduce the DR from accidents by one fifth and serious injuries by two-fifths	• providing a health skills programme for 14–16 year-olds and adults • implementing a road safety strategy • funding research programmes
Mental health To reduce the DR from suicide and undetermined causes by one-fifth	• setting up initiatives such as the NHS Direct • modernising Mental Health Services

Table 1 *Our Healthier Nations national priorities.*

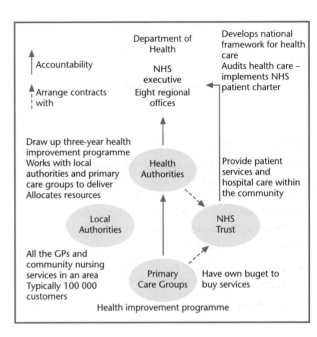

Figure 1 *The organisation of the National Health Service (1999). The aim is to both provide and improve health care in the future.*

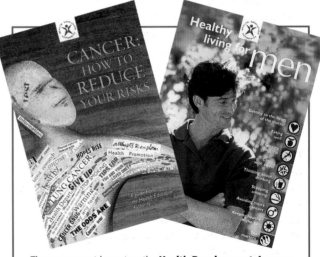

The government has set up the **Health Development Agency** to take a lead role in developing and implementing 'Health improvement programmes' which target community needs.

Figure 2 *There is a lot of health information available in hospitals, health care centres and similar places.*

What do **you** know?

You should now be able to:

- Review the ways in which you are responsible for your own health.
- List the health related services provided by the local authorities in England.
- Explain precisely the role of the Environmental Health Officers and Public Health Inspectors.
- Outline what a Primary Health Care Group is and what it does.
- Explain the aims of health education.
- Discuss the role of the WHO in the management of world health.
- List 6 more organisations involved in world health issues.

13.12 Safe water and refuse

How do humans affect the water cycle?

Water covers about two thirds of the Earth's surface and can form up to 90% of an organism's body. It is constantly being recycled between these. The main processes involved are shown in figure 1.

Human beings are also involved in the recycling of water. The average person in the UK uses about 120 litres of water every day for cooking, cleaning, washing and drinking. This means an average sized city (300 000 people) will need to find 36 million litres of water every day. Most of this comes from our fresh water rivers, lakes, reservoirs and underground sources. These are the same places we return our used water into (chapter 16.7).

Humans interfere with the water cycle in several ways:

- **deforestation** reduces the amount of water re-entering the atmosphere (see chapter 16.2)

- **dams** and **reservoirs** interfere with the natural flow paths of water

- artificial **drainage systems** reduce the flow of water into rivers and streams.

How is water made safe to drink?

To be of drinking quality, water should be clear, neutral, low in mineral content, free from harmful chemicals and micro-organisms (pollution). Very few sources of water provide clean, safe water suitable for drinking straight away. To make it safe to drink it must undergo a series of treatments. The extent of these will depend on where the water came from. Water taken from underground sources or mountain springs is usually already fairly clean and so does not undergo many processes.

The possible water treatments are described in figure 2, however, these treatments do not remove many of the chemicals found in water as a result of pollution. The effects of these are described in chapter 16.7.

The biological filter contains a range of different sized particles from sand to small stones. As the water trickles through these, any organic matter present is trapped and digested by **saprophytic micro-organisms** which live between the particles. **Protozoa** also help to remove many of the bacteria, including some of the pathogenic bacteria.

Which diseases are spread in water?

Diseases which are spread in water include **cholera**, **typhoid**, **dysentery** and **food poisoning**. Samples of treated water are routinely tested for these as part of the quality control procedures.

Water which has not been treated, can usually be made safe by boiling for 10 minutes to kill all the microbes.

What is refuse?

Refuse is the rubbish that we all produce during our day-to-day living. It includes things like empty cans, plastic containers, potato peelings, newspapers and wine bottles. Millions of tonnes of refuse are produced every year and the hygienic disposal of it presents a big problem for local authorities. The refuse is usually collected on a weekly basis by council workers and taken to areas where it can be dealt with.

At present most refuse is either burnt in large incinerators or compacted and tipped into holes in the ground at special **rubbish tips** or **land fill** sites. It is then covered by at least 0.5 metres of soil to prevent rats, mice and flies getting at it and to bring it in contact with the soil micro-organisms. These **decomposers** break down the biodegradable materials producing a gas (**bio-gas**, chapter 16.4). At some sites, this gas is collected and used as fuel. Eventually the land is re-used, usually for recreational purposes.

An alternative way of dealing with refuse is to recycle it. This involves sorting through the refuse to remove items which can be re-used. Some items can be re-used in their original form, such as bottles, whereas others may need to be processed and turned into new products. For example, recycled paper is used to make newspaper, cardboard and toilet paper (see chapter 16.4).

What do **you** know?

You should now be able to:

- Draw a diagram to show how water is recycled.
- Explain how we interfere with this recycling.
- Name 4 diseases which can be spread in water.
- Describe the desirable quality of drinking water.
- List the possible treatment processes which can be used to produce safe drinking water.
- Explain what happens in the biological filter.
- Explain why chlorine is added to water.
- List the 3 methods used to dispose of refuse.
- Explain what happens to refuse at rubbish tips.

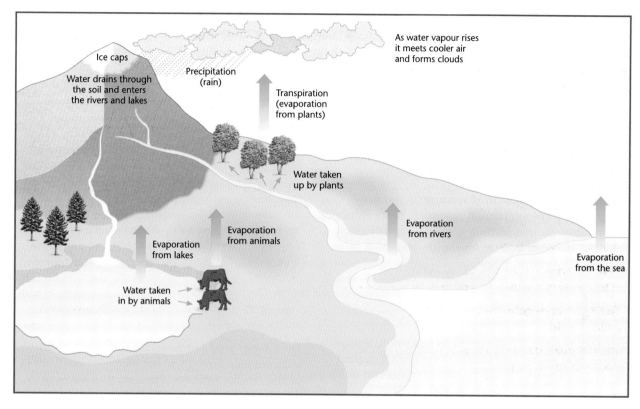

Figure 1 *The recycling of water involves both physical and biological processes.*

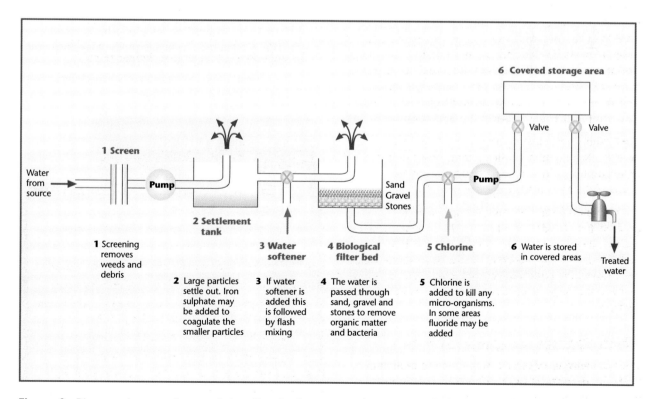

Figure 2 *River water usually needs treating before you drink it. These are some of the possible treatments.*

13.13 Sewage treatment

What is sewage?

Sewage is the wet waste from houses, factories, farms and the streets. **Domestic sewage** may consist of:

- human urine and faeces containing organic matter and bacteria, some of which could be pathogenic

- waste water from the kitchen and bathroom, containing organic matter and detergents

- rainwater from roads and roofs, containing grit and debris.

Industrial and **agricultural sewage** (slurry) may also contain unpleasant liquids containing heavy metals left over from the manufacturing processes and farming practices. These two kinds of sewage are often dealt with separately from domestic sewage.

In some countries, untreated sewage is discharged directly into the waterways causing many problems for the organisms that live there (see chapter 16.7).

In the UK, before it is discharged into waterways, sewage is taken from houses to treatment works in underground pipes called **sewers**. Houses that are not connected to the sewers have to use a **septic tank**.

Sewage treatment

The aim of sewage treatment is to produce much cleaner water which is safe to discharge into waterways. The stages in a typical treatment process include:

- The removal of solids such as grit, other debris (e.g. plastic bags) and large particles of organic matter. This is done by an **initial screening**, followed by a **settlement tank** and then the **first sedimentation tank** (see figure 1).

- The breaking down of the organic matter and removal of pathogens. There are two ways this can be achieved. Most modern sewage treatment works use an **activated sludge method**. The sewage effluent (liquid) is passed into large tanks which contain a complex mixture of **aerobic micro-organisms**. These use the sewage for food. Bacteria and fungi start the digestion of the organic matter producing simpler substances. For example, some of the bacteria breakdown proteins releasing ammonia. Others convert this ammonia into **nitrates**. Protozoa (ciliates) and roundworms also feed on the organic matter, but also take some of bacteria (including some pathogens) and fungi. It is important to maintain a high oxygen level for respiration by bubbling air through. This prevents the build up of pathogens.

- The production of a sludge which is low in organic matter, but high in micro-organisms. Some of this is used to 'seed' the next batch of sewage, the rest is passed on to an **anaerobic digester** (figure 3). The effluent produced is passed into another settlement tank.

The alternative method makes use of a **biological filter**, sometimes called a **trickling filter** (figure 3). Sewage is sprayed onto a bed of porous rocks (clinker). These rocks are covered in slime containing bacteria, fungi, protozoa, roundworms and insect larvae. As the sewage percolates through the clinker, the bacteria and fungi feed on the organic matter. The protozoa feed on the bacteria and fungi and the insects and worms eat the protozoa. A food web exists in the filter, for example:

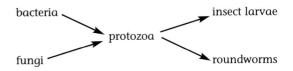

The effluent produced passes into another sedimentation tank where the remaining small bits of organic matter settle out. These are then removed to the **anaerobic digester**. The effluent is eventually discharged.

- The **anaerobic digester** where the sludge and humus is mixed with anaerobic bacteria which feed on any remaning organic matter, producing methane gas. This is often used as fuel to produce electricity for the sewage works. The sludge is then dried and because it contains a lot of minerals, especially **nitrates**, it is used as a fertiliser.

What do **you** know?

You should now be able to:

- Outline the possible contents of untreated domestic sewage.
- List the processes involved in treating domestic sewage.
- State which of the processes remove solids and large particles of organic matter.
- Explain what happens in an activated sludge tank.
- Describe how a biological filter works.
- Draw the food web in a biological filter.
- Explain what happens to sludge and humus in the anaerobic digester.
- Suggest why treated sludge would make a good fertiliser.

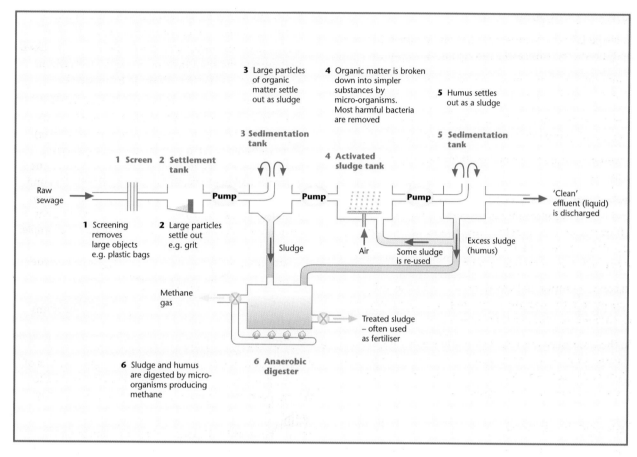

Figure 1 *The treatment of sewage can involve many different processes.*

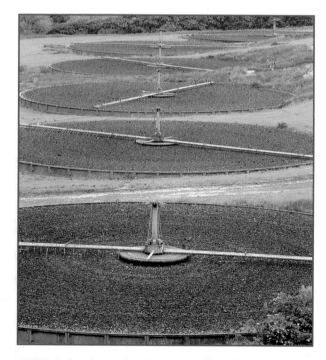

Figure 2 *'Trickling filters' at a modern sewage plant.*

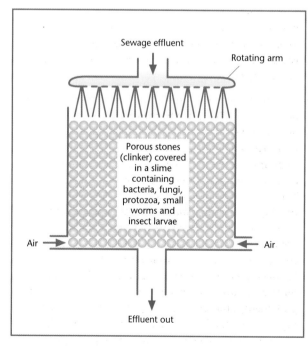

Figure 3 *A biological 'trickling filter'.*

13.14 Safe food

When is food not safe?

Our food can be infested by a variety of micro-organisms, some of which are pathogenic and can cause **food poisoning**.

What is food poisoning?

Food poisoning is the term used to describe a range of infections of the alimentary canal. These are caused by a variety of micro-organisms including bacteria, viruses and protozoa. They cause disease by:

- excreting **toxins** into the food which will poison your body when you eat it

- infecting your body after being taken in with the food.

The symptoms of food poisoning range from sickness and diarrhoea to abdominal bleeding, severe dehydration and even death.

Treatment may involve pain killers or antibiotics and, in severe cases, a saline drip is used to replace lost body fluids.

The World Health Organisation has estimated that over one thousand million people suffer some form of food poisoning every year. Every year there are over 40000 reported cases in the UK, making it the second most common illness. Even so, it is increasing as more and more people use convenience foods and fast food outlets. Figures 1 and 2 show some of the main bacterial causes of food poisoning.

How can food poisoning be prevented?

We can all reduce our chances of food poisoning by taking a few simple precautions during food preparation.

1 **Preventing the contamination of food** during the preparation and handling by:
   - always washing your hands and cleaning your nails before handling food.
   - cleaning utensils with hot soapy water
   - wiping work surfaces with antibacterial preparations
   - keeping flies and pets out of the work area.

2 **Destroying any harmful bacteria** in the food. Many animals already have harmful bacteria in their bodies as part of their normal **bacterial flora** and others are contaminated at the slaughter houses. These need to be destroyed by:
   - thoroughly cooking the food, especially meats and meat products
   - defrosting completely before cooking
   - pre-warming the oven to the cooking temperature
   - re-heating food for long enough.

3 **Preventing bacteria already in the food from multiplying** during the storage and serving of the food. All micro-organisms require food, water and warmth to live and reproduce. Some also require oxygen. The bacteria in food left in these conditions will quickly build up their numbers to levels which could cause disease. Situations to avoid are:
   - leaving food at room temperature for a few hours
   - leaving food uncovered
   - covering the food with dirty cloths or container lids
   - keeping food warm in warmed containers for long periods
   - allowing food to cool too slowly or for too long before serving.

4 **Storing food safely** by:
   - not storing cooked and uncooked meats next to each other (see figure 4)
   - refrigerating at less than 4 °C
   - using before the 'best by date'.

In 1995 the **Food Safety (General Food Hygiene) Regulations** were published. These are a set of guidelines for anyone who is preparing or selling food to the public. They require these businesses to:

- identify food safety hazards and take measures to minimise these

- train and supervise all staff who are involved in handling food

- make sure food is prepared and stored in hygienic conditions

- make sure food is supplied and sold in hygienic conditions.

These are enforced by the Environmental Health Department and help to make sure that food sold in supermarkets, restaurants, pubs, fast food outlets and take-aways is safe.

What do **you** know?

You should now be able to:

- Describe how micro-organisms in food can cause food poisoning.
- Outline the general symptoms of food poisoning.
- Describe the specific symptoms and reasons for *Salmonella* and *Botulinum* food poisoning.
- List and explain the precautions which can be taken to reduce your chances of catching food poisoning.
- Outline the standards which have to met by establishments who sell food to the public.

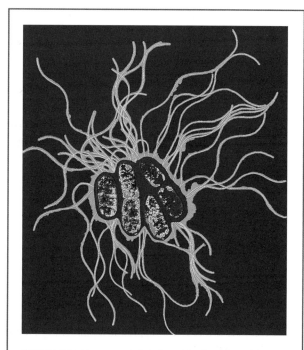

Caught from raw eggs and undercooked poultry.

Symptoms appear 24–48 hours after being ingested with food.

The bacteria invade the cells lining the intestine and produce a toxin which causes inflammation.

Symptoms include fever, diarrhoea, vomiting, dehydration and abdominal pain. These may last several days and can lead to septacaemia (blood poisoning).

Figure 1 Salmonella *food poisoning can be serious.*

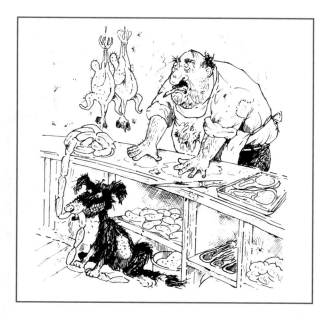

Figure 3 *Would you shop here?*

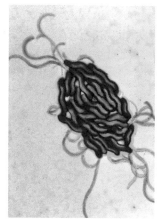

Clostridium botulinum

Rare but often lethal.

Incubation period 2 hours.

Symptoms include vomiting, diarrhoea and muscle paralysis.

Death comes from respiratory failure.

Caught from a variety of sources – canned fish to yoghurt.

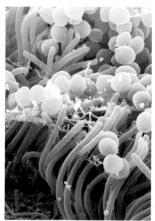

Staphylococcus aureus

Incubation period 1–6 hours.

Symptoms include diarrhoea, vomiting and pain.

Caught from contaminated dairy products, cooked meats and poultry.

Very common – 40% of people carry the bacteria.

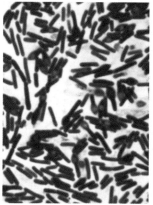

Campylobacter

Most common cause of stomach upsets.

Incubation period 1–11 days.

Symptoms can reoccur.

Symptoms include fever, headache, dizziness, diarrhoea and pain.

Caught from undercooked meats, untreated water and milk contaminated by birds.

Figure 2 *There are many causes of food poisoning.*

Can the natural life of food be extended?

Foods go off for several reasons:

- Because of the feeding actions of **saprophytic** organisms such as bacteria and fungi (chapter 15.2). Some of these are responsible for causing food poisoning.

- Fresh foods such as fruit continue to ripen. This involves **chemical changes** brought about by **enzymes**, some of which cause deterioration.

- Some chemicals in the food are **oxidised** causing changes in consistency and flavour. When fats are oxidised, they become rancid.

Trying to make food last longer has now developed into a multi-million pound industry. It is because of this industry that we can now enjoy some foods out of season, and exotic fruits from abroad.

Food preservation methods

These methods aim to reduce the level of micro-organisms in the foods by removing their growth requirements (chapter 2.2), destroying the enzymes which cause chemical changes and/or preventing oxidation. Unfortunately many methods also alter the flavour, texture and nutrient value of the foods.

- **Sterilisation** involves heating the food to high temperatures. The food is usually first sealed into cans or jars and then using steam, it is heated to 100 °C (for most foods) or 115 °C (for meats and vegetables). This kills most of the microbes and denatures the enzymes which cause chemical changes.

  Unfortunately, sterilisation does not always work as some microbes can produce heat resistant forms called **spores**. As the food cools, these spores grow into new microbes and re-contaminate the food. Many of the toxins which some microbes produce are also unaffected by heat. *Clostridium botulinum* produces both spores and deadly toxins. These toxins cause the deadly disease **botulism**.

  Sterilising food also alters its flavour. You will know this if you have tried UHT (ultra high temperature) or sterilised milk. UHT milk is heated to 132 °C for two seconds. This kills all micro-organisms and their spores.

- **Pasteurisation** is a milder form of heat treatment, used to kill pathogenic bacteria in foods without altering the flavour. One method involves heating the food quickly to 72 °C and holding it there for 15 seconds before cooling it rapidly. This treatment is used on cow's milk to kill the bacteria which cause TB and reduce the number of spoilage bacteria. Much of the wine we drink is also pasteurised.

- **Freezing** of food works because most microbes are incapable of reproducing at very low temperatures and the action of enzymes is slowed down or stopped. To freeze most foods, the temperature must be below −5 °C. Most domestic freezers store food at −18 °C. Some industrial ones can store food at −80 °C.

  A method known as **quick freezing** is sometimes used to avoid any damaging of texture and altering of taste. This involves bringing the overall temperature of the food to below −18 °C very quickly. The speed of the process is essential to prevent large ice crystals forming which could damage the food and lead to the loss of nutrients.

  Before freezing, many foods are **blanched** to denature the enzymes. To blanch food, it must be put into hot water (90–100 °C) for 1 to 5 minutes.

- **Dehydration** is the removal of water. Many micro-organisms stop growing below a certain water content. Removing the water is usually done by passing hot air over the food. The more quickly the water is removed, the less damage there is to the food. The fastest method currently used is called **accelerated freeze drying** (AFD). AFD involves freezing the food and then heating it inside a vacuum. The ice turns directly into steam and leaves the food. Coffee, milk and eggs are preserved in this way.

Some more methods of preserving food are shown in figure 2. Table 1 shows how preserving food can affect the nutrients.

What do **you** know?

You should now be able to:

- Explain 3 reasons why foods go 'off'.
- List the methods which could be used to prevent microbial degradation of food and explain why they work.
- Describe the effcets of different temperatures on bacterial growth.
- Suggest the temperatures at which you can safely store food.
- List the methods which could be used to prevent enzymic degradation of food and explain why they work.
- List the methods which could be used to prevent oxidation of food and explain why they work.
- Suggest how the various methods of food preservation can affect the flavour, texture and nutritive value of a food.

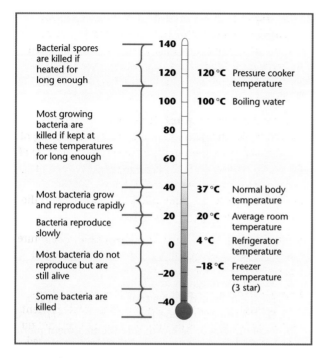

Figure 1 *How safe your food is often depends on the temperature it was stored at.*

	Using heat	Freezing
Proteins	Can alter the structure/texture	Can alter the structure/texture
Fats	May cause rancidity	May cause rancidity
Vitamins	Destroys vitamins A, some B and C	Blanching results in loss of vitamin C and some B vitamins
Minerals	No effect	Losses of water soluble minerals on thawing

	Dehydration	Altering pH
Proteins	No effect	Can alter the structure/texture
Fats	No effect	No effect
Vitamins	Losses of vitamins C and D	Losses of vitamin C
Minerals	Losses of water soluble minerals such as calcium	No effect

Table 1 *Nutrients are affected by preserving. Some foods can lose up to 25% of their water-soluble vitamins.*

Method	Why it works	Types of food used on	
Pickling	Soaking in acids like vinegar inactivates many enzymes and stops microbes reproducing	Fruits and vegetables	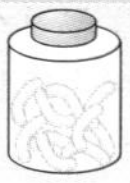
Curing	Salt injected into the food helps draw water from the bacteria	Meats and fish	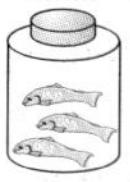
Smoking	The food is covered with chemicals which inhibit microbial growth	Meats, fish, cheeses	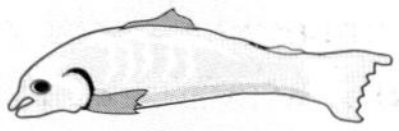
Adding chemical preservatives	Chemicals like sulphur dioxide inhibit the growth of microbes	Soft drinks, fruit juices, sauces	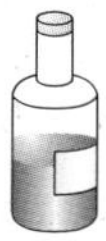
Irradiating	Radiation inactivates or kills micro-organisms (not spores)	Fruit grains	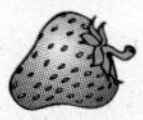
Vacuum packing	Removes air so oxidation cannot occur. Also prevents some microbes feeding	Poultry, meats, fish	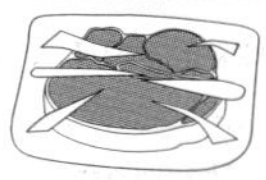
Cook chilling	Heat kills microbes and denatures enzymes. Chilling prevents microbes reproducing	Prepared meals	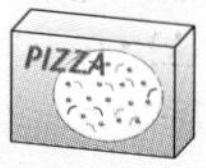

Figure 2 *Some methods of making food last longer.*

Chapter 13: Questions

1   The table gives some information about several diseases.

Disease	Caused by	Method of spread
Influenza	virus	through the air
Tuberculosis		through the air
Athlete's foot	fungus	
Rabies		

a Copy and compete the table by filling in the blank spaces.   *(4 marks)*

b Read the passage and answer the questions which follow.

> Cholera is caused by a pathogen transmitted in water. The faeces of people with cholera cause the water to be contaminated. Usually, cholera occurs as an epidemic in a particular area. The death rate may be 50%. Epidemics of cholera indicate poor sanitation and poor living conditions.
>
> The pathogens infect the large intestine and the incubation period is about six days. The most obvious symptom of the disease is severe diarrhoea, which occurs almost non-stop. Fluid loss can be as high as twenty litres per day. Death may occur in 24 hours.
>
> Treatment includes the transfusion of a saline solution and the use of antibiotics.

i Name the type of pathogen which causes cholera.   *(1 mark)*

ii Explain how cholera causes death.   *(2 marks)*

iii Explain why the transfusion of a saline (salt and water) solution is an essential treatment for cholera.   *(2 marks)*

iv Why are cholera sufferers given antibiotics?
                                                         (1 mark)

c In countries where cholera is common, tourists are advised to drink only boiled water. Suggest one reason for this advice.   *(1 mark)*

d Name two types of white blood cell. For each type, explain how it protects the body against diseases.
                                                         (4 marks)
                                              (NEAB June 1998)

2   The diagram shows an activated sludge sewage treatment plant.

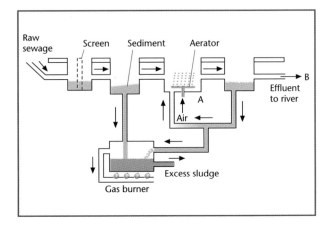

a Sketch the diagram and label
  i the activated sludge tank;   *(1 mark)*
  ii the anaerobic digester.   *(1 mark)*

b Explain why air is blown into the treatment plant at A.   *(2 marks)*

c Explain why the effluent leaving the treatment plant at B contains more nitrate than the liquid entering.   *(2 marks)*

d Give one advantage of activated sludge treatment compared to biological filtration.   *(1 marks)*

e When untreated sewage is discharged into rivers it may result in pollution. The table shows river quality classifications.

Class	Chemical properties	Biological properties	Potential uses
1	dissolved oxygen greater than 80%	non-toxic to fish	drinking water coarse fishing
3	dissolved oxygen greater than 60%	non-toxic to fish	suitable for drinking after treatment coarse fishing
5	dissolved oxygen greater than 20%	fish absent	suitable for low grade industrial purposes

i Explain why an increase in sewage pollution could lead to a decrease in the dissolved oxygen content of a river.   *(3 marks)*

ii In class 3 rivers pollution may cause discolouration of water. Suggest why untreated sewage may cause this.   *(1 mark)*

iii A sign of sewage pollution in class 5 rivers may be excessive growth of plants on the surface of the water. Explain why this may happen.   *(2 marks)*
                                              (NEAB June 1998)

3 The graph shows the number of cases of whooping cough in England and Wales between 1940 and 1990. Whooping cough is caused by a bacterium.

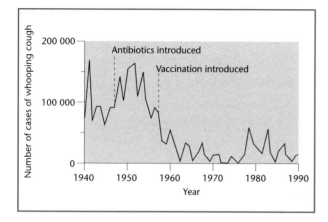

a What evidence is there in the graph to suggest that:
  i the antibiotics used had no effect on the whooping cough bacterium; *(1 mark)*
  ii vaccination is a good way of controlling the whooping cough bacterium? *(1 mark)*

b Some time after vaccination against whooping cough was introduced, there was public concern that brain damage was a possible side-effect of using the vaccine. Many parents did not have their children vaccinated around this time. Give evidence from the graph to suggest when this occurred. *(2 mark)*

c How does vaccination prevent a person becoming ill with a particular disease? *(4 marks)*

d Whooping cough is spread by *droplet infection*. What does *droplet infection* mean? *(2 marks)*
(SEG June 1999)

4 The table shows antibody production in the human body in response to injections with dead disease-causing bacteria.

	Time in days	Concentration of antibody in the blood in arbitrary units
First injection	0	0
	5	0
	10	3
	20	10
	30	15
	40	14
Second injection	50	11
	60	18
	70	29
	80	36
	90	36

a Plot the data as a line graph. Join the points with straight lines. *(5 marks)*

b Use the terms antigen, antibody and white blood cell, and information from the graph, to explain how artificial immunity can be caused. *(5 marks)*
(You will be awarded up to one mark if you write your ideas clearly)
(SEG June 1996)

5 a i What is a tumour? *(2 marks)*
  ii Describe how cancer may spread from one organ of the body to another part. *(2 marks)*

b The following pieces of advice are taken from a leaflet about cancer prevention. For each explain why it is given.
  • "Don't smoke"
  • "Take care in the sun" *(3 marks)*

c Some research has shown a link between nuclear power stations and the number of cases of leukaemia.
Suggest two possible reasons why there may be more cases of leukaemia in areas around nuclear power stations. *(2 marks)*

d There are approximately 5.9 million new cancer cases in the world each year and 1 in 10 deaths is caused by cancer. The table shows some differences between industrialised countries and developing countries.

	Industrialised countries	Developing countries
Number of new cancers	2.9 million	3.0 million
Number of deaths due to cancer per year	1 in 5	1 in 16
Life expectancy	70+ years	50–60 years
Age range with greatest number of cancer cases	60+ years	30–40 years

The number of cancer cases and deaths due to cancer are different in industrialised and developing countries. Suggest two reasons for these differences. *(2 marks)*
(NEAB June 1998)

6 a i Describe how the body responds to infection by a pathogen. *(4 marks)*
  ii How does this response protect the body from further infections by the same pathogen? *(2 marks)*
  iii Certain viruses such as the common cold are constantly able to change their outer surface. Suggest one reason why this makes it impossible to vaccinate a person against the common cold. *(1 mark)*

14 Biotechnology

Biotechnology is one of the most exciting developments of the last few decades. It is based on both old and new techniques which together promise to change our lives forever. In this chapter you will learn about these techniques and see how they are going to affect your life.

After you have worked through this chapter, you should be able to:

- Describe how uncontaminated cultures of bacteria can be grown in a laboratory.
- Discuss what biotechnology is and outline how some of the techniques are being used.
- Describe a modern industrial fermenter.
- Describe the processes involved in transferring genes from one organism to another.
- Describe how enzymes can be obtained and made use of in the home and by industry.

- Describe the use of micro-organisms in the traditional fermentation processes of baking, brewing and yoghurt production.
- Explain what GM foods are.
- Describe how genetic engineering is being used to improve crop plants and animals.
- Outline some of the medical uses of biotechnology.

Gene therapy

Gene therapy is the medical use of genes to treat genetic diseases such as **cystic fibrosis, muscular dystrophy** and **severe combined immune deficiency syndrome** (**SCIDS**). The possibilities are:

- replacing faulty genes by normal working genes, e.g. cystic fibrosis
- introducing genes which inhibit the replication of infectious agents, e.g. HIV
- introducing genes which result in the destruction of abnormal cells, e.g. cancer.

Gene therapy promises to be the next major step in eliminating disease. The first success came in 1990 when a four-year-old girl, Ashanti Desilva, was treated for a rare inherited disease which leads to SCIDS. A defective gene results in T lymphocyte destruction and therefore impairs the immune system.

Lymphocytes were removed from her body and a working copy of the gene inserted. The lymphocytes were allowed to proliferate before being transfused back to her body. Ashanti was able to live a relatively normal life with a functioning immune system.

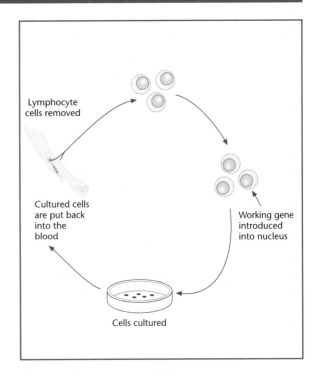

Lymphocyte cells removed

Working gene introduced into nucleus

Cells cultured

Cultured cells are put back into the blood

Figure 1 *Treatment for SCIDS.*

In 1999 gene therapy was used to introduce a working gene into blood stem cells (blood producing cells in the bone marrow) removed from a baby unable to produce lymphocytes. When transfused back, these re-seeded the bone marrow which starting producing normal lymphocytes. A future step may involve attempts in an unborn foetus so that the baby can be born without the condition.

Gene therapy techniques

Gene therapy is a very complex procedure and has many requirements (see figure 2).

A successful method of delivering genes to cells is by using a virus – the **virus vector** method. The therapeutic gene is spliced into the viral DNA replacing the viral replication genes, but not its infection genes. This way the gene is not only delivered to the cell, but also enters it and is incorporated into the cell's chromosomes (chapter 13.1). All new cells produced from this cell by mitosis will also contain the therapeutic gene.

There are three ways of making sure the correct cells are targeted:

● Remove the cell and insert the gene, then put it back. This is the same technique as used for SCIDS.

● Insert the gene into a virus vector which infects the target cell. This has been successfully achieved to treat cystic fibrosis. Cystic fibrosis is an inherited disorder (chapter 11.5) in which the mucus membranes produce extra thick and sticky mucus. In the bronchial passages this can reduce air flow and lead to infection, which may produce complications and early death. It is now possible to deliver a normal working gene to the mucus producing cells by a virus. The virus spliced with the normal working gene for mucus production can then be delivered to the cells using an inhaler.

● Attach the gene to a **designer antibody** (chapter 14.7) which will deliver it to the target cell. This is a variation of the viris vector method and may, one day soon, be used to help fight cancer. Cancer cells have different signals on their surfaces. Antibodies with suicide genes attached can be targeted to these.

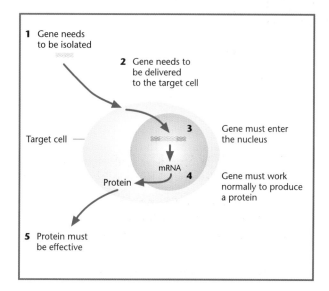

Figure 2 *Gene therapy is a complex process.*

Fears for the future

The new **germ line gene therapy** technique has concerned many people! The technique involves introducing a gene into the zygote so that all the cells of the forthcoming baby will contain it, as will some of its future offspring. This permanently alters the genome and some say interferes with nature. Once the human genome project is complete and all the genes on human chromosomes have been identified it should be possible to swap any number of genes and produce designer babies.

Another worry is that no one really knows what happens during the development of a foetus and interfering with a chromosome may have disastrous and unknown effects.

14.1 Growing micro-organisms

Micro-organisms are everywhere, in the soil, water, air and even in other organisms. **Bacteria** and **fungi** will grow wherever there is food, water, warmth and an absence of hostile conditions, such as an acid pH. Some may require oxygen (aerobic bacteria), others grow better if there is no oxygen (anaerobic bacteria). **Algae** make their own food providing there is carbon dioxide, light and a source of nitrates. To grow micro-organisms in the laboratory, we must supply them with all of these essential requirements.

Growing bacteria

To grow a culture of bacteria, you need to supply nutrients, water and warmth. The nutrients and water are usually supplied as a nutrient medium called a **nutrient broth**. Bacteria can be grown in this, but usually, the solidifying agent **agar** is added to turn it into a jelly. This is set in a petri-dish to form an **agar plate** (see figure 1). To provide warmth, the agar plate is placed in an **incubator** set at a suitable temperature, usually 30 to 40 °C (25 °C is used in school laboratories).

A growth medium which contains the full range of nutrients is called a **complete medium**, on which any species of bacteria can be grown. A **selective growth medium** is formulated to contain only those nutrients required by a particular species.

The growth medium and equipment must be **sterile** (free from all micro-organisms) before the bacteria are transferred to it.

Sterilising the materials

Sterilisation means the complete destruction of all micro-organisms, including spores. There are various methods of achieving this:

- **Dry heat** produced in a hot air oven can be used to sterilise glassware. Equipment used to transfer micro-organisms to the growth medium can be sterilised by passing it through a naked flame.

- **Moist heat** produced in an **autoclave** or pressure cooker can be used to sterilise the culture medium before use, and when disposing of it after use. Steam is produced at a pressure of 100 kPa, which raises its temperature to 121 °C, hot enough to kill all bacteria and their spores. The microbes are killed because the hot steam denatures the proteins in their cytoplasm. However, sufficient time must be allowed for the heat to penetrate the cells. This will usually be 25 minutes in a small pressure cooker.

- **Chemicals** such as **disinfectants** can be used to sterilise contaminated glassware and other materials after use. Strong disinfectant is often used to dispose of used cultures.

Transferring the bacteria to the agar

There are two main methods used to transfer bacteria (**inoculate**) onto an agar plate. These are illustrated in figure 1.

Because micro-organisms are found almost everywhere, there is always the chance of these contaminating the growth medium when you inoculate it with the required micro-organisms. It is also possible that you could contaminate the atmosphere, or even yourself. To minimise this threat, some precautions can be taken. This is called the **aseptic technique** and includes:

- wiping the work area with disinfectant

- using sterile equipment

- working around a Bunsen burner flame

- **flaming** all equipment used in the transfer

- immediately placing used equipment into disinfectant

- sealing the inoculated petri-dishes with adhesive tape

- washing your hands with a bacteriocidal solution before and after preparing the agar plate.

Bacterial colonies

Every single bacterium transferred onto the surface of an agar plate will grow into hundreds of bacteria during the incubation period. These will show up on the agar plate as **colonies** (see figure 1). Each separate colony is formed from one bacterium. A **confluent lawn** is formed when the colonies merge together.

Bacterial colonies vary in shape, colour and form depending on the type of bacteria. This is one way to identify them (chapter 13.3).

Growing fungi and viruses

Fungi can be grown in much the same way as bacteria, using a growth medium containing carbohydrates, minerals and vitamins. Yeasts will normally grow in a solution of sugar and minerals. They prefer a lower incubation temperature, usually around 25 °C. Fungal colonies are usually easy to recognise because they are less compact. Much more of the growth takes place below the surface of the agar.

Viruses will only multiply inside other living cells. This makes it difficult to grow them. Hen's eggs are often used, but other animal and plant cells can also be used if they have been isolated and grown by a process called **tissue culture**. A tissue culture can then be inoculated with a virus.

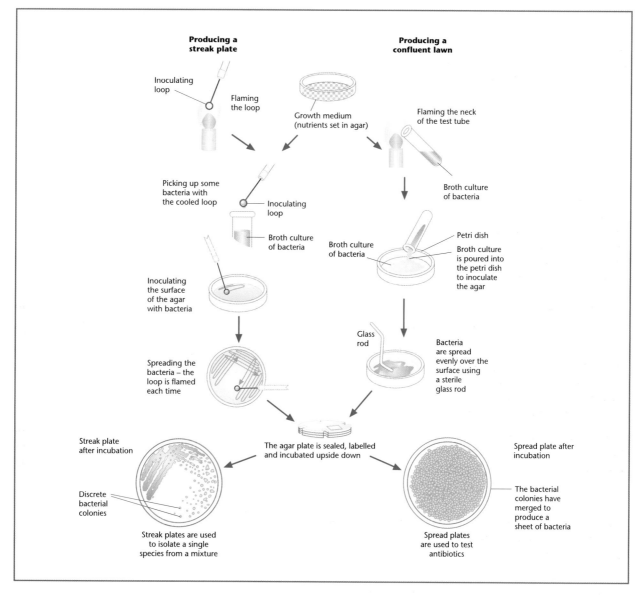

Figure 1 *Producing a streak plate and a confluent lawn.*

What do **you** know?

You should now be able to:

- Describe what bacteria need in order to grow.
- Distinguish between selective and complete growth media.
- Describe an agar plate.
- Outline the 3 methods of sterilising materials and state examples of their uses.

- Using diagrams, describe how you would produce a streak plate of bacteria.
- Explain the difference between a streak plate and a confluent lawn of bacteria.
- Outline the aseptic technique.
- Explain how fungi can be grown in a laboratory.
- Explain why viruses can not be grown in the same way.

14.2 Biotechnology

What is biotechnology?

Biotechnology is the word used to describe the way we make use of living organisms, especially micro-organisms, to produce useful substances.

Humans have been using micro-organisms in the production of bread, cheese, yoghurt, alcohol and vinegar for hundreds of years. The industry has suddenly grown because of the development of new techniques which have enabled us to make better use of the organisms. Two of the most important of these techniques are:

- genetic engineering (GE)
- fermentation technology.

Genetic engineering is about altering the **genome** of an organism usually by inserting new genes. This will add new genetic instructions. The processes involved in genetic engineering are described in chapter 14.3.

What is fermentation technology?

Fermentation technology is the process of growing micro-organisms on a large scale in carefully controlled conditions, and using them to produce substances of value to us. Most biotechnology processes use this technique to produce the product.

The micro-organisms are grown in vessels called **fermenters** (see figure 1). A fermenter is a container which provides a suitable environment for the growth of the micro-organism and the production of the product. A controller can alter the environment (e.g. pH, temperature, oxygen/carbon dioxide concentrations) to produce optimum conditions.

Some fermenters allow the substrate to be fed in continuously and the product to be extracted. This is called a **continuous system**. Others must be set up and sealed, then re-opened to extract the product after growth is completed. This is a **batch system**.

In both systems, the product will have to be separated from the cells and growth medium. This separation, purification and packaging of the product is called **downstream processing**.

Which products are produced?

Table 1 shows some of the products currently being produced in fermenters. A selection of these are described in the next few chapters.

Why use micro-organisms?

The use of micro-organisms in industrial processes has developed for several reasons:

- They have a relatively simple structure, most consisting of only one cell.
- They have simple metabolism which has been extensively studied.
- They have simple food requirements and some will even feed on our wastes.
- They contain some useful enzyme systems.
- They have a very rapid reproductive rate.
- They can be easily cultured in easily maintained conditions.
- It is relatively easy to genetically modify them, i.e. insert or remove genes.

Producing substances by biotechnology

The advantages of producing products by biotechnology are that:

- the product is always the same high quality and free from impurities
- it can be made species specific, e.g. human insulin
- it will be free from contamination, e.g. HIV
- production is not dependant upon animal experimentation.

Table 2 illustrates the variety of products produced through biotechnological methods.

What do you know?

You should now be able to:

- Explain the term biotechnology.
- List some of the techniques modern biotechnology makes use of.
- Draw a flow diagram to show how GE and fermentation technology link together in biotechnology processes.
- Draw and fully label a typical fermenter and describe what happens in it.
- Distinguish between a batch and a continuous fermentation process.
- Explain why downstream processing is necessary.
- List 2 advantages and 1 disadvantage of using biotechnology to produce products.

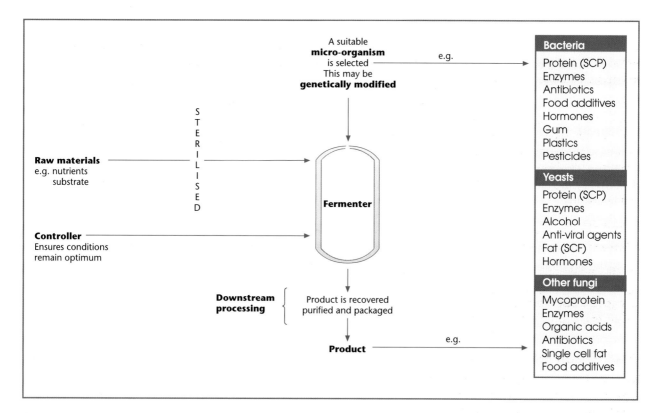

Figure 1 *A typical biotechnology process.*

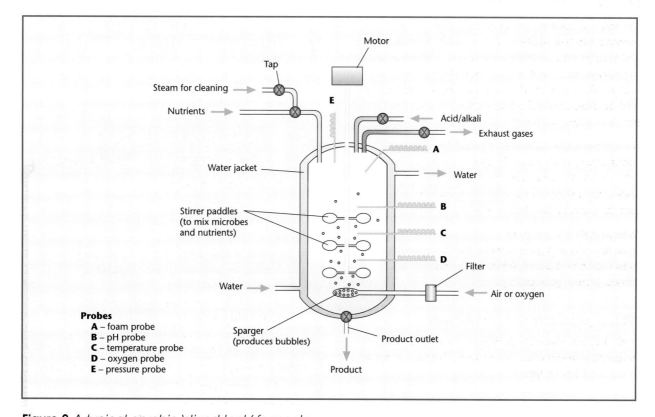

Figure 2 *A typical aerobic 'stirred tank' fermenter.*

14.3 Genetic engineering

What is genetic engineering?

The genes control the functions of a cell and the products it makes. Scientists can now transfer genes from one organism to another and thereby add or take away functional instructions. The technique is called **genetic engineering** (GE). It is also called **recombinant DNA technology** because you are changing the DNA molecule.

Genetic engineering is an extension of **genetic breeding**. Organisms with favourable characteristics are bred together in the hope that some of the offspring will inherit these characteristics. Most of our crop plants and domestic animals have been produced in this way. Some of them bear no resemblance to the wild stock they originally came from. Genetic engineering has simply taken the guesswork out of genetic breeding.

The process of gene transfer

Most genetic engineering involves transferring genes into micro-organisms by a process that involves:

- Obtaining the gene to be transferred from the DNA of the donor organism. Genes can be cut from donor DNA using special enzymes called **restriction enzymes**. These cut the DNA at specific base sequences leaving a few exposed bases called '**sticky ends**' (see figure 1).

  These enzymes cut the DNA into sections, one of which will contain the gene required. A **gene probe** is used to find this. A gene probe is a single strand of DNA which has been made specially so that it will attach to the required gene. It is also made slightly radioactive so you can detect it.

  Genes can also be made from messenger RNA (mRNA) or using a special machine called an automatic polynucleotide synthesiser (APS).

- Inserting the isolated required gene into a vector. The main vector used is the **plasmid**. Plasmids are short pieces of circular DNA found in the cytoplasm of some bacterial cells. They can easily be removed from the bacterial cell and cut open. If the same restriction enzyme which was used to cut the donor DNA is used, this will leave complementary 'sticky ends'. The donor gene can now be joined to the plasmid using another type of enzyme called **DNA ligase**.

  Viruses are also used to transfer genes into bacteria. (see figure 2 on page 223).

- Transferring the required gene into the host organism. Bacteria can be treated so that they take up the plasmid containing the donor gene.

- Cloning of the required gene. The bacterial cells containing the new plasmid are selected and placed in favourable conditions so that they reproduce. They are usually grown in a **fermenter** (chapter 14.2). Because all the new bacterial cells produced come from the same original parent, they are called **clones**. Each clone will contain a copy of the new plasmid and therefore a copy of the inserted gene.

- Supplying the bacteria with the conditions and materials they require to produce the product coded for on the inserted gene.

How are cells with the inserted gene selected?

One technique involves the insertion of two genes, the required gene, and a gene which gives the bacterium resistance to an antibiotic such as penicillin. When the bacteria containing the two genes are transferred onto a growth medium containing the antibiotic, only those with the resistance will grow. These are the ones which will contain the inserted gene. Of course, putting antibiotic resistant genes into bacteria is a cause for some concern (see page 188). Another way is to test for the product that is produced as a result of the inserted gene.

How is genetic engineering being used?

Some of the many current applications of genetic engineering are:

- To produce high quality products. Human genes have been transferred into micro-organisms so that they can make hormones, enzymes, antibiotics and blood clotting factors.

- To make micro-organisms more efficient so that they will increase yields or work in adverse conditions, such as high temperatures.

- To enable micro-organisms to use specific substrates, such as our wastes or pollutants like oil.

- To introduce useful genes into animals and plants so that they are more productive or capable of withstanding disease.

- To introduce or replace faulty genes in humans, i.e. gene therapy for cystic fibrosis.

Many of these applications are described in the next few chapters.

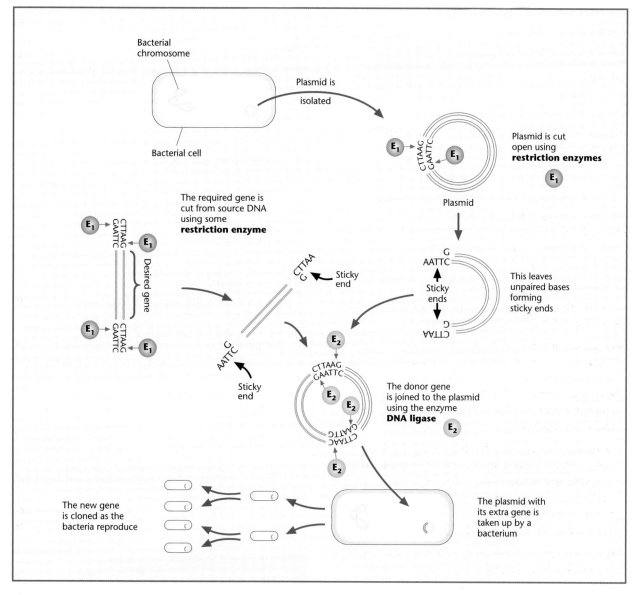

Figure 1 *The process of gene transfer.*

What do **you** know?

You should now be able to:

- Discuss why GE can be seen as an extension of genetic breeding.
- List 3 current uses of GE.
- Explain what a plasmid is and how it is used in GE.
- List in sequence, the stages in a GE process.
- Outline what 'sticky ends' are and how they can be produced.

- Explain why it is important to use the same type of restriction enzyme to cut the gene from the host and to open the plasmid.
- Explain how copies of the spliced gene are made.
- Describe how you can select the bacterial cells which have received the gene.

14.4 Enzyme technology

What is enzyme technology?

The traditional processes of baking and brewing make use of the **enzymes** *within* yeast. Making yoghurt uses the enzymes *within* bacteria. **Enzyme technology** is about extracting the enzymes and using them in isolation from the cells which produced them. Enzymes produced in this way are now used extensively in the baking, brewing, dairy, pharmaceutical, starch, detergent and waste industries among others (see table 2).

How are the enzymes obtained?

Enzymes can only be produced inside living cells. Most enzymes used in industry are produced by micro-organisms. For example, the enzymes added to biological washing powders are produced by the bacterium *Bacillus licheniformis*. This is grown in a fermenter using a mixture of potato starch, soy meal and minerals as food. As it grows, it produces the required enzymes. These are then removed, dried and added to washing powder.

Enzymes from animal and plant cells are also used. **Rennin**, used in the manufacture of cheese, is still extracted from the stomach of young calves, although this is gradually being replaced by rennin produced by genetically modified bacteria and fungi. Proteases, such as **papain** used to tenderise meats, are obtained from exotic fruits such as the papaya and pineapple.

Table 1 shows the main source of some important enzymes.

Immobilised enzymes

Enzymes can be expensive to produce and so most manufacturing processes attempt to recycle them. The main problem is separating an enzyme from the product it has just taken part in making. However, if the enzyme is **immobilised**, by trapping it in a jelly-like bead or fibre – it can be easily collected and used again.

Producing lactose-free milk uses an immobilised enzyme. The enzyme lactase, which breaks down lactose into glucose and galactose, is immobilised by bonding to fibres of cellulose acetate. This is stacked in a column and milk is poured through. As the milk passes through the column, the lactose is broken down by the enzyme lactase, which also remains bonded to the cellulose acetate. The enzyme remains separated from the product of the reaction and can be reused (see figure 1).

Enzymes and genetic engineering

Many of the enzymes required for medical applications have to be of human origin. If they are not, they could result in an immune response and place further stress the body. By using genetic engineering techniques, human genes coding for specific enzymes can now be inserted into micro-organisms and cloned. The micro-organisms can then be used to produce the human enzymes.

Genetic engineering can also be used to redesign enzymes to improve their characteristics. For example, proteases used in washing powders can be made more heat stable so that they work at a higher temperatures. Altering enzymes in this way is often called **enzyme engineering**.

Enzymes in biosensors

Biosensors can be used to monitor the presence of specific chemicals accurately and rapidly. They combine the chemistry of micro-electronics and enzymes.

Because enzymes are very specific to one chemical reaction they can be used to detect specific molecules. Sometimes a product, such as hydrogen, can change the colour of a dye. And if energy is released in a chemical reaction it can be **transduced** into an electrical signal.

Biosensors containing enzymes are now used to detect blood glucose and cholesterol levels, pollutants in the air or water and nutrient levels in water. They are also used to indicate the presence of disease. For example, diabetes mellitus results in excess glucose in the urine. This can be detected by a simple dipstick (or clinistix) which changes colour (see figure 2). The detecting enzyme is glucose oxidase which is immobilsed in cellulose fibres.

Blood tests always measure enzyme levels because they are strong indicators of liver, kidney and heart functions. For example, high levels of creatine kinase indicate a heart attack.

What do **you** know?

You should now be able to:

- Discuss what you understand by enzyme technology.
- Describe some of the uses of amylase, protease, isomerase and catalase enzymes.
- Outline how the enzymes used in washing powders are obtained.
- Explain what immobilised enzymes are and how they are so useful to industry.
- Describe how the process of GE is used in enzyme technology.
- Explain why enzymes can be used as biosensors.
- State two examples of the diagnostic use of enzymes.

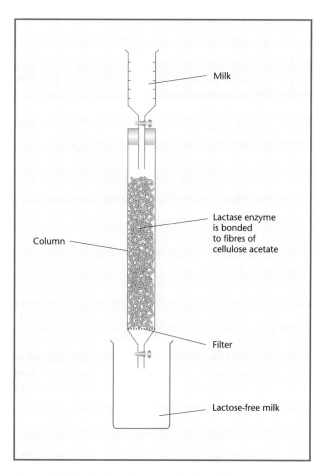

Figure 1 *Producing lactose-free milk.*

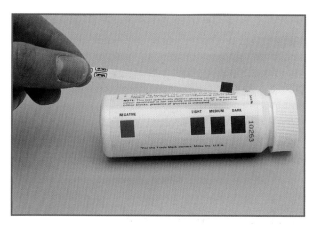

Figure 2 *Testing for glucose is easy with a clinistix. Glucose is converted by enzymes into hydrogen peroxide. The hydrogen peroxide changes the colour of the pigment.*

Enzyme	Source(s)	What it does	Industrial application
Amylase	Fungi/bacteria	Splits starch into maltose	Baking – to improve ??? by converting starch to sugar Brewing – to produce sugars from cereal starch, e.g. malt Medicine – given as an aid to digestion Syrup – to produce sugar syrups from starch
Catalase	Bacteria	Converts hydrogen peroxideto water and oxygen	Drinks – as a preservative in soft drinks Rubber – in the conversion of latex to foam rubber
Cellulase	Fungi	Breaks down cellulose	Agriculture – to produce animal feed from straw Drinks – to increase the yield of fruit juice from fruits
Isomerase	Bacteria	Changes glucose into fructose	Syrup – to convert glucose into fructose
Lactase	Fungi (yeast)	Breaks down lactose	Dairy – to remove lactose from milk
Lipase	Fungi	Breaks down fats and oils	Dairy – to ripen cheeses Detergent – to break down fatty stains
Protease	Bacteria/fungi	Breaks down proteins	Food – to predigest proteins in baby food Baking – to reduce gluten in flour Brewing – to remove cloudiness in beer Detergent – to break down protein based stains Medicine – to clean wounds and remove blood clots

Table 1 *Some applications of enzymes.*

Biotechnology and traditional processes

Micro-organisms have been used for centuries in the traditional processes of brewing, bread making and yoghurt production. Whilst the essentials of these have changed very little, new techniques such as genetic engineering are making them more efficient and increasing productivity.

Brewing

Brewing of beer is based on the **anaerobic fermentation** of sugars by yeast. Barley provides starch and the enzyme amylase. Amylase converts the starch into sugars which the yeast can use. An outline of the full process is shown in figure 1.

Genetic engineering is used to produce strains of yeast which can produce amylase to make use of cheaper starch sources. It is also difficult to produce high alcohol content beers because yeast is killed at alcohol levels of 6.5%. Again, genetic engineering may one day provide a solution.

Baking bread

Baking bread is also based on the anaerobic fermentation of sugars by yeast. In this case flour provides starch and enzymes. The yeast supplies several enzymes, some to breakdown the sugars and produce the carbon dioxide which makes the dough rise, and others which alter the flour proteins giving the bread a better texture. An outline of the process is shown in figure 2.

Genetic engineering is used to produce yeast strains, which can make the enzyme amylase. This helps the yeast to use the starch in flour to produce fermentable sugar. Yeast strains which can ferment sugars, and produce the carbon dioxide gas to make the dough rise at lower temperatures are also being produced.

Yoghurt production

Yoghurt is produced by the fermentation of milk sugars by a mixture of bacteria. This mixture contains two kinds of bacteria, each of equal importance in the process because each one produces growth factors needed by the other. The bacteria are added as a **'starter culture'**. Genetic engineering is being used to produce better strains of bacteria for this starter culture.

The characteristic consistency of yoghurt is produced by the coagulation of milk proteins. This is caused by the lactic acid produced during fermentation of lactose. The flavour is mainly due to another product of fermentation called acetaldehyde.

New sources of food

One of the more recent applications of biotechnology has been the production of new foods, in particular, new sources of protein, which take a lot of energy to produce by traditional means. There are two main developments:

- **Single cell protein** (SCP) is protein produced by micro-organisms such as bacteria, fungi and algae. This is a particularly exciting source of food because of the high protein content and rapid reproductive rate of many micro-organisms. For example, one bacterium can give rise to over a million others in as little as 24 hours, and 80% of this new growth is protein.

  The main SCP currently available for human consumption is a **mycoprotein** (fungal protein) sold as Quorn. This can be textured, shaped and flavoured to taste like beef, chicken or lamb (see figure 3).

- **Textured vegetable protein** (TVP). Plant protein has often been dismissed as a good source of human protein because plants generally contain less protein than animals and much of it is deficient in some of the essential amino acids. However, soya bean protein is an exception and is now being sold as an alternative to animal protein (see table 1).

Genetic engineering can of course be used to increase the yields of both SCP and TVP.

What are genetically modified foods?

Genetically modified (GM) foods are foods which:

- have been altered by genetic engineering, e.g. tomatoes which have had a gene from an Arctic fish spliced into them to make them frost resistant

- contain ingredients which come form organisms which have been altered by genetic engineering, e.g. soya flour from soya beans which have had a gene inserted to make them resistant to a herbicide.

Animal/plant	Protein (% dry weight)	Protein yield (kg/ha)
Beef	68	25
Pork	35	30
Chicken	50	40
Sunflower	32	380
Soya bean	43	510

Table 1 *Soya is a good alternative to meats as it has a high protein content and a high land area to protein yield.*

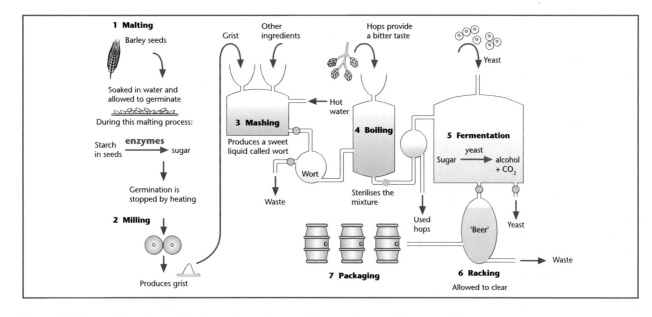

Figure 1 *The methods used to brew beer have changed very little over the years.*

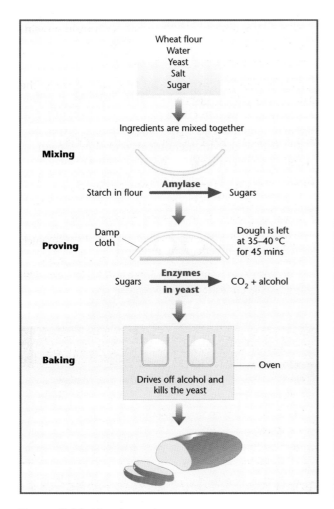

Figure 2 *Making bread.*

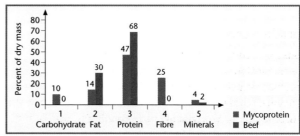

Figure 3 *Mycoprotein compares favourably to beef.*

What do **you** know?

You should now be able to:

- Draw a flow diagram to outline how bread is made.
- Explain the roles of the flour and yeast in the process.
- Explain how genetic engineering may eventually improve the bread making process.
- Describe in outline the stages in brewing beer.
- Explain why it is difficult to produce a high alcohol beer and suggest how this may be solved.
- Explain what is responsible for the characteristic texture and flavour of yoghurt.
- Explain what single cell protein is and comment on its nutritional value.
- Explain what GM foods are.

Selective breeding

Many of the recent exciting advances in agriculture have been due to biotechnology and, in particular, genetic engineering (GE).

For years agriculturalists have tried to improve crop plants and animals by selecting ones with the most desirable characteristics and interbreeding them. This is both time consuming and unpredictable. For example, it has taken hundreds of years to produce modern varieties of wheat and involved a lot of setbacks as useful genes have been lost in the attempt to introduce new ones. Another problem is that only organisms of the same, or closely related, species (plants only) can interbreed, so limiting the available **gene pool**.

Genetic engineering has taken the guesswork (and time) out of interbreeding. If a useful gene can be identified, it can usually be isolated and transferred into another organism, simply adding this characteristic to the organism. It is even possible to transfer genes from unrelated species (which would stand no chance of interbreeding in nature). This is called **transgenics** and the organisms are called **transgenic organisms**.

Some examples of these applications are described below.

Improving crop plants

Moving genes has enabled us to produce:

- **frost resistant crops** such as strawberries and tomatoes

- fruit and vegetables with a **longer shelf life** allowing us to transport them, e.g. tomatoes

- cereals which can **grow in high salt conditions**, such as land reclaimed from the sea

- crop plants which are **resistant to viral, bacterial and fungal diseases**, e.g. tomatoes and tobacco which are resistant to tobacco mosaic virus

- crop plants which **produce their own natural insecticide** against a specific pest, e.g. tobacco against caterpillars

- crop plants which are **resistant to certain herbicides** so the whole field can be sprayed without affecting the crop, e.g. soya beans

- crop plants such as oil seed rape and wheat, which have **increased yields**.

These new techniques are environmentally friendly in that they reduce the reliance on pesticides and allow us to make better use of our food, and even reduce food shortages. Figure 1 illustrates the technique of gene transfer in plants.

So far it has not been possible to transfer nitrogen fixing genes from bacteria to plants, but once this is accomplished, it will reduce the need for fertilisers and the pollution this causes.

Can farm animals be improved?

Animals are being made healthier by being given **vaccines** against fatal diseases such as foot and mouth. These new vaccines are produced by bacteria growing in fermenters. An anti-worming agent first isolated from fungi is now also being produced by bacteria.

When cows are given a hormone called **bovine somatotropin** (BST), they produce more milk and leaner meat. Cows produce this BST naturally, but only after calving. The gene responsible for production of BST has now been isolated and transferred into bacteria. It can be produced and given to cows at any time. The result is more milk and leaner meat. Figure 2 illustrates the technique of gene transfer in plants.

Micropropagation

Micropropagation, also called **tissue culture**, describes the technique used to **clone** plants from pieces of plant tissue or individual cells. The plant extract is grown on a solid medium containing nutrients and plant growth regulators such as **auxins**. The new plants are exact genetic copies of the parent plant, making the technique very useful for mass production of ornamental and rare plants.

The technique is also used to grow plants from cells which have been genetically modified.

What do **you** know?

You should now be able to:
- Explain the term transgenic organism.
- Describe the technique for inserting foreign genes into crop plants.
- List 7 reasons why you would use this technique.
- Describe how biotechnology is helping to improve farm animals.
- Explain how foreign genes can be inserted into animals.

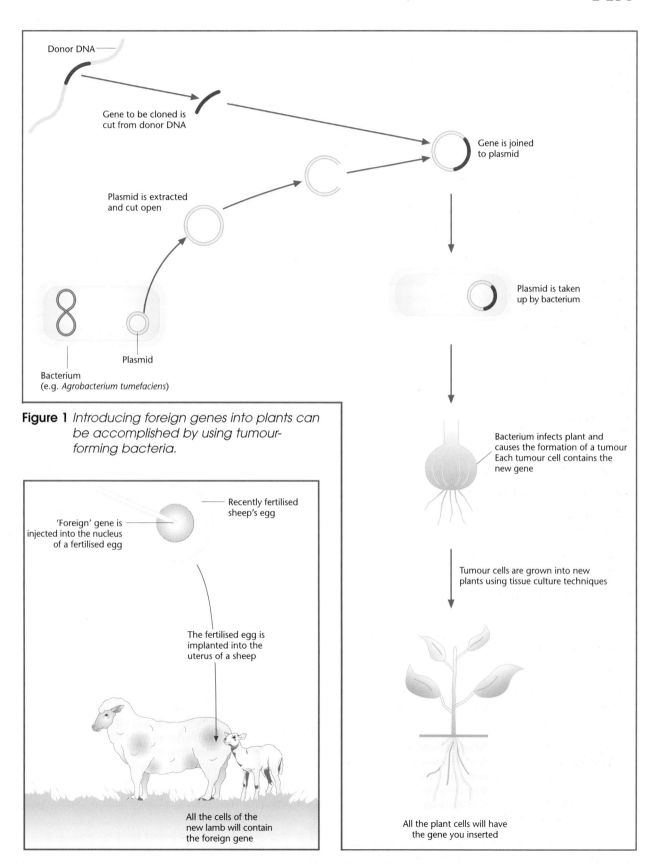

Donor DNA

Gene to be cloned is cut from donor DNA

Gene is joined to plasmid

Plasmid is extracted and cut open

Plasmid is taken up by bacterium

Bacterium
(e.g. *Agrobacterium tumefaciens*)

Plasmid

Figure 1 *Introducing foreign genes into plants can be accomplished by using tumour-forming bacteria.*

Bacterium infects plant and causes the formation of a tumour Each tumour cell contains the new gene

Recently fertilised sheep's egg

'Foreign' gene is injected into the nucleus of a fertilised egg

The fertilised egg is implanted into the uterus of a sheep

Tumour cells are grown into new plants using tissue culture techniques

All the cells of the new lamb will contain the foreign gene

All the plant cells will have the gene you inserted

Figure 2 *Introducing foreign genes into animals.*

Human insulin from bacteria

One form of **diabetes mellitus** is controlled by daily injections of insulin. Until recently this insulin was obtained from the pancreas of pigs which had been slaughtered for meat. However, the yields were low and because the insulin was not of human origin it often caused side effects.

By using genetic engineering, it is now possible to insert a synthetic human insulin gene into the bacterium *E. coli* so that it produces human insulin. The process is similar to that described in chapter 14.3.

Human growth hormone (HGH), used to treat children who are not growing properly, is produced in much the same way.

Commercial production of antibiotics

It has been known for a long time that some micro-organisms produce chemicals that inhibit the growth of other micro-organisms. We call these **antibiotics** (chapter 13.10). However, the commercial production of antibiotics is relatively new, having been developed over the last 50 years or so.

The antibiotic **penicillin** is produced in a batch fermentation process by the mould *Penicillium*, which grows on the waste produced from soaking corn (see figure 1).

Many micro-organisms are becoming resistant to antibiotics (see page 150), especially ones which have been established for some time, such as penicillin. Genetic engineering is being used to produce modified forms to which the bacteria have no resistance. Enzymes produced by enzyme technology are even used to modify the antibiotic after it has been produced.

Better vaccines

Vaccines (chapter 13.9) are normally produced from weakened or dead forms of the pathogen. The problem has always been getting enough of the pathogen, but now new methods are being used to obtain these. For example, viruses such as influenza, polio, and herpes can be produced by animal cells grown in **tissue cultures**. Figure 2 shows how a vaccine for Hepatitis B can be produced by yeast cells.

Designer antibodies

Normally antibodies can only be produced when antigens enter an organism (chapter 13.8). Until recently any attempt to grow the antibody producing lymphocytes outside an organism have failed. But now modern **cell fusion** techniques have successfully combined the lymphocyte with a cancer cell. The hybrid cell, called a **hybridoma** can be cloned in culture vessels and made to produce antibodies. Since all the cells are the same (clones), the antibodies they produce will all be the same. They are called **monoclonal antibodies** (see figure 3).

The production of monoclonal antibodies is one of the most exciting developments in biotechnology in recent years. They can be made to respond to almost any antigen and are therefore often called designer antibodies. The uses include:

- Diagnosis of specific diseases by detecting the presence of the antigen, e.g. chlamydia.

- Locating cancer cells/tumours by attaching to the antigens on the cancer cell surface. It is hoped that in the future they can be used to deliver drugs to these cells.

- Pregnancy testing by responding to hormones produced during the early stages of pregnancy.

- Manufacturing of new vaccines.

- Destroying the specific T lymphocytes which attack transplanted cells. This reduces the need for immunosuppressant drugs and leaves the rest of the immune system intact.

What is gene therapy?

Gene therapy is a technique which replaces a faulty gene with a normal one. This restores the normal cell function and thereby eliminates the disease or disorder. The gene therapy techniques used to treat cystic fibrosis and severe combined immune deficiency syndrome are described on page 222.

What do **you** know?

You should now be able to:

- Suggest 2 reasons why it is better to produce human insulin by genetically engineering bacteria.
- Describe in outline how bacteria can be used to produce human insulin.
- Outline the fermentation process used to produce penicillin and when and how the penicillin should be extracted.
- Explain how genetic engineering is helping to improve the process of antibiotic production.
- Outline the process used to produce a vaccine for Hepatitis B.
- Explain what monoclonal antibodies are and list some of their uses.
- Explain how gene therapy is helping cure cystic fibrosis.

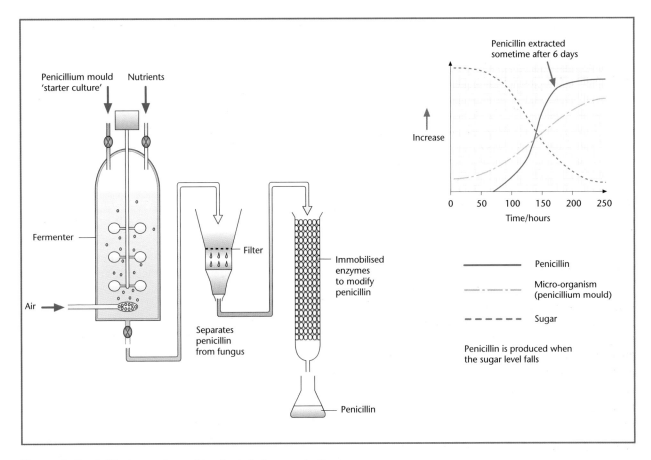

Figure 1 *Penicillin is produced by batch fermentation.*

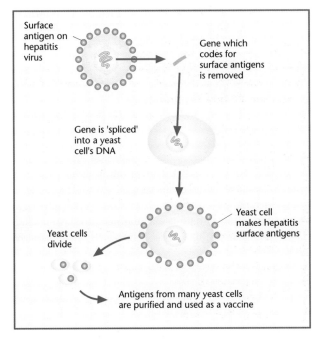

Figure 2 *Vaccines can now be produced by genetic engineering.*

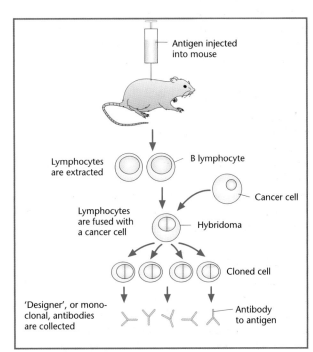

Figure 3 *Making designer antibodies.*

Chapter 14: Questions

1 a A student decided to investigate the connection between houseflies and disease. The following shows the main stages of an experiment that was carried out.

A – Sterilisation of food medium and glass dishes.

B – Preparation of a food medium containing nutrients suitable for the growth of micro-organisms.

C – Housefly placed on surface of food for several minutes.

D – Food medium melted by heating and poured into dishes. Allowed to set to a jelly.

These four stages are not given in the correct order. Give the correct order using the letters A, B, C and D. *(1 mark)*

b Suggest a suitable control for this experiment. *(1 mark)*

c The diagram below shows the appearance of the surface of the food medium on which the housefly was placed. This result was obtained after the dish had been left in a warm place for several days.

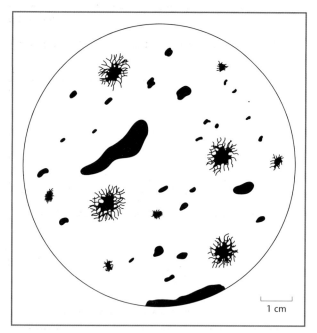

1 cm

How would you expect the result of the control experiment to differ from that shown in the diagram? *(1 mark)*
(SEG June 1992)

2 Genes can be transferred from one species to another by genetic engineering. The diagram shows how the gene for human growth hormone (HGH) can be put into bacteria. The bacteria can then be used to manufacture the hormone. E_1 and E_2 are two different enzymes.

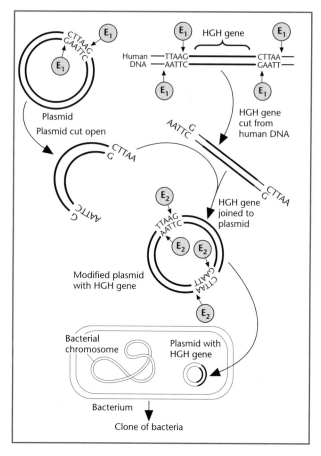

a i The HGH gene and the bacterial plasmid are made of DNA. Give a brief description of a DNA molecule. You may include a diagram if you wish. *(4 marks)*

ii Why is it important to use the same enzyme to break open the plasmid and to cut the human DNA? *(2 marks)*

iii The diagram shows that a clone of bacterial cells will be formed. Will all the bacteria in the clone be genetically identical? Explain your answer. *(2 marks)*

b In humans and in other mammals, growth hormone is made by the pituitary gland. Suggest two advantages of making growth hormone by genetic engineering rather than extracting it from the pituitary glands of slaughtered mammals like sheep or cattle. *(2 marks)*
(SEG June 1998)

3 DNA is the substance which forms genes.

a i Describe the structure of DNA. You may answer this question by a fully labelled diagram. *(5 marks)*

ii Describe how a DNA molecule is copied during cell division. You may answer this question by a fully labelled diagram. *(5 marks)*

b i Give one example of a vaccine produced by genetic engineering. *(1 mark)*

ii Copy and complete the diagram to explain how this vaccine is produced. *(3 marks)*

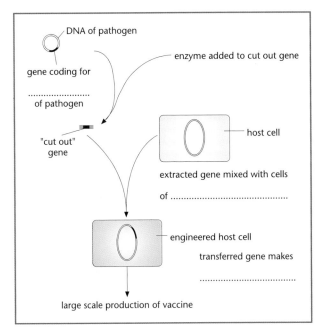

DNA of pathogen

gene coding for

....

of pathogen

enzyme added to cut out gene

"cut out" gene

host cell

extracted gene mixed with cells

of ....

engineered host cell

transferred gene makes

....

large scale production of vaccine

c Genetic engineering can be used to transfer genes to the cells of an organism at an early stage of their development. Suggest two reasons why this may be done. *(2 marks)*

(NEAB June 1997)

4 Penicillin is an antibiotic produced by fermentation. The graph shows changes in the growth of the microorganism, the amount of sugar and the amount of penicillin produced during fermentation.

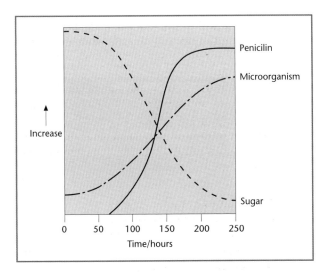

Increase

Penicilin

Microorganism

Sugar

0   50   100   150   200   250

Time/hours

a Name the microorganism used to produce penicillin. *(1 mark)*

b i What is the relationship between the growth of the microorganism and the amount of sugar? *(1 mark)*

ii Give one reason for your answer *(1 mark)*

c At what time should the penicillin be removed from the fermenter?
Give a reason for your answer. *(2 marks)*

d How is penicillin separated from the contents of the fermenter? *(2 marks)*

e i From the following list of diseases choose two that can be treated using antibiotics. *(2 marks)*

ii Explain why the other two diseases cannot be treated by antibiotics. *(2 marks)*

tuberculosis cholera rabies influenza

f Some disease organisms have become resistant to the effect of certain antibiotics. This means that these antibiotics no longer kill these disease organisms. Resistance is due to a change in the characteristics of the disease organism.

i Suggest how resistance could have arisen in the disease organisms. *(1 mark)*

ii Suggest one way in which the development of resistance might be prevented. *(1 mark)*

(NEAB June 1999)

5 The diagram below shows the main stages in making bread.

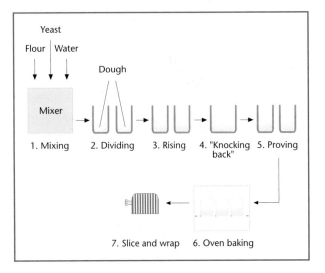

Yeast

Flour   Water

Dough

Mixer

1. Mixing   2. Dividing   3. Rising   4. "Knocking back"   5. Proving

7. Slice and wrap   6. Oven baking

a Describe how the yeast makes the bread rise. *(3 marks)*

b The main constituent of flour is starch.
Yeast needs to absorb sugar.
Flour contains some enzymes, but bakers often add extra enzymes to the flour.

i What type of enzyme would you expect the bakers to add? *(1 mark)*

ii Suggest why this enzyme is added. *(1 mark)*

(NEAB Sample Assessment)

15 Ecosystems

Ecology is the study of living things in relation to their environment. The planet Earth is too large to be studied as a single environment, so smaller sections of it, called ecosystems are studied. In this chapter you will learn all about ecosystems, what they are, how the organisms interact with one another and with their environment. You will also learn about the underlying processes that maintain ecosystems and just how easy it is to disrupt these.

After you have worked through this chapter, you should be able to:

- Describe the components of and interactions within an ecosystem.

- Explain the process of succession.

- List the nutritional types in an ecosystem and describe their feeding relationships.

- Describe how energy enters and flows through an ecosystem.

- Describe the processes involved in recycling the nutrients in an ecosystem.

Organic farming - a managed ecosystem

Modern farming methods may produce a lot of food on the limited land available, but at what cost.

- Soil is being degraded by growing the same crop year after year.

- Species are declining as habitats such as hedgerows are removed. Between 1970 and 1990, 24 of the 28 species of farmland bird disappeared (chapter 16.3).

- The gene pool of crops and livestock is narrowing as 'superbreeds' take over. Pig farming in the UK is dominated by just two breeds.

- Many of our waterways are heavily polluted with nitrates due to the overuse of fertilisers.

- Animal populations are declining because of the use of chemical pesticides. These also leave poisonous residues on food.

- More and more bacteria are becoming resistant to antibiotics because they are being used as growth promoters (see page 150).

- Livestock have to suffer horrendous conditions created by the intensive rearing techniques.

Not at all eco-friendly!

How is organic farming different?

Organic framing is a method of food production which does not use artificial fertilisers or chemical pesticides, uses crop rotation rather than monoculture and inputs only those natural resources available locally. It makes room for the other organisms within the ecosystem and uses humane production techniques for livestock rearing. Organic farming could be renamed **ecological farming** because it is extremely eco-friendly. It is also **sustainable** in that

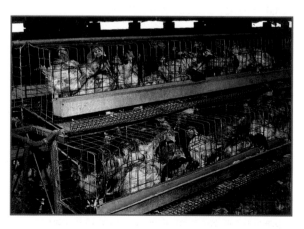

Figure 1 *Chickens in a battery house.*

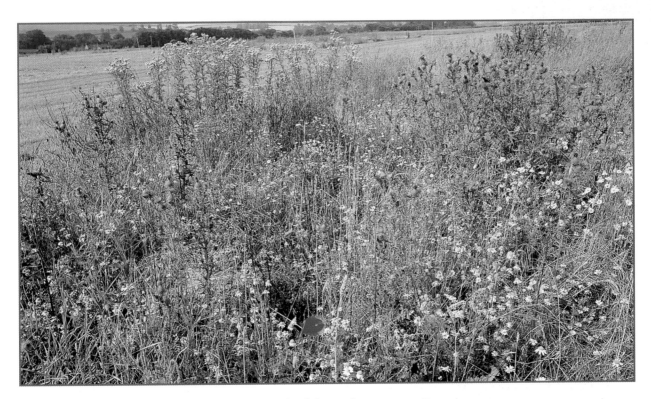

Figure 2 *Land that has been set aside so that wild species can continue to grow.*

it utilises techniques which do not deplete the natural resources or disrupt the ecological cycles which replenish them. The farm is treated as an ecosystem in which the soil, minerals, humus, micro-organisms, animals, plants and humans all interact to create a stable self-supporting unit which should last forever.

Features of organic farming

Some organic farming methods are outlined below.

- Food is produced using only the natural materials available locally, e.g. fertiliser from the farm animals.

- Other nutrients, e.g. minerals, are provided in a form which are made available to the plants by the action of the soil micro-organisms, and cannot be washed out of the soil into the waterways.

- A useful level of soil micro-organisms is maintained by adding organic matter.

- Each field is sown with a different crop each year to prevent the build up of pests and stop disease becoming established.

- Legumes are used as part of the crop rotation cycle to increase the nitrate content of the soil.

- Crops with a natural resistance to pests and disease are used rather than 'superbreeds'.

- Biological control methods replace pesticides, i.e. the natural predators of pests are encouraged.

- Areas of land are set aside to preserve and create habitats for wildlife, e.g. hedgerows, field margins, ponds, woods (see figure 2).

- Livestock are allowed to roam freely and are fed on organically grown fodder. The use of antibiotics and other drugs is kept to a minimum and never used as growth promoters.

Are there drawbacks to organic farming?

The main disadvantage is expense. Organic farming is costly, mostly due to the high labour costs, but also because less food is produced in the same amount of land. This cost is passed onto the consumer who must choose whether or not pay to protect the environment.

What determines where an organism lives?

The place where an organism lives is called its **habitat**. The habitat it selects depends on many things, for example, where its food is, where the best shelter is or where it is safe from predators. Examples of habitats include ponds, woods, seashores and grassland.

The different organisms that live in each of these form a **community**. Within this community, the organisms of a particular species are known as a **population**. The populations of organisms that live in a pond will make up the pond community, and the organisms that live in a wood will make up the woodland community.

Each habitat will also have its own physical environment made up of all the non-living factors such as the soil, water and temperature. These may vary within the habitat.

What is an ecosystem?

An **ecosystem** consists of a community of organisms living in a particular area (habitat), with its own physical environment, all interacting as a self-contained unit.

The inhabitable part of the Earth, the **biosphere**, is composed of many different types of natural ecosystems. Most of these are balanced, stable and self-supporting, having their own feeding structure and nutrient cycles. Unfortunately, human interference, all too often, can upset these.

The pond ecosystem

The pond ecosystem illustrated in figure 1 is an example of a natural ecosystem. It has its own community made up of all the plants, animals, fungi and micro-organisms that live there. This forms the **biotic component** of the ecosystem.

It also has a physical environment formed from the water, soil, rocks and stones, temperature, the oxygen dissolved in the water, the aspect, etc. This is the **abiotic component** of the ecosystem.

The biotic and abiotic components constantly affect each other. For example, some of the organisms will use others as food, or excrete wastes into the water which will alter the physical environment. If the temperature goes up, the amount of dissolved oxygen in the water will fall. These interactions generally work for the benefit of the organisms and result in a **balanced**, **stable**, **self-supporting unit**, i.e. the pond ecosystem.

Managed ecosystems

We as humans do not just live in any one ecosystem, we interact with many. By our farming practices, we change ecosystems to produce food for our consumption. Traditional farming methods strive to do this without disturbing the delicate balance within the ecosystems, but unfortunately many modern farming practices are disruptive. The consequences are described in chapter 16.3.

We sometimes create our own **artificial ecosystems** to produce food, e.g. the greenhouse. Greenhouse ecosystems have the advantage that we can manipulate both the biotic and abiotic components to maximise food production. These of course, unlike natural ecosystems, are not stable or well balanced. It is however, possible to create a fish pond or aquarium which is self-sustaining.

Interactions within ecosystems

The organisms within an ecosystem will be affected by many things. Most will be food for other organisms. They will compete for living space, shelter, mates and so on. The organisms will also be affected by many aspects of their environment. Plants, for example, can not live where there is insufficient light. Many animals can not withstand extremes of temperature or humidity.

The organisms will also affect their environment. For example, animals will excrete waste, enriching the soil with nutrients. Plants will remove water from the soil, making it drier.

All these interactions may cause changes to the habitat and the community which lives there. This could result in one ecosystem changing into another, for example, a pond turning into a wood. It could also result in an ecosystem developing from a purely physical environment, such as bare rock.

Can an ecosystem develop from rock?

The bare rock is first colonised by lichens, then mosses as more water is retained. Weathering will break the rock down into small particles, which together with the nutrients from the dead bodies of the organisms forms soil. With soil present, the grasses and ferns start to become established followed by small shrubs and eventually trees.

Along with the plants come the animals. Just small insects and mites to start with, then the worms and other invertebrates, and eventually mammals. The full process is shown in figure 2.

This series of changes taking place, one after another, is called **succession**. Each new species will alter the environment in such a way that other new species can move in, thereby changing the community. The final stable community is called the **climax community**. In the UK, this is generally oak woodland.

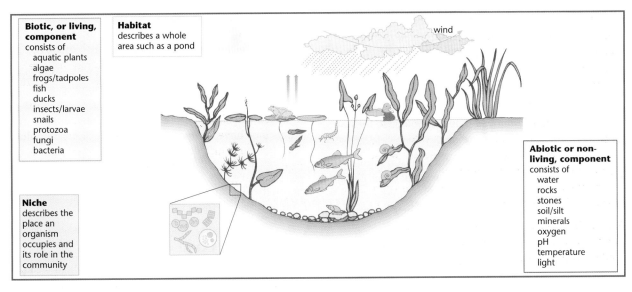

Figure 1 *A pond ecosystem.*

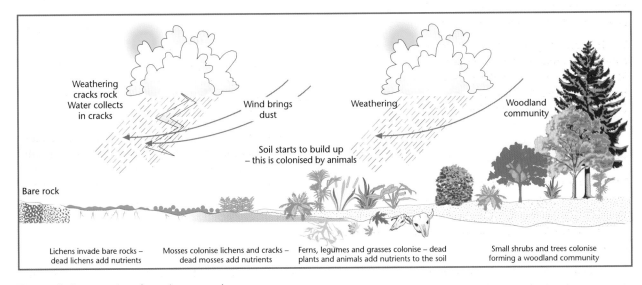

Figure 2 *Succession from bare rock.*

What do **you** know?

You should now be able to:

- Explain the terms habitat, population and community.

- Describe the term ecosystem.

- List the biotic and abiotic components of a pond ecosystem.

- Explain why an ecosystem such as the pond is described as a balanced, self-supporting unit.

- Describe 3 ways the organisms in a pond ecosystem will interact (affect) with one another.

- Describe 3 ways the organisms in a pond ecosystem will interact with their environment.

- Describe how these sort of interactions can result in succession from bare rock to woodland.

How do the organisms get their food?

Organisms obtain the food they need in two ways:

- Green plants (and some bacteria) make it from simple substances and energy which they can obtain from their environment. The process is called **photosynthesis**. Green plants are the producers of the ecosystem. The food they produce ultimately supplies energy to the rest of the organisms in the ecosystem.

- Animals can not make food, so they must obtain it by eating ready made sources in the form of other living organisms or dead organic matter from these organisms. The animals are therefore the **consumers** in the ecosystem.

A balanced ecosystem will always contain a mixture of producer and consumer organisms.

What is photosynthesis?

Photosynthesis is the process by which the green parts of plants make glucose. It requires:

- **carbon dioxide**, usually obtained directly from the air
- **water**, obtained via the roots from the soil
- **light energy** to power the reactions, usually obtained from sunlight
- **chlorophyll**, a green pigment which absorbs light energy.

The process takes place in oval shaped structures called **chloroplasts**. These are in the cytoplasm of most leaf cells. Although really a very complex series of chemical reactions, photosynthesis can be summarised by the equation in figure 1. The oxygen produced is released into the air. The glucose produced is used in three ways:

- some is used by the plants cells in respiration to **provide energy** for the plant to grow, reproduce, etc.

- some is converted to substances needed for **growth**, such as cellulose for cell walls, lipids for cell membranes and amino acids for proteins. Amino acid production also requires a source of nitrogen which the plant can usually obtain from its environment (chapter 15.4).

- most is converted to starch or lipid and **stored** for use later.

The consumers

Any organism which eats another organism, is called a consumer. Animals which eat plants, are called **primary consumers**. They are also **herbivores**.

Animals which eat the herbivores are called **secondary consumers**, and animals which eat these are called **tertiary consumers**. Animals which prey (predators) on other animals are also **carnivores**. Some animals eat both palnts and animals and are called **omnivores**.

These different feeding relationships can be summarised as a **food chain** (see figure 2). The different feeding levels are called **trophic levels**. Often, the same organism will crop up in several food chains linking the chains together to form a **food web**.

A special kind of consumer is the **parasite**. A parasite can feed anywhere in the food web because it lives in or on another living organism and removes food from it, usually without killing it (chapter 13.4).

Decomposers and detritivores

Decomposers are the bacteria and fungi which feed on dead organic matter such as dead plants and animals, fallen leaves or excreted waste. They usually live in or on the organic matter, secreting digestive enzymes into it, and then absorbing the products of digestion. In this way the organic matter disappears. This method of feeding is called **saprophytic nutrition** and the organisms are called **saprophytes**. Their action brings about decay and decomposition.

Detritivores are small animals which feed on small pieces of decaying organic matter called detritus.

All ecosystems need decomposers and detritivores because they stop dead organic matter building up, and their feeding methods help recycle useful minerals. They are also food sources for other consumers.

What do **you** know?

You should now be able to:

- Explain the difference between a producer and a consumer.
- Write a word equation for photosynthesis and explain why only green plants can photosynthesise.
- Describe what happens to the glucose made in photosynthesis.
- Describe the different trophic levels in a food chain.
- Draw 3 different food chains from a pond ecosystem and link these together to form a food web.
- Describe what decomposers are and how they feed.
- Explain why decomposers are such essential organisms in ecosystems.

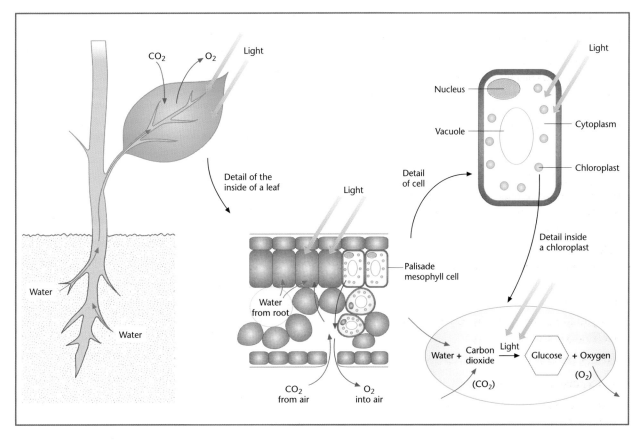

Figure 1 *Photosynthesis takes place within the chloroplasts in the mesophyll cells of a leaf.*

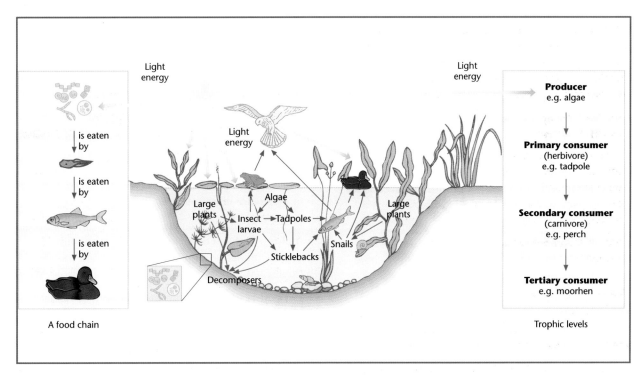

Figure 2 *The feeding structure of a pond ecosystem.*

15.3 Energy and ecosystems

Energy requirements

All living things need energy. They need this energy to power life processes such as:

- **growth and repair**, i.e. to build new proteins, fats, carbohydrates, etc.
- **movement**, i.e. movement of substances in and out of cells or around an organism and locomotion
- **reproduction**, to produce sperms, eggs or pollen grains
- **excretion** of metabolic wastes
- **heating effects**, i.e. many animals need to keep warm.

They get this energy in the form of food. Food is a way of transferring energy as well as materials. The producers (green plants) convert the energy from sunlight into the chemical energy of food. The consumers obtain this energy when they eat the plants and other organisms. Energy is therefore passed through the food web in the form of food.

Energy transfers

Only a very small amount of the light energy striking a green plant (less than 2%) is actually absorbed by the chlorophyll in the plant and used in photosynthesis to make food. Some of this food is used as material for growth, and will therefore increase the mass (**biomass**) of the producer. The rest is used in respiration to provide energy for its life processes.

When the producer is eaten by a consumer, again only part of the food is used for new growth, to increase the biomass of the consumer. Much of the food is used in respiration to provide energy for movement, excretion, transporting materials around the body, keeping the body warm and so on. This energy is 'lost' at this stage in the food chain. It is not really lost, but used and therefore, no longer available to the other consumers. Energy is also 'lost' when one consumer is eaten by another consumer (see figure 3).

Every time an organism eats some food, some of this food is not digested and passes out with the faeces. This provides food and energy for the decomposers.

The 'loss' of energy at each feeding stage puts a natural limit on the number of links a food chain can have. When you get to the top carnivores, there is very little energy left to pass on. This is why there are fewer of these than the smaller organisms at other trophic levels. Most food chains have only three or four links.

What happens to the food you eat?

When you eat food, only a small proportion of it is used to produce new tissue, that is to increase your size. Some of it will be lost in your faeces, but most of it will be used to provide energy for your daily living. When the energy in the food is released in respiration, about 50% of it is turned into heat. This heat enters your blood and is used to warm your body. It is the heat for your 'central heating'.

When you reach adulthood and have stopped growing, your food only has to supply materials for repair and energy to power your daily activities. If you overeat at this time of your life, you will continue to grow as the extra energy is stored as fat!

Humans and food chains

Humans use both plants and animals as food, but which is the most efficient in terms of energy used to produce it and energy supplied? For the same area of land, you can produce a lot more crops than meat. In fact you can produce ten times as much. This is because you are cutting out a trophic level and therefore not losing so much energy as figure 2 shows. So in countries with food shortages, it makes sense to grow more crops rather than graze lots of animals.

Ecological pyramids

Ecological pyramids are a visual way of displaying the feeding relationships and structure in an ecosystem. There are three kinds (see figure 1):

- **Pyramids of numbers** show the relative number of organisms at each trophic level in an area at a particular time. Generally, as you move from one trophic level to the next, the numbers decrease. This is partly because of the 'losses' in energy during the transfer and partly due to the 'higher' consumers being larger. There are exceptions to this as illustrated in figure 1.

- **Pyramids of biomass** show the total biomass of all the living organisms at each trophic level in a particular area (or unit area, e.g. m^2), at a particular time. Dry mass (all the water removed) is usually used in preference to wet mass.

  Biomass diagrams are nearly always pyramid shaped, showing that you always need a larger amount of organic matter to support the organisms in the next trophic level.

- **Pyramids of energy** show the amount of energy converted to biomass (productivity), at each trophic level over a period of time, e.g. a year. This can be used to calculate energy transfers (and losses) between trophic levels. It can also be used to show growth from one year to the next.

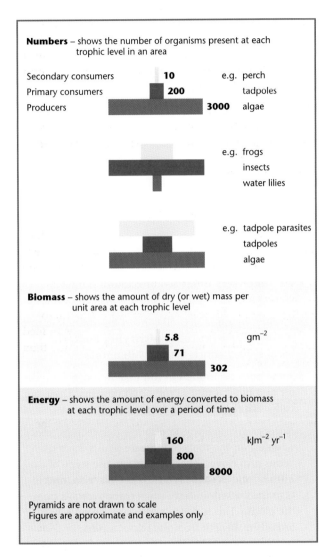

Numbers – shows the number of organisms present at each trophic level in an area

Secondary consumers	**10**	e.g. perch
Primary consumers	**200**	tadpoles
Producers	**3000**	algae

e.g. frogs
insects
water lilies

e.g. tadpole parasites
tadpoles
algae

Biomass – shows the amount of dry (or wet) mass per unit area at each trophic level

5.8 gm^{-2}
71
302

Energy – shows the amount of energy converted to biomass at each trophic level over a period of time

160 $kJm^{-2} yr^{-1}$
800
8000

Pyramids are not drawn to scale
Figures are approximate and examples only

Figure 1 *Ecological pyramids are used to show feeding relationships and energy flow.*

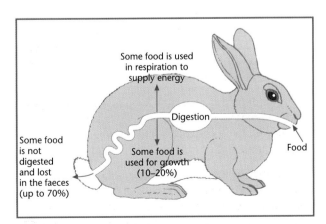

Figure 2 *What happens to food after it has been eaten.*

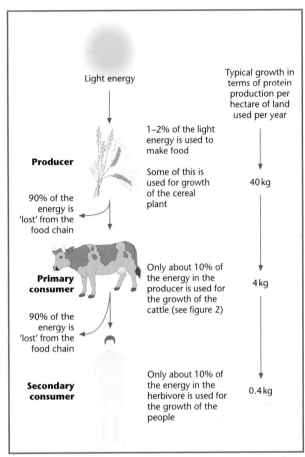

Figure 3 *How energy passes through a food chain.*

What do **you** know?

You should now be able to:

- List 5 ways we make use of the energy in our food.
- Explain how energy enters a food chain.
- Draw a food chain to show how this energy is passed from one organism to another.
- Explain what happens to the food eaten by a consumer.
- Explain why there is a loss of energy at each trophic level.
- Discuss why, in energy terms, humans would be better eating more plants rather than animals.
- Explain where decomposers get their energy from.
- Draw examples of the 3 kinds of ecological pyramids and explain what they show.
- Explain how pyramids of energy can be used to calculate productivity and growth.

How do plants keep producing food?

Plants must get all the substances they need to make food from their environment. For example, they get carbon dioxide from the air, and nitrogen (as nitrates) and water from the soil. So why doesn't this supply run out? As these substances are removed by the plants, they are put back by other organisms such as the decomposers. This is called recycling. All the basic nutrients which green plants need to make their food are recycled in this way.

How is water recycled?

Water is crucial to all living things, not just plants. It also plays an important role in the recycling of other nutrients. The way water is recycled is described in detail in chapter 13.12.

Humans can affect the water cycle in several ways.

How is carbon dioxide recycled?

Carbon dioxide is recycled as part of the carbon cycle. This involves carbon-containing organisms and materials:

- the carbon compounds in plants, animals and decomposers
- the carbon compounds in dead organisms and excreta
- fossil fuels such as coal, gas and oil
- as carbon dioxide gas in the air.

The main processes involved in recycling carbon dioxide are:

- respiration releases carbon dioxide into the air
- photosynthesis removes carbon dioxide from the air
- combustion (burning) releases carbon dioxide into the air.

The links between all these elements are shown in figure 1.

How do humans affect the carbon cycle?

Humans can affect the recycling of carbon in two main ways:

- by the burning fossil fuels, such as coal, oil and gas, we increase the amount of carbon dioxide released into the air
- by deforestation (massive removal of trees) we reduce the amount of carbon dioxide being taken out of the air.

The possible effects of these practices on the ecosystems are described in chapter 16.

How is nitrogen recycled?

Animals get the nitrogen they need from eating other organisms. Plants get nitrogen from the soil, but they can only take it up into their roots in the form of **nitrate**. Soil nitrates are replenished in several ways:

- through the high temperatures created by **lightning** which can combine gaseous nitrogen and oxygen in the air. This dissolves in rain to form nitrates.
- by artificial **fertilisers** containing nitrates that can be added to the soil.
- by the activities of bacteria and fungi, as follows:

  1 **Decomposers** in the soil breakdown nitrogen compounds in organic wastes and release ammonia.

  2 Bacteria living in the soil convert this ammonia into nitrates. These are called **nitrifying bacteria** because they enrich the soil with nitrates.

  3 Some bacteria in the soil can take nitrogen from the air and build it into nitrates and proteins. These are called **nitrogen fixing bacteria**.

  Nitrogen fixing bacteria also live in swellings (root nodules) on the roots of **legume** plants, such as beans and clover. These plants can use some of the nitrates and proteins made by the bacteria, and in turn the bacteria receive some carbohydrates from the plants. This is called **symbiosis** because both organisms benefit from the relationship.

  Unfortunately, there are also some bacteria living in the soil which convert nitrates back into atmospheric nitrogen and oxygen. These are called **de-nitrifying bacteria** because they remove nitrates from the soil. They are particularly active in waterlogged soil.

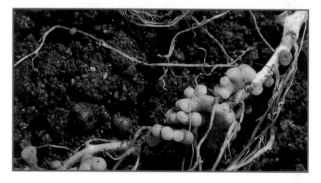

Figure 3 *Nodules on legume roots contain nitrogen fixing bacteria.*

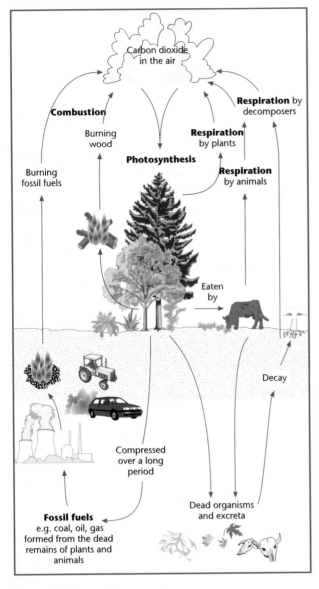

Figure 1 *The carbon cycle.*

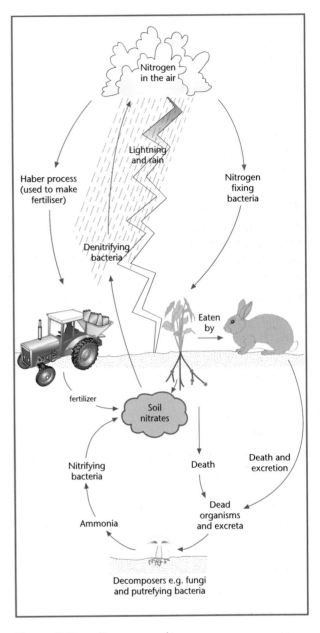

Figure 2 *The nitrogen cycle.*

What do **you** know?

You should now be able to:

- Review the water cycle and explain how the activities of humans can affect it.
- List the compounds in plants and animals which contain carbon and nitrogen.
- List the other sources of carbon in the biosphere.
- Draw a diagram to show how carbon is recycled between organisms and name the processes.

- Name the form of nitrogen taken up by most plants.
- Draw a diagram to show how soil nitrates can be replenished.
- Name the 4 kinds of micro-organisms involved and describe what they do.

Chapter 15: Questions

1 The diagram shows a simple food web.

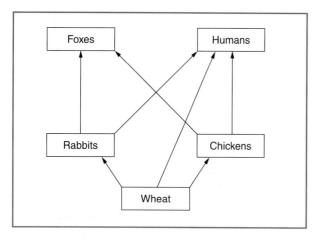

a Use the diagram to name:
  i a herbivore;
  ii an amnivore;
  iii a producer. *(3 marks)*
b i The animals in the food web get their energy from the food they eat. From where do the wheat plants gets their energy? *(1 mark)*
  ii Draw a pyramid of energy for the following food chain.
    Wheat → Rabbit → Fox *(2 marks)*
    (SEG June 1998)

2 A compost heap was built up as shown in the diagram. After a few days, steam was seen rising from the heap and the temperature in the centre had risen from 16 °C to 45 °C. This was due to decomposition of the plant material.

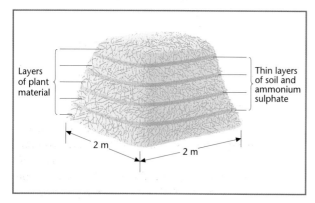

a Name two types of organism, present in soil, which cause decomposition. *(3 marks)*
b Name the process which occurs in these organisms which releases heat energy. *(1 mark)*
c The ammonium sulphate added to the compost heap supplies the decomposers with the element nitrogen. State one use of nitrogen to the decomposers. *(1 mark)*
    (SEG June 1993)

3 The following pyramid shows the amounts of energy (in kilojoules per m² per year) in different types of organisms which lived in a freshwater habitat.

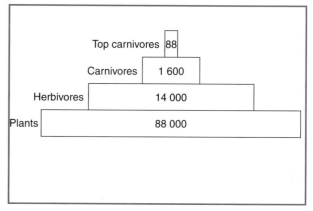

a Sketch the pyramid and write the following terms on the correct lines next to the sketch:
  first-order consumer   second-order consumer
  third-order consumer   producer *(1 mark)*
b i From where do the plants get their energy? *(2 marks)*
  ii What percentage of the plants' energy is passed to the top carnivores? Show your working. *(2 marks)*
  iii Suggest two ways in which energy is lost from these organisms. *(2 marks)*
    (SEG specimen 1998)

4 The diagram below shows how much energy is lost as it passes along a food chain.

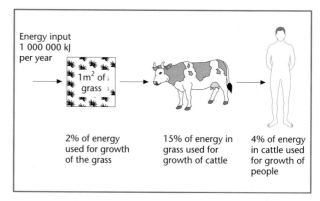

a Where does the 'energy input' come from? *(1 mark)*
b i 1 m² of grass receives 1 million kJ of energy per year.
    How many kJ of this energy are used by the grass. (Show your working.) *(2 marks)*
  ii Use your answer from part (i) to calculate how much of this energy is used for growth of the cow. *(2 marks)*

c Humans may obtain food by the following routes:
Route A Cereal crop → bread → people
Route B Cereal crop → meat → people.
Which route provides more of the energy in the cereal crop for people?
Explain fully the reason for your answer.

(6 marks)
(NEAB Sample Assessment)

5 a The diagram below shows some features of the circulation of nitrogen in natural conditions.

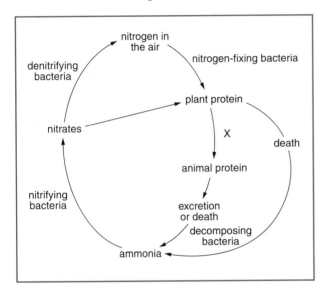

i How many different types of bacteria are shown in this diagram? *(1 mark)*

ii What is the name of the type of bacteria which produce nitrates? *(1 mark)*

iii Give the name of one compound which contains nitrogen and which is shown in this diagram. *(1 mark)*

iv What process happens at the part marked X to cause the change shown? *(1 mark)*

v Denitrifying bacteria are most commonly found in waterlogged soil in which water has filled the air spaces of the soil. Suggest how the digging of drainage ditches round a field can help to keep a suitable amount of nitrates in the soil. *(2 marks)*

vi In agriculture, crops such as potatoes or wheat are harvested and removed from the field. How does the diagram help to explain why farmers need to add fertilisers or manure to the soil? *(2 marks)*

6 The diagram shows a pond and some of the animals and plants which live there.

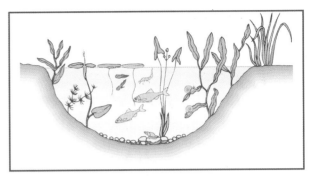

a The following words are used to describe different relationships in the pond.
community   habitat   ecosystem
Match one of these words to the following.
i the pond and the animals and plants

_____ *(1 mark)*

ii the animals and plants

_____ *(1 mark)*

b The pond is close to a farm.
The farmer uses pesticides to kill insects on his crops.
Suggest how the use of pesticides can affect the animals and plants in the pond. *(4 marks)*
(NEAB June 1998)

7 The figure shows the flow of energy through the trees in a forest ecosystem. The numbers represent inputs and outputs of energy in kilojoules per m^2 per year.

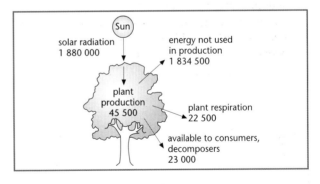

a i Write down the number which indicates the energy entering the system via photosynthesis. *(1 mark)*

ii The total energy available to the plants in the ecosystem is 1 880 000 kJ per m2 per year. Calculate the efficiency of photosynthesis. Show your working. *(2 marks)*

b Suggest four reasons why so much solar energy is not used in production in the forest ecosystem. *(4 marks)*

c In what form will energy from plant respiration escape from the ecosystem? *(1 mark)*
(SEG sample assessment)

CHAPTER 16 The environment

The human population is increasing. In the past, the effects of the population on the environment were small and local. The ecosystems could absorb the effects without too many long term problems. But now the effects of the increasing population can be very damaging and often global. This chapter will help you identify these effects, find out why they are happening and how we can prevent them.

After you have worked through this chapter, you should be able to:

- Outline the factors which affect the size of human populations.
- Interpret population pyramids and relate these to the change in population size.
- Outline the implications of rapid human population growth.
- Describe the environmental problems associated with changing land use.

- Explain the consequencies of massive deforestation.
- Explain the environmental consequences of keeping food production at a high level.
- Discuss the concept of sustainability with respect to renewable and non-renewable resources.
- Discuss the need for conservation.
- Describe some of the techniques used to maintain genetic resources and species diversity.

Energy from biomass

What is biomass?

Biomass is the material produced by plants. Plants use the Sun's energy to make organic compounds such as sugars, starches and cellulose. The energy trapped in just a fraction of the organic compounds produced every year by plants far exceeds the total energy needs of the human population currently on the planet. This represents a sustainable energy source that we are already tapping into.

Energy from trees

Wood has been used for energy since humans discovered fire. It is still the most used fuel in many parts of the world. To be a sustainable energy source, trees which are chopped down must be replaced and given time to grow to maturity. This does not happen in some parts of the world, creating a shortage of mature trees and problems from soil erosion.

Wood is heavy to carry because it contains moisture. This moisture can be driven out by heating it in the absence of air. The product is charcoal, which is a very light and energy-dense material.

Energy from crops

In Brazil they produce **alcohol** by the fermentation of sugar from sugar cane. Volume for volume, this alcohol produces as much energy as petrol and much less pollution. Car engines can be modified to use it. If the alcohol is added to petrol to make a 20 : 80 mixture, a substance called **gasohol** is produced. Cars can run on this without any modifications.

In the USA, alcohol is being produced from starch in surplus grains. This is possible because the grains supply amylase enzymes to degrade the starch to fermentable sugar. Biotechnologists are attempting to engineer strains of yeast which produce their own amylase enzymes, potentially allowing any source of starch to be used.

Oil from rapeseed

In Britain and Italy rapeseed oil is being used to produce a diesel substitute called rape methyl ester

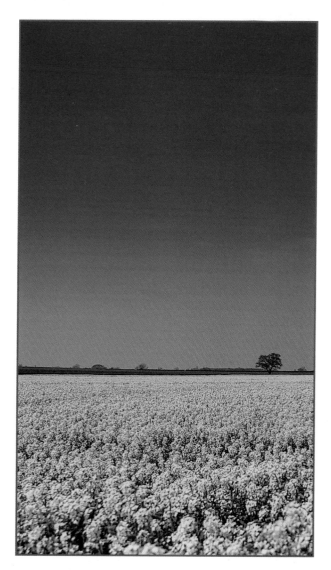

Figure 1 *More than a million tonnes of rapeseed oil is produced in the UK every year.*

(RME). This is simple to produce and has the advantage of not producing any sulphur dioxide when burned. But it would take half a million acres of land to grow the rape to replace all the diesel used in the UK in one year.

Almost any plant oil can be used as a fuel, but not all are as good as rapeseed oil. Brazil is adding 20% palm oil to a mixture of diesel and alcohol to make an efficient alternative fuel.

Even algae can be used to produce oil. The same area of algae will yield twice as much oil as rape.

What is biogas?

When organic wastes rot in the absence of air, they produce a gas. This gas, called **biogas**, is a mixture of **methane** and carbon dioxide. The **anaerobic** process that produces it is the same process as happens naturally in the intestines of cows.

The use of biogas for fuel was first developed in China. Plant, animal and human wastes are fed into a special container called a **digester**, which is then sealed. Once the air has been used up, the bacteria start to ferment the organic compounds and after a week or so, enough biogas has collected to fuel a small stove and light sources (see figure 2).

In the UK we collect biogas from **landfill sites**. Pipes are put into the sites to allow any gas produced to escape. This prevents the dangerous buildup and escape of these greenhouse gases into the atmosphere.

Energy from sewage

Another potential source of energy is the **sludge** produced when sewage is treated. This can be transferred into anaerobic digesters where bacteria and other micro-organisms convert it to useful products such as alcohols, organic acids, hydrogen and methane. The gases can be drawn off and used to generate electricity. There are a number of power stations in the UK which operate in this way.

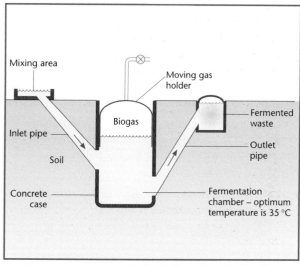

Figure 2 *A simple biogas digester.*

16.1 Human populations

How do populations grow?

A population is a group of organisms of the same species, living in an area or community.

All animal populations tend to grow (increase in numbers) in a similar way, even humans. Imagine a few rabbits moving to a new area where food and space are plentiful and there are no competitors or predators. The population would grow as illustrated in figure 1. The size of the population would increase slowly at first, but as more organisms are born and then breed themselves, the numbers would start to increase much more rapidly. The birth rate would far exceed the death rate. Soon the population could be doubling in size every month. This kind of growth rate is called **exponential growth**.

Very few populations can go on increasing at this rate – usually because food, water and space start to run out. These are called **limiting factors** because they affect the ability of a population to increase in size. Limiting factors may affect the rabbits, they may not breed as much and many may die from starvation. The population increase will start to slow down as the death rate catches up with the birth rate. Their numbers may even start to decline, but generally a balance is reached, where the birth rate equals the death rate and the population size stays the same. All habitats have a limit to the number of organisms they can support. This is called the **carrying capacity**.

How is the human population growing?

The world population reached 6000 million people in 1999. It has doubled over the last 50 years and although this growth rate shows signs of slowing down, it is still increasing by 78 million people per year. This is a lot of people! Figure 2 shows how the human population has grown over the years and how it is predicted to grow in the future. The United Nations has predicted that growth will probably continue into the middle of the 22nd century, at which time the world population will stabilise. However, by this time it will be seriously overcrowded.

Why is the population increasing so much?

Humans, unlike any other animal, can control their environment to minimise or even eliminate many of the limiting factors which most animal populations experience. For example:

● we can produce food almost anywhere on the planet and transport it to where it is needed

● we can build living space upwards and underground

● we can prevent and even cure many diseases and better medical care has resulted in increased life expectancy (see figure 4).

Everything is still far from perfect, and many of the limiting factors do still affect the population growth of many countries in the world. Another factor unique to humans is war. Over recent years this has seriously affected many populations.

How is the growth rate determined?

The rate at which a population is growing is worked out from the difference between the **birth rate** and **death rate** for the population. These are usually expressed as numbers per thousand people in the population. Of course, in calculating the population size, **immigration** and **emigration** also have to be taken into account.

It is also sometimes useful to know the structure of a population in terms of age and gender. This can be drawn as a population pyramid. Figure 4 is the population pyramid for the UK in 1997.

The problems of overpopulation

Many environmental issues are a result of trying to cope with the ever increasing population. The increase in population has created:

● the need for more living space

● the need for more food

● the need for more resources, especially energy

● more pollution.

These are discussed in the rest of this chapter.

What do **you** know?

You should now be able to:

● Draw a typical growth curve for a population and explain each stage.

● List 3 things which determine how fast a population grows.

● Explain the term limiting factor and give 3 examples for humans.

● State 3 reasons why the human population is still growing rapidly.

● Outline the pressures this growth is going to put on our environment.

● Explain why population statistics are useful to local authorities and governments.

● Explain what the population pyramid for the UK shows.

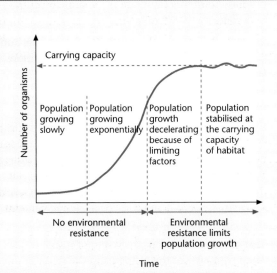

Figure 1 *The graph shows how a typical population grows.*

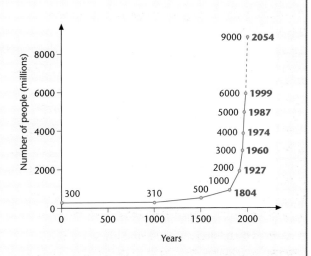

Figure 2 *After a slow start the world population is now growing exponentially.*

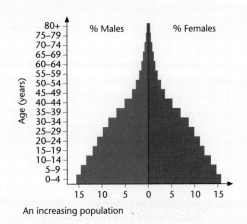

An increasing population

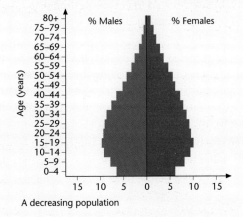

A decreasing population

Figure 3 *Population pyramids show the age and gender distribution.*

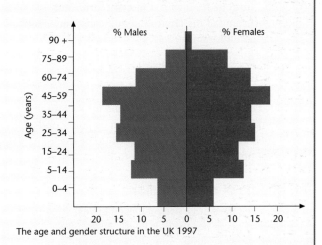

The age and gender structure in the UK 1997

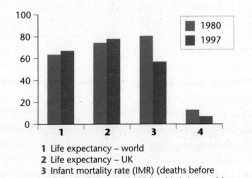

1 Life expectancy – world
2 Life expectancy – UK
3 Infant mortality rate (IMR) (deaths before the age of one per 1000 live births) – world
4 IMR – UK

Life expectancy and infant mortality rate

Figure 4 *Population statistics for the UK.*

16.2 Land use

More land

An increasing population demands more land for:

- growing food
- grazing animals for food and resources, such as wool
- building houses to live in and roads for commuting.

Where is this land going to come from?

This land could potentially come from several sources:

- The **sea**, but this would be no good for growing crops because of its high salt content. Salt can be removed from seawater, but this is very expensive.

- The **deserts**, but sand has no nutrients or water and is very unstable for building on. This again can be resolved by adding nutrients and irrigation, but this is very, very expensive.

- From **under-used land** or land which is being used for something else, i.e. hedgerows and wetlands. This is current policy. Figure 1 in chapter 16.3 compares a typical farm in 1950 with a modern farm and highlights some of the environmental consequences of the changes in land use.

- The **woods** and **forests,** which could provide land suitable for building on, grazing animals and growing crops with very little effort or expense. Also the chopped down trees can provide wood for building, and making furniture, resources such as paper and even fuel. This would, therefore, seem to be the cheapest option, but at what cost to the planet?

The effects of deforestation

In recent years trees have been removed in vast quantities, so many in fact, that nearly 50% of the natural tropical rainforests and natural woodlands have now gone. Forests are still being chopped down at the rate of 12 million hectares per year (1999 figures). What are the consequences of this? Figure 2 shows the value of trees to the Earth's ecosystems. Removal of them has led to:

- **Climatic changes**. Less trees means less photosynthesis and therefore an increase in the atmospheric carbon dioxide concentrations. The burning of these trees as fuel also releases carbon dioxide into the air. Carbon dioxide is a **greenhouse gas**. It absorbs heat and thereby contributes to the warmth of the atmosphere. If the carbon dioxide level increases, more heat will be absorbed and the atmospheric temperature will go up resulting in **global warming** (chapter 16.5).

  Fewer trees will also affect the water cycle. Transpiration will be reduced so less water will enter the atmosphere leaving it drier. Less rain will be produced and this could affect the growth of our crops, i.e. productivity will be lower.

  The bare soil will quickly absorb heat from the Sun resulting in thermal gradients and therefore more **wind**. This could mean more hurricanes.

- Changes in **species diversity**. Forests and woods are habitats for many different species. Destroy these, and some of the species may become extinct. In the last 400 years, 36% of all extinctions have been due to habitat removal through, for example deforestation. Estimates have put this at 5000 species a year. More than 50% of our medicines come from plants, and new ones are still being discovered. These valuable resources will also disappear for good.

- **Soil erosion**. In forests, recycling of nutrients is very rapid with 80% of the nutrients in the trees (at any one time)! Removing these will remove these nutrients from the area, leaving the soil relatively infertile and very poor for growing crops. The nutrients will be further depleted by the rain which will now reach the soil. The rain will **leach** (dissolve them and take them with it as it passes through the soil) the nutrients.

  The soil will also contain less organic matter (humus) to bind it together. Heavy rains can wash this loose soil away causing mud slides.

  The heat from the Sun will dry it more quickly and ultimately the structure will be destroyed. This loss of soil is called **soil erosion** and taken to the extreme, could result in a desert.

The effects of quarrying

Quarrying is the process of extracting stone or rock from the surface of the Earth. This is used for building.

Coal can be extracted by a process similar to quarrying called open cast mining. This has serious consequences for the environment.

Removal of top soil also removes the vegetation. The subsoil is generally piled up into unsightly mounds. Finally extracting the coal stirs up a lot of harmful dust and leaves large holes in the ground. The noise also frightens animals in the area.

The coal is often washed before transporting away. The 'dirty' water drains through the land and enters the waterways where it is toxic to the organisms.

Urbanisation

The changes in agriculture and industry over the last 100 years have resulted in the development of large static communities such as towns and cities. This is described as **urbanisation**.

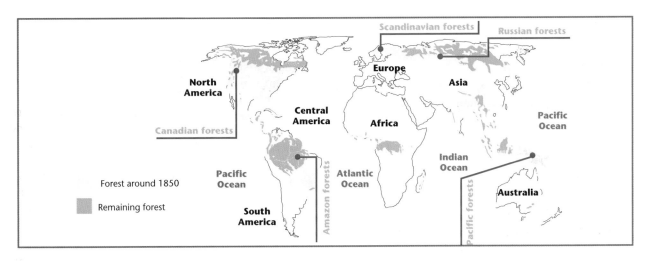

Figure 1 *Since 1850 we have destroyed 50% of the world's forests.*

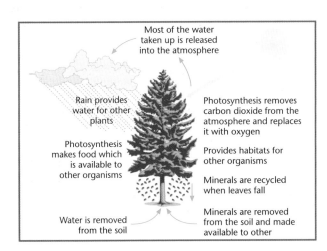

Figure 2 *Trees are a vital part of many natural cycles.*

Most of the water taken up is released into the atmosphere

Rain provides water for other plants

Photosynthesis makes food which is available to other organisms

Water is removed from the soil

Photosynthesis removes carbon dioxide from the atmosphere and replaces it with oxygen

Provides habitats for other organisms

Minerals are recycled when leaves fall

Minerals are removed from the soil and made available to other

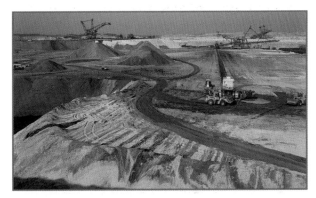

Figure 3 *Quarrying for natural minerals often devastates ecosystems.*

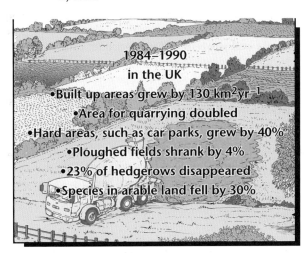

1984–1990 in the UK
- Built up areas grew by 130 km^{2}yr^{-1}
- Area for quarrying doubled
- Hard areas, such as car parks, grew by 40%
- Ploughed fields shrank by 4%
- 23% of hedgerows disappeared
- Species in arable land fell by 30%

Figure 4 *Some of the findings in a recent countryside survey.*

What do **you** know?

You should now be able to:

- Explain why humans require more land.
- List 4 possible places this land could come from.
- Describe the problems of using land from the sea or deserts.
- Explain how and why the changes in farming have affected species diversity.
- Outline the value of trees to ecosystems.
- State 4 reasons why trees are being cut down.
- State 5 major problems caused by the loss of trees.
- Explain why soil becomes less fertile and how this could result in soil erosion.
- Describe the effects of quarrying on the environment.

16.3 Food production

More food

An increasing population will need to produce more food. Although food production has increased over the last 40 years, the amount of food per person has fallen.

Traditionally if you needed more food, you simply planted more land. But now land is in short supply and so the land available has to be made more productive. There are many ways of achieving this, but few come without problems.

Use of machinery

Machines now do the jobs of horses and people. They help make food production quicker, more efficient and more cost effective, but they also cause more damage to the ecosystems. For instance, large machines need large fields, so hedgerows, ponds and rough margins have to be sacrificed as small fields are joined up to make larger fields. The result is a loss of habitats and therefore a decline in species diversity (see figure 1).

Using fertilisers

Fertilisers are used to put nutrients, such as nitrates and phosphates, back into the soil so it can be re-used, often for the same crop. Traditionally farmland manure was used, but this has largely been replaced by artificially produced chemical fertilisers. The production of these uses energy equivalent to 100 gallons of oil per tonne. This high energy demand is only half the problem. Up to 10% of the fertiliser applied to soil is often washed out into the waterways – more if too much was applied or if it rains soon after application. This can lead to **eutrophication** in waterways and excessive nitrates in drinking water (chapter 16.7).

Using pesticides

Pesticides are chemicals which are usually sprayed onto crops to reduce the competition from other organisms or prevent infection. There are three main types of pesticides:

- **Herbicides** are used to kill weeds which would remove valuable nutrients from the soil.
- **Fungicides** are used to kill disease causing fungi.
- **Insecticides** are used to kill insects which could eat the crops or spread disease-causing organisms.

Unfortunately some of the pesticides may kill organisms they are not intended for, even those high up in the food chain.

Many pesticides are **biodegradable**, that is they can be broken down by microbes into harmless substances.

Some pesticides like **DDT** and **dieldrin** are not biodegradable and may stay (persist) in the soil for many years. These may enter living organisms they were not intended for and accumulate in their tissues. DDT, for example, builds up in the fat tissue. This build up in living tissue is called **bioaccumulation**. Once in an organism, the pesticide can be passed along a food chain and become concentrated in organisms (see figure 3). Notice that the larger organisms higher up the food chain get a massive dose, often large enough to kill them.

Using new or improved crops

The alternative to making the land more productive is to make the crops and animals more productive.

- Genes can be transferred into crops from nitrogen fixing bacteria, enabling them to use atmospheric nitrogen to make proteins. This would reduce the need for fertilisers.

- Genes can be transferred into plants which give them resistance to certain diseases or pests. for example, rice has been genetically modified to resist a serious viral disease which threatened to dramatically reduce productivity.

- New varieties of crop plants can be bred or genetically modified to grow on soil high in salt concentration or very dry land so that land reclaimed from the sea and deserts can be used.

- Food animals can be selectively bred or genetically altered to increase their growth rate and produce more milk and meat. Modern wheat has been bred over the centuries from wild grasses, taking their best features. The use of genetic engineering has accelerated this process.

- **Single cell protein** and single cell fat can be produced by growing micro-organisms such as bacteria, fungi and algae in large containers called fermenters. Many of the micro-organisms can be genetically altered to increase yields.

Some of these practices are described more fully in chapter 14.6. Using genetic engineering to increase food production is still in its early development. Whilst it has many economic and environmental benefits, some also see many pitfalls and ethical problems.

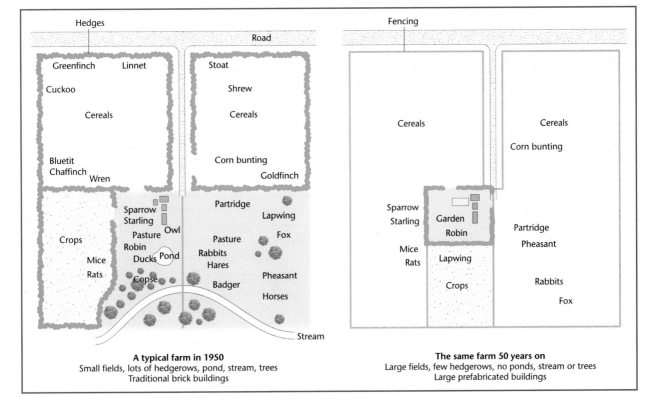

Figure 1 *Modern farming methods reduce the number of habitats available.*

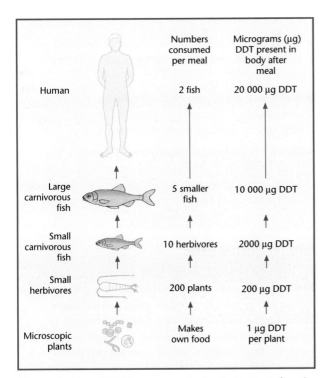

Figure 2 *How DDT is concentrated along a food chain.*

What do **you** know?

You should now be able to:

- Discuss the advantages and disadvantages of the 3 main methods of getting food.
- Describe how changes in farming practices have affected the species diversity on farms.
- Describe how the use of fertilisers and pesticides can make land more productive.
- Explain why farmers have to be very careful about how much fertiliser they use.
- Draw a diagram to explain how a pesticide can build up in a food chain.
- Describe 5 modern ways of increasing food production.

16.4 Natural resources

More natural resources

An increasing population will require more natural resources, such as iron, copper, coal, oil, cotton, wool, paper and so on.

Renewable and non-renewable resources

We can think of resources as being of two kinds:

- **Renewable resources** are those which can be replaced and consist of growing organisms, such as plants and animals or the products they produce. With good management these should never run out. Each will have a sustainable yield, usually equal to the rate of production. For example, if a population of fish produce 50 new fish every three months, then 50 older fish can be removed every three months. This is good management because the size of the original population does not decrease or become unbalanced (also see chapter 16.8).

  Of course, we can also affect renewable resources by interfering with the ecosystem in which they live, e.g. pollution.

- **Non-renewable resources** are present in the environment in fixed amounts and once used can never realistically be replaced, e.g. fossil fuels and minerals. Alternatives have to be found or they have to be **recycled**.

What is already being recycled?

Recycling is not always the cheapest method of dealing with waste materials, but as resources run out and prices go up, it is becoming an attractive option. For some resources it is already **cost effective** and **energy efficient**. For example, the recycling of glass saves the equivalent of 30 gallons of oil energy per tonne on the manufacturing cost. Figure 2 shows the extent of current household recycling in the UK.

Energy resources – how much energy is left?

So far, most of our energy has come from the non-renewable energy sources such as coal, oil and natural gas, but these will not last forever. The World Energy Council has predicted a 50% increase in energy use over the next 30 years. Even without this expected growth, estimates suggest that the known oil reserves will be used up by the year 2035, gas by the year 2050 and all the coal will have been used by 2250. This also does not take into account the amount needed to produce industrial products such as plastics and medicines.

Another non-renewable energy source being used more and more, is uranium. When atoms of uranium are split in two by bombarding them with neutrons, a great deal of energy is released. This energy can be used to produce electricity. A nuclear power industry has developed to do just this, and it promises to go on producing 'clean' electricity for many years to come. Uranium is found in the Earth's crust and although stocks are limited, one tonne of uranium will produce as much energy as one million tonnes of coal. At this rate it will last a lot longer than existing coal reserves, possibly for another 2000 years or more.

Can we use natural forms of energy?

Energy from the Sun, wind, water and rocks can all be harnessed. These are all renewable and unlike burning fossil fuels, they do not create any pollution, that is, they are clean. Unfortunately, they are very expensive methods and it is unrealistic to expect them to replace fossil fuels in the near future (see figure 4).

- **Energy from the Sun** (**solar power**). The energy in sunlight can be absorbed by solar panels and used for heating purposes. **Photo-voltaic cells** can be used to turn solar energy directly into electricity. They can be used to power isolated items, such as telephone boxes.

- **Energy from the wind** (**wind power**). Large windmills can be used to rotate turbines and generate electricity (see figure 3).

- **Hydro-electric power**. When water moves from high ground to lower ground, it can be used to rotate huge turbines and thereby generate electricity (see figure 3).

- **Tidal power**. The tidal movement of river and sea water can be used to turn turbines and generate electricity.

- **Wave power**. The up and down action of waves contains a lot of potential energy which can be used to turn turbines and generate electricity.

- **Energy from rocks** (**geothermal power**). The rocks below the Earth's surface contain a lot of heat. Water pumped through bore holes deep in these rocks can be extracted as hot water and used for heating purposes or to produce electricity.

Energy from wastes

We can also produce energy from natural wastes and **biomass**. Organic wastes such as manure and vegetable matter can be used to produce a fuel called biogas. Wood can be used directly as a source of fuel, or to produce charcoal. Sugar cane can be fermented to produce ethanol. When added to petrol this produces a mixture called gasohol. More details about these processes can be found on page 252.

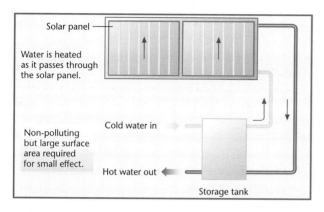

Solar panel

Water is heated as it passes through the solar panel.

Non-polluting but large surface area required for small effect.

Cold water in

Hot water out

Storage tank

Figure 1 *Energy from the Sun can be harnessed directly using solar panels.*

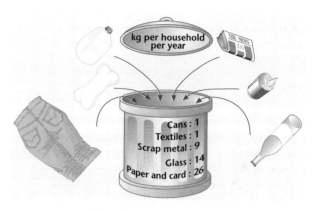

kg per household per year

Cans : 1
Textiles : 1
Scrap metal : 9
Glass : 14
Paper and card : 26

Figure 2 *Household recycling in the UK, 1996–97.*

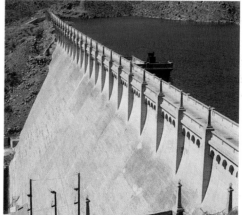

Non-polluting but spoils areas of natural beauty.

Non-polluting but flooding areas of land destroys more habitats than it creates and devastates ecosystems.

Figure 3 *Some alternative forms of energy.*

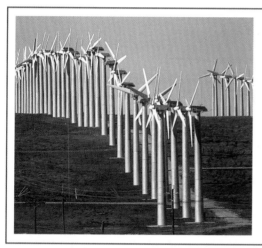

A 1000 megawatt (medium sized) coal power station can be replaced by:

25 km tidal barrage

20 km wave generators

100 km² of solar panels

20 000 tonnes of biomass

100 × 50 m diameter windmills

1 tonne of uranium generates the same energy as 1 million tonnes of coal

Figure 4 *Just how realistic are the renewable energy sources?*

What do **you** know?

You should now be able to:

- Distinguish between renewable and non-renewable resources.
- Discuss sustainable yields with respect to renewable resources.
- Review how fossil fuels are formed and explain why they are considered to be non-renewable.
- Describe the advantages and disadvantages of some of the natural forms of energy we can use.
- Explain why it is unlikely that these natural forms will ever replace our present forms.
- Discuss the advantages and disadvantages of producing energy from uranium.
- Explain how fuel can be produced from wastes.
- Describe how biomass is used for fuel.

16.5 Polluting the environment

More pollution

Pollution is created when potentially harmful substances are added to the environment at a rate faster than the environment can deal with. These substances, called **pollutants** build up in the atmosphere, rivers, lakes, sea and soil, and interfere with natural ecological systems. They can also cause disease and harm to ourselves. Some pollutants are natural substances already present in the environment, but in much smaller quantities, e.g. carbon dioxide. Others are manmade, some of which are known to be toxic, such as DDT.

In our efforts to cope with an increasing population, we are unfortunately also increasingly polluting the environment. Some of the ways are detailed below.

How we pollute the air

There are three main ways we are polluting the air:

- By burning fossil fuels such as coal and oil. This releases **carbon dioxide**, **sulphur dioxide** and **nitrogen oxides** into the atmosphere. The extra carbon dioxide is causing **global warming** (chapter 16.6). Sulphur dioxide and nitrogen oxides result in **acid rain**.

- Burning petrol also produces nitrogen oxides and carbon dioxide as well as **carbon monoxide** and **ozone**. Carbon monoxide is a colourless, odourless, but deadly gas. In your body, it is taken up by the haemoglobin in your blood in preference to oxygen. This reduces your ability to obtain oxygen which can lead to drowsiness and even death.

  Faulty gas appliances burn natural gas in the absence of oxygen producing carbon monoxide. This can quickly build up in a room to levels which can kill.

  The exhaust fumes from cars that still use leaded petrol will contain **lead vapours**. These can interfere with the development of the nervous system of children and result in a lower IQ.

  Ozone is a respiratory irritant which can cause asthma.

- The release of **CFC's** (chlorofluorocarbons) by aerosols, refrigerators, air conditioning units and in the manufacture of polystyrene is resulting in the **destruction of the ozone layer** (chapter 16.6).

Acid rain

Acid rain is rain with a pH of less than five. It is formed when sulphur dioxide and nitrogen oxides are released into the atmosphere from burning coal, oil and petrol.

These dissolve in rain to form dilute acids which can be very damaging to the environment:

- It damages the leaves of some plants, especially slow growing evergreens such as conifers.

- It acidifies waterways killing many of the organisms that live there. Fish and small crustaceans, in particular, are affected.

- It reacts with chemicals in the soil releasing many of the toxic metals such as aluminium, calcium and magnesium. These are washed into the streams, rivers and lakes seriously affecting the organisms that live there. Aluminium for example, kills the fish by interfering with their gill function. Plants die from lack of calcium and magnesium.

- It erodes stonework ruining many old buildings and monuments.

- It is a respiratory irritant.

Sometimes the gases are carried hundreds of miles away before forming acid rain. The tall chimneys favoured by the UK power industry pump them high into the air where air currents can take them into other countries. Much of the damage to Germany's Black Forest (conifers), Sweden's lakes and Norway's lakes has been blamed on the UK.

The main gas involved is sulphur dioxide. Many plants absorb this directly and it kills them. **Lichens** in particular are sensitive, some species more than others. They are therefore used as indictors of the level of sulphur dioxide pollution.

Reducing acid rain

The only way to reduce acid rain is to stop releasing sulphur dioxide and nitrogen oxides into the air. This can be achieved by:

- Fitting '**scrubbers**' to power stations. These contain calcium carbonate which reacts with sulphur dioxide. The problem is that carbon dioxide is formed, and this is also a pollutant.

- Fitting **catalytic converters** to car exhausts. These remove oxides of nitrogen from the exhaust fumes.

- Using low sulphur (pure) coal.

- Converting to cleaner fuels such as natural gas.

Much of the damage already done to the environment is irreparable. The aim must be to prevent any more damage in the future by choosing our future energy sources carefully.

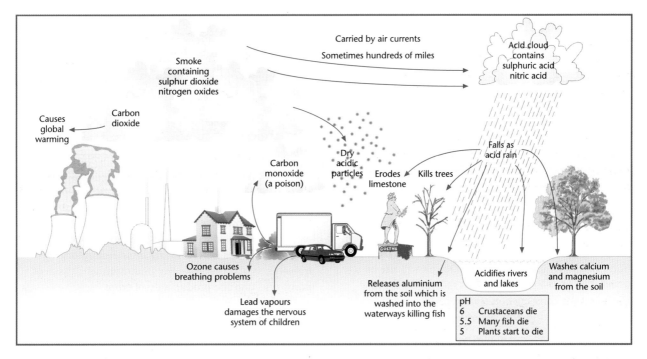

Figure 1 *Some of the ways in which we pollute our air.*

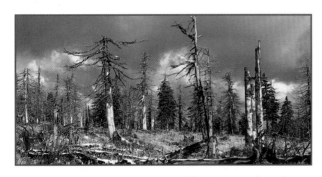

Figure 2 *Acid rain damages the leaves of trees.*

What do **you** know?

You should now be able to:

- Define the terms pollution and pollutant.
- List the ways we are polluting our environment.
- Explain how acid rain is produced and describe the damage it is causing to our environment.
- Explain why we are damaging Germany's forests.
- Describe 4 ways to reduce acid rain levels.
- Explain why carbon monoxide is poisonous.
- Discuss why lead-free petrol is more environmentally friendly.

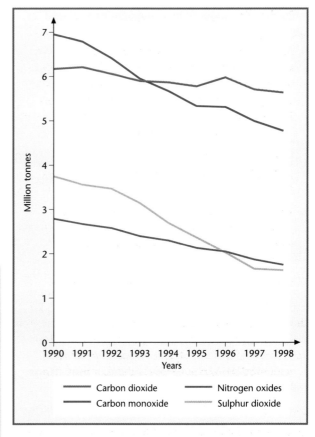

Carbon dioxide — Nitrogen oxides
Carbon monoxide — Sulphur dioxide

Figure 3 *The amounts of air pollutants (gases) we produce in the UK every year is falling.*

Global warming – the greenhouse effect

Some of the gases in the atmosphere around the Earth have the ability to absorb and retain much of the heat radiated from the Sun and land. They are called **greenhouse gases** and without them the surface temperature would be at least 30 °C cooler and considerably more hostile to most living things. The effect of retaining this heat has been called the **greenhouse effect**, because the gases prevent much of the heat escaping in much the same way as the glass in a greenhouse (see figure 1).

The two main greenhouse gases in the atmosphere are carbon dioxide and methane. Recent measurements have shown that the volume of these is increasing. The atmospheric temperature is therefore rising. Over the last 100 years, it has risen by 0.5 °C and predictions by the World Health Organisation suggest that it will rise by a further 1 °C by the year 2030. This may not seem very much, but the consequences, some of which we are already experiencing, can be devastating:

- Polar ice caps will start to melt raising the sea level. A 1 °C rise is sufficient to melt enough ice to raise sea levels by 20 cm. This would flood much of the world's lowlands, including considerable parts of the UK (see figure 3).

- Increases in evaporation, changes in rainfall and temperature differences. This could result in more droughts, flooding, winds, storms and hurricanes.

- Climatic changes will affect vegetation and changes to the rates of photosynthesis will alter agricultural productivity.

- Some organisms will become extinct as they fail to adapt to the changes in ecosystems.

- Diseases like malaria, once confined to warmer areas, will become endemic in more countries as the insects that spread them survive in more places.

The other greenhouse gases are shown in figure 2.

Ozone destruction

Ozone is a form of oxygen (O_3) formed naturally in the atmosphere. At ground level, it is a respiratory irritant responsible for problems like asthma, but about 25 km above the Earth's surface it forms a protective layer which filters out harmful ultra violet (UV) **radiation** from the Sun. This is high level ozone. UV radiation damages the DNA in our cells resulting in **mutations** and **cancers** (see figure 4).

Ozone can be destroyed by chlorofluorocarbons (**CFC's**) released into the air by aerosols and air conditioning units. There is already a large hole which appears above Antarctica every Spring. Research has suggested that as

little as a 2.5% reduction in the ozone layer could result in 40 million more cases of skin cancer every year.

A thinning of the ozone layer also allows more infra-red (IR) rays through to cause global warming.

Although most countries have now agreed to limit the use of CFC's, those already in the atmosphere will go on damaging the ozone layer for many more years.

Low level ozone

Low level ozone comes from burning fossil fuels such as petrol. There are large amounts of it in cities which have a lot of cars, and in the summer months it forms part of the **petrochemical smog**. This ozone is responsible for headaches, coughs, sore throats, and eye, throat and lung irritation, as well as many more respiratory problems. It also damages the photosynthetic tissue of plants affecting the productivity of crops.

Other forms of pollution

- **Radioactivity**. Radiation is all around us in the form of heat, light, sound radio-waves and so on, and is mostly harmless. **Ionising radiation** comes from radioactive materials and can be damaging to living tissue, causing mutations, cell damage and tissue destruction. This is the radiation we usually call radioactivity.

  Most of the radioactivity in the atmosphere is from natural sources, but about 13% is manmade – released during medical procedures such as X-rays, body scans and so on. The nuclear power industry also produces radioactive wastes.

- **Noise**. The effects of noise pollution are described in chapter 12.2.

What do **you** know?

You should now be able to:

- Explain why the Earth's atmosphere is warming up.
- Name the 2 main greenhouse gases, explain how they are produced and why they are increasing.
- Describe 4 consequences of global warming.
- Suggest how global warming can be reduced or even eliminated.
- Explain what ozone is and where it is found.
- Explain why high level ozone is beneficial to health.
- Explain what CFC's are, where they are from and what damage they are causing.
- Describe radioactivity, explain where it comes from and what damage it can cause to living tissue.

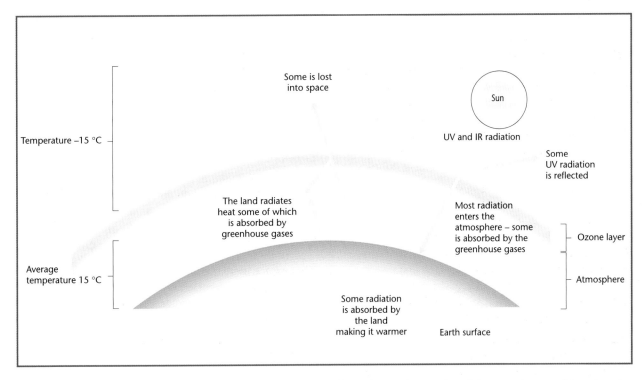

Figure 1 *The greenhouse effect is caused by gases in the atmosphere absorbing and re-emitting heat.*

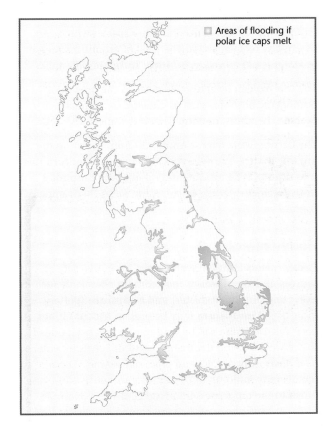

Areas of flooding if polar ice caps melt

Figure 3 *How global warming could affect the coastlines of the UK.*

Carbon dioxide	From burning fossil fuels
Methane	From the action of anaerobic bacteria in swamps, paddy fields and the guts of cattle
Nitrogen oxides	From burning fossil fuels and denitrifying bacteria
CFCs	From aerosol propellants and refrigerant coolants
Water vapour	Part of the Earth's natural cycles

Figure 2 *The sources of the main greenhouse gases.*

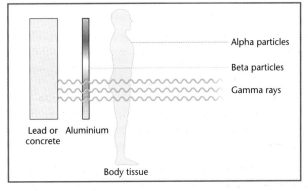

Alpha particles
Beta particles
Gamma rays

Lead or concrete   Aluminium

Body tissue

Figure 5 *Radioactivity can cause mutations and damage living tissue.*

Polluting the water

How we pollute our water

Water is essential to us and all other living organisms. By polluting sources of water we are doing immediate harm to the fish and other organisms that live there and long term harm to the balance of nature and to ourselves.

There are several major ways we pollute water supplies:

- By **discharging untreated sewage** into it. This creates a **biochemical oxygen demand** (BOD) and leads to **eutrophication**.

- By using **fertilisers** on agricultural land. These can be washed by rain into the natural waterways resulting in eutrophication. Agricultural **slurry** (natural manure from the farm animals) and silage (rotted grass used as animal feed) also supply nitrates.

- From **pesticide use** on crops. These are washed into the waterways and build up in the food chains (see chapter 16.3).

- By **discharging industrial wastes** containing heavy metals and heat into the waterways. Many of the heavy metals are toxic and can build up in the food chains. Heat kills many organisms directly and accelerates the growth rates of many others, upsetting the ecological balance in the ecosystems. Warm water also holds less oxygen.

- From **acid rain** created by burning fossil fuels. This changes the pH of water killing many of the organisms and unbalancing the food chains.

What is eutrophication?

Eutrophication is the term used to describe the build up of large amounts of minerals such as nitrates and phosphates in fresh water. This happens for several reasons:

- Bacteria in the water produce nitrates from the organic matter in any sewage discharged into the water.

- Detergents in the sewage contain phosphates.

- Excess nitrates and phosphates are washed from fertilisers applied to agricultural land.

The excess nitrates and phosphates enable unicellular algae in the water to grow more rapidly producing an **algal bloom**. The algae prevent light from reaching the plants below which then die. As nutrients become scarce the algae also die, thereby adding to the organic matter for the aerobic bacteria in the water. This sequence of events seriously upsets the ecology of the ecosystem resulting in the death of many organisms.

If drinking water is extracted from a polluted river or lake, the high nitrate content could cause harm, especially to babies (see figure 2). The European Union (EU) has set an upper safety limit of 50 mg dm^{-1} of nitrates. Much of the natural water in the UK is dangerously close to this.

Disposal of untreated sewage

Sewage contains:

- organic matter from human excrement and food residues

- detergents

- bacteria, some of which may be **pathogenic**.

The organic matter becomes food for aerobic decomposers (mainly putrefying bacteria). As they break it down, they use up oxygen from the water. The amount of oxygen needed by these decomposers is called the biochemical oxygen demand (see Table 1). The more organic matter in the water, the higher the BOD. The BOD is, therefore, sometimes used to indicate the level of pollution.

The removal of oxygen from water leads to the death of many of the organisms which require high levels of oxygen, such as insect larvae and fish. These are replaced by sludgeworms and other species which can live in low oxygen levels. The level of organisms present in water is often used as a **biotic index** of pollution.

The low oxygen level also encourages the growth of pathogenic bacteria, such as cholera, salmonella, typhoid, hepatitis, meningitis and dysentery.

The decomposers release ammonia from digesting the organic matter. Nitrifying bacteria in the water turn this into nitrates. The nitrates and additional phosphates from detergents results in eutrophic water (high mineral content water).

Heavy metals

Heavy metals found in water come from a variety of sources. Industrial wastes may contain chemicals such as **mercury** (tinning industry) and **cadmium** (pottery industry). **Aluminium** may be present because it has been released from soil by acid rain or has been added to the water during treatment. **Lead** dissolves in water as it flows through old lead pipes and sewers. These metals may build up to concentrations which can cause harm to the top feeders in a food chain. For example, high concentrations of mercury cause blindness, deafness and joint deformities in humans. Aluminium has been linked with Alzheimer's disease.

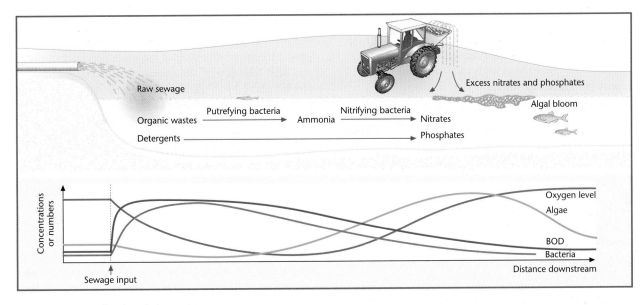

Figure 1 *The effects of dumping raw sewage.*

NITRATES IN DRINKING WATER

Nitrate levels have been increasing.
The safe level is 50mg per litre

Nitrate levels below 50mg per litre can
be dealt with in the body and excreted

Levels above 50mg per litre cause problems
because nitrates are converted to nitrites

In infants nitrites combine with haemoglobin
reducing its oxygen carrying capacity

In adults nitrites are converted to
carcinogens called nitrosamines

Figure 2 *Nitrates in drinking water can be dangerous.*

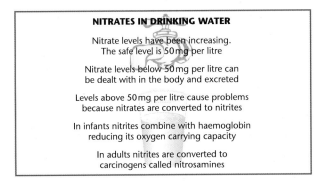

Organisms which live in low oxygen water (polluted)

Tubifex worm

Midge larvae
e.g. *Chironomus*

Organisms which live in medium oxygen water

Alderfly larvae

Caseless Caddis
fly larvae

Water slater

Organisms which require a lot of dissolved oxygen (clean)

Cased Caddis
fly larvae

Mayfly larvae

Stonefly larvae

Freshwater
shrimp

Figure 3 *The organisms that live in water can be used as an indicator of whether water is polluted.*

What do **you** know?

You should now be able to:

- List 5 ways we are polluting the water.
- Describe the effects on a body of water of dumping raw sewage into it.
- Describe 2 ways of assessing the level of organic pollution.
- Explain the term eutrophication.
- Describe the effects on humans of excessive nitrates in drinking water.
- Explain why even though heavy metals are dumped in such small quantities, they can still harm the top carnivores.

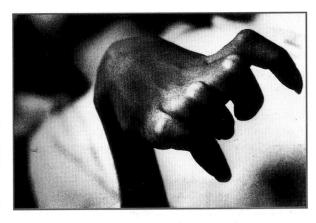

Figure 4 *Deformed hand from mercury poisoning.*

16.8 Conservation

The need for conservation

We share the planet with many other species. Whilst our needs are great we must consider the needs of other species. Let's look at what we have done so far to the planet and these organisms:

- Destroyed nearly half of all the rain forests, previously home for about half of all known species of living things.
- Drained over half of the world's wetlands with the loss of hundreds of species.
- Hunted many whales to near extinction.
- Over-fished resulting in such dangerously low fish stocks that they may never recover.
- Created a large hole in the protective ozone layer allowing damaging radiation through.

These are just a few of our achievements. Due to our neglect, one species becomes extinct every hour on our planet. It has to stop. We really are in a privileged position on the Earth – you could say its future is in our hands. Fortunately, we appear to have now recognised this and realized that we can still use the Earth's resources without endangering other species or destroying the planet. This is what conservation is all about.

What should we do?

Every few years, many of our nations leaders get together to talk about conservation. They discuss the past and the present, and set goals for the future. You could say they put together a **World Conservation Strategy**.

The ultimate aim of any strategy is to ensure the continued existence of all the species on the planet, not just ourselves, and the genetic diversity within these species. This can only be achieved by protecting the ecosystems where they live to preserve their habitats, and avoiding over-exploitation.

Protecting the ecosystems

Ecosystems are complex. They have complex feeding structures, energy flow and nutrient cycles. The organisms in the communities interact in complex ways to produce stable, balanced self-supporting systems. It does not take much to de-stabilise them. We need to study them to try and work out how they function. Only then will we know why, for example using a specific pesticide to kill one type of organism can cause the whole ecosystem to crash. Protecting ecosystems is not simple. It is about maintaining the processes which can drive the nutrient cycles; stopping practices like deforestation which will alter the rainfall and stopping the use of toxic chemicals which can devastate the food webs.

Avoiding over-exploitation

The problem is how do we increase food production yet protect the environment, plus maintain species diversity, and keep costs down? The answer is by good management, by changing to a form of agriculture which is **sustainable** (see chapter 16.3). There will have to be a bit of give and take. Integrating farming with conservation may, in the short term, reduce yields but at least by preserving the ecosystems we will be able to continue producing food in them for many years to come.

What has happened to the fish stocks is a good example. For many years now the fish populations have been decreasing mainly due to overfishing. In Europe this has been recognised as a major problem and a **Common Fisheries Policy** has been designed. The aim of this is to ensure that fish are not taken at a rate greater than they can be replaced by reproduction. The policy is backed by research into the life cycle of the fish and the ecological requirements of the fish and its spawning areas. This information has been used to set fishing **quotas** (limit the number of fish allowed to be caught); make sure that the breeding grounds are not fished, especially during the spawning season; and set net sizes so that the smaller, younger fish are not taken. With good management like this, the fish stocks should be there forever.

Suggestions for conservation

- Provide and protect habitats by setting up **national parks** and **nature reserves** such as the North York Moors and Dartmoor (see figure 1).
- Maintain and protect **sites of special scientific interest** (SSSI) such as Twyford Down and **areas of outstanding natural beauty** (AONB) such as the Cotswolds
- Create **green belts** which cannot be built on or farmed. Pay farmers not to grow food on sensitive areas of their land, such as areas near to hedgerows or rivers.
- Encourage more **urban regeneration** schemes such as London docklands.
- Provide legal protection for **endangered species** such as the badger, osprey (see figure 2) and lizard orchid.
- Set up **gene banks,** such as those at Kew Gardens, to keep samples of seeds from all plants, especially those used for breeding purposes and those replaced by new varieties, e.g. wild wheat.
- Set up **zoos** to breed endangered species such as black rhinos and giant pandas.

The **Nature Conservatory Council** is the government body which promotes and advises on nature conservation in the UK.

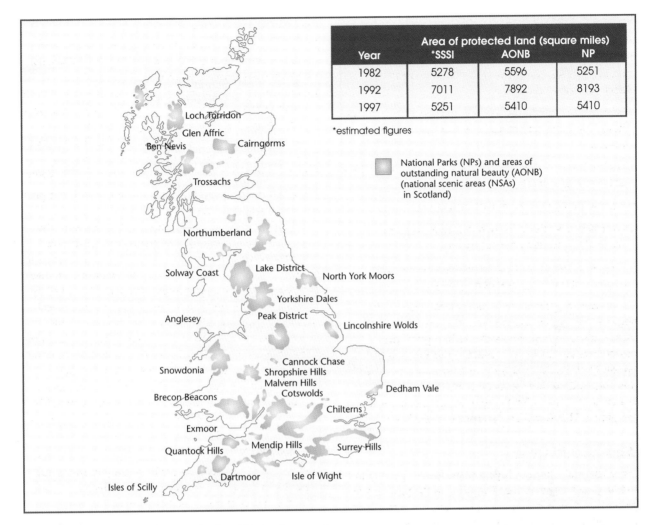

| Year | Area of protected land (square miles) | | |
	*SSSI	AONB	NP
1982	5278	5596	5251
1992	7011	7892	8193
1997	5251	5410	5410

*estimated figures

National Parks (NPs) and areas of outstanding natural beauty (AONB) (national scenic areas (NSAs) in Scotland)

Figure 1 *The protected areas in the UK are increasing.*

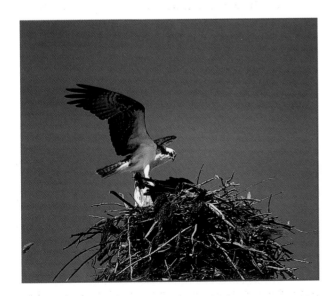

Figure 2 *Many endangered species are protected.*

What do **you** know?

You should now be able to:

- Define the term conservation.
- Explain why we need conservation measures.
- List some of the practices we are using which are helping to destroy ecosystems and their support systems.
- Explain how we can protect the ecosystems.
- Suggest how farming practices can be integrated with conservation practices.
- Explain how careful management of fish stocks can reverse the decline in fish populations.
- Describe some of the ways we can help to maintain genetic resources and species diversity.

Chapter 16: Questions

1 a The diagram shows the age distribution of a population in a country.

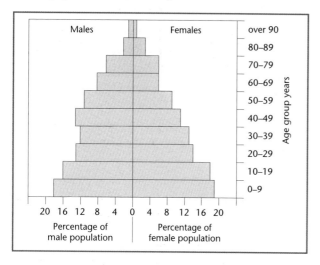

i Give the percentage of females aged 20–29.

(1 mark)

ii Which age group has an equal percentage of males and females? *(1 mark)*

b "Infant mortality" is the number of deaths of children aged from birth to 1 year. In a population there is a fall in infant mortality. Suggest how this may affect the population. Give a reason for your answer. *(2 marks)*

c The fall in infant mortality may be due to improvements in health measures. Suggest two examples of these improvements.

(2 marks)

d In countries with increasing populations there is a greater demand for energy and an increase in pollution.

Explain how the demand for more energy has resulted in
i acid lakes and rivers; *(3 marks)*
ii global warming. *(3 marks)*
(NEAB June 1999)

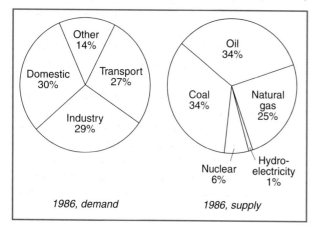

1986, demand   1986, supply

2 The pie chart shows the energy demand and supply in Britain in 1986.
a Which group of users used the most energy?

(1 mark)

b i Coal, oil and gas are 'fossil fuels'.
Describe how fossil fuels were formed.

(2 marks)

ii Describe how the burning of fossil fuels can affect the environment. *(3 marks)*

c Hydroelectricity is known as a "renewable" source of energy.
i Explain what is meant by a renewable energy source. *(2 marks)*
ii Suggest one reason why so little of our energy needs are supplied by hydroelectricity.

(2 marks)
(NEAB sample assessment)

3 a DDT was once commonly used as an insecticide. The diagram shows concentrations of DDT in organisms in food chain in a lake.

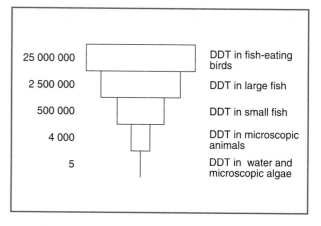

i DDT was sprayed on crops around the lake. How might DDT have reached the lake water?

(1 mark)

ii DDT is stored in the body and not excreted. What is excretion? *(1 mark)*

iii 1 How many times more concentrated was the DDT in the fish-eating birds than the DDT in the microscopic algae? Show clearly how you get to your final answer.

(2 marks)

2 Only a very low concentration of DDT was present in the water. Using information given earlier in the question, explain why the fish-eating birds might be killed by DDT. *(2 marks)*

b The table shows how quickly DDT and another insecticide called Aldrin are broken down in the soil. *(2 marks)*
(SEG June 1998)

Time in years	Percentage remaining in the soil	
	Aldrin	DDT
0	100	100
2	8	60
4	2	34
6	0.5	22
8	0	15
10	0	8

Suggest why Aldrin is a safer insecticide to use than DDT.

4 The ice-caps of Greenland and Antarctica are very deep and build up in layers from snow that falls every year. They can be used to estimate the amount of carbon dioxide in the air from pockets of gas trapped in the ice.

Results from some of these measurements are shown in the table.

Age of sample (thousands of years)	Carbon dioxide concentration (parts per million)
0	290
10	180
20	200
40	230
60	200
80	230
100	245
120	270
140	190

a **i** Suggest why gas pockets trapped in the ice can be used to estimate the carbon dioxide content of the atmosphere. *(1 mark)*

ii The temperature of the atmosphere can also be estimated from the gas pockets. At which two sample ages would you expect the temperature to have been highest? Explain your answer. *(4 marks)*

b Measurements have been made on the rate of addition of carbon dioxide to the atmosphere from 1930 until the present time. They show a rapid increase in this rate.

Describe how human activities have contributed to this rapid increase in the rate of addition of carbon dioxide to the atmosphere. *(5 marks)*

c Suggest two ways in which the rate of carbon dioxide addition to the atmosphere could be reduced. *(2 marks)*

(NEAB June 1998)

5 The table shows the different ways in which the world's land is used today, compared to the way the world's land was used 100 years ago.

Land	Percentage land use	
	Present day	100 years ago
Waste/desert	23	10
Forest	27	44
Built on	13	7
Farming	30	23
Unused	7	16

a Which land use shows the least percentage change over the last 100 years? *(1 mark)*

b The percentage of forest has greatly reduced.

i Suggest two reasons why human activity has brought about this change. *(2 marks)*

ii Explain the effect of this reduction on the gases in the atmosphere. *(3 marks)*

c Despite a great increase in demand for food, only 7% more land is now used for farming. One of the reasons for this is increased productivity, i.e. a higher yield per hectare due to more intensive farming methods.

State one way in which each of the following helps to increase productivity

i using fertilisers;

ii using pesticides;

iii using herbicides. *(3 marks)*

d In the last 10 years people have become more aware of the use of chemicals in farming. Some people are concerned about the effects of these on their health and choose to buy 'organically grown' produce. The farmers who use 'organic' methods to produce food, do not use any chemicals on their crops.

i Suggest one way in which the use of chemicals in farming may be a danger to the health of people buying these foods. *(1 mark)*

ii Suggest one reason why 'organically grown' food is usually more expensive. *(2 marks)*

e The use of pesticides may also cause damage in natural ecosystems. For example the use of selective herbicides in wheat fields can lead to a fall in the numbers of small insect-eating birds living nearby.

i Suggest how this use of herbicides may have affected the bird population. *(3 marks)*

ii Suggest one way in which farmers who continue to use herbicides may reduce their effects on the natural environment. *(1 mark)*

(NEAB June 1997)

Answers

Chapter 1

1 a A = red blood cell
B = ciliated epithelial cell
C = nerve cell/(neurone)
D = muscle cell/(striated muscle fibre) *(4 marks)*
b A Function – carries oxygen/transports oxygen.
Feature – contains haemoglobin/large surface area for
diffusion of oxygen in or out. *(2 marks)*
B Function – move mucus/deloris/fluids.
Feature – surface covered by cilia which can move.
(2 marks)

2 a cytoplasm
nucleus
cell membrane *(3 marks)*
b chloroplasts/large vacuole/cell wall/starch grains *(4 marks)*
3 a i amino acids/peptides *(1 mark)*
ii clear/colourless/not cloudy *(1 mark)*
b i doubles *(1 mark)*
ii *On graph paper:*
orientation of axes (temperature horizontal and time
vertical) *(1 mark)*
scale (half of each axis used for spread of data) *(1 mark)*
axes labelled and units *(1 mark)*
points plotted correctly *(1 mark)*
line drawn neatly *(1 mark)*
(If **wrong** extrapolation – subtract 1 mark
iii enzyme denatured *(1 mark)*
4 A lung – used for breathing/gas exchange/taking in
oxygen/getting rid of carbon dioxide/water (vapor)
(2 marks)
B heart – pumps blood *(2 marks)*
C liver – stores vitamins/stores minerals/makes bile/
deamination/destroys old red blood cells/ destroys
poisons or alcohol/produces heat/helps keep blood
glucose level steady/stores glycogen *(2 marks)*
5 a 3.9% no cells visible cells have taken up water
and burst (lysed);
0.9% normal cells have taken up and lost
the same amount of water;
0.09% crenated cells have lost water and
shrivelled up *(6 marks)*
b Isotonic solutions have the same osmotic concentration as
blood. *(2 marks)*
6 a A = nucleus
B = (cell surface) membrane *(2 marks)*
b white blood cell correctly drawn – partially engulfing
bacterium *(1 mark)*
7 a amylase breaks down starch
increased temperature increases rate of reaction
enzyme denatured at 70 °C
enzyme does not work at 70 °C *(4 marks)*
b Use same quantities (amounts) of starch
suspension/amalyse/use same concentration of amalyse/
allow solutions to reach the temperature before mixing.
(1 mark)
c Control – set up another tube at each temperature but do not
add the amylase. *(2 marks)*

Chapter 2

1 *In table, in following sequence:*
protein
fibre/roughage
water *(3 marks)*
2 a *In table*
amylase
stomach
fat *(3 marks)*
b *Any two from:*
• makes food soluble
• makes food easier to absorb
• to break it down into smaller units/molecules
• to provide substances for synthesis *(2 marks)*
3 a i *Any two from:*
• warmth
• growth/reproduction/protein synthesis/cell production/repair

• movement/contraction of heart/breathing/peristalsis
• active transport or absorption/nerve impulse/
(*Reject:* digestion/excretion/sensitivity/respiration) *(2 marks)*
ii 3255 kJ *(1 mark)*
iii fat *(1 mark)*
iv protein *(1 mark)*
v *In table:*
bread
potato *(2 marks)*
vi *1st:* add iodine (solution):
2nd: blue–black, black, *dark* blue *(2 marks)*
b i A = stomach
B = small intestine or duodenum or ileum *(2 marks)*
ii amylase/ptyalin *(1 mark)*
iii maltose, glucose of sugar *(1 mark)*
iv *On diagram:*
Small intestine *(1 mark)*
v diffusion *or* active transport *(1 mark)*
4 a small intestine, duodenum, ileum *(1 mark)*
b large surface area;
many capillaries, capillary network, good blood supply;
thin surface *or* capillaries near surface; *(3 marks)*
c diffusion, active transport, facilitated diffusion
(*Reject:* absorption) *(1 mark)*
5 a i production of acid
fatty acid *(2 marks)*
ii pH drops faster (with bile salts)/in flask 1/faster reaction
(1 mark)
iii lower pH denatures the enzyme
(all) fat digested/reaction is complete *(2 marks)*
b liver (*Reject:* gall bladder) *(1 mark)*
6 a food molecules too large/have to be made smaller;
cannot be absorbed/small enough for absorption *(2 marks)*
b i smell (of food) *(1 mark)*
ii chemicals (in food)
detached by receptor cells in (nose lining)
impulses/signals sent to brain *(3 marks)*
iii release of saliva *(1 mark)*
c i amylase *(1 mark)*
ii breaks down starch
into maltose/sugars
(*Reject:* glucose) *(2 marks)*
d i acid/enzymes (in gastric juices)
destroys/erodes/damages (cells in) stomach lining *(2 marks)*

Chapter 3

1 a biconcave disc/no nucleus/contains haemoglobin;
irregular shape/large nucleus/does not contain
haemoglobin/contains granular cytoplasm;
b transports oxygen/carries oxygen;
defense against disease/micro-organisms/phagocytosis.
(4 marks)
2 *Any five from:*
• bacteria cannot pass through epidermis/can pass through
damaged epidermis/through wound
• white blood cells can get out of capillaries
• white blood cells engulf/eat/kill/digest/destroy bacteria
(*Reject:* fight/attack/swallow bacteria – no mark)
• platlets stick/come/hold together (*Reject:* clot/clump together –
no mark)
• formation of fibrin/fibres
• blood cells caught in fibres/correct reference to a clot forming or
its method of formation or its structure as shown in the diagram
(*Reject:* platlets or red blood cells only forming a clot – no mark)
• clot will stop bacteria entering capillary/blood *(5 marks)*
3 a A = vein *(1 mark)*
D = artery *(1 mark)*
b prevent backflow/cause one way flow/cause flow in correct
direction *(1 mark)*
c correct arrows *(2 marks)*
d i increases: up to 100/105/110/ 5.9 litres; then decreases
(3 marks)
ii decreases *(1 mark)*
e oxygen and carbon dioxide named;
correct direction of movement for both;
reference to alveoli;

reference to capillary walls;
reference to passage through walls of alveoli and capillaries;
(5 marks)

4 a i A = aorta
B = left ventricle (2 marks)
ii lung (1 mark)
b i 280
ii *Any five from:*
- fat (/cholesterol) deposited in blood vessels
- blood clot formation
- blocking of coronary artery
- reducing blood flow
- less food/less oxygen to heart muscle (/cells)
- less respiration/less energy release (5 marks)
iii A *Any two from:*
- allows blood passage
- heart muscle received oxygen/food
- allows respiration (2 marks)
B avoid rejection (1 mark)
5 a pumps blood (1 mark)
b A = vein
C = artery (2 marks)
c towards heart (1 mark)
d i red blood cells (1 mark)
ii white blood cells (1 mark)
iii plasma (1 mark)

Chapter 4

1 a i A = diaphragm
B = alveoli or alveolus (2 marks)
ii *In sequence:*
downwards
rib cage
decrease
oxygen
carbon dioxide (5 marks)
b i 10 (1 mark)
ii e.g. $\dfrac{2180 - 650}{3}$
$500 - 533$ cm^3 min^{-1} (based on figures used) (1 mark)
iii breathing rate increases
depth of breathing increases (2 marks)
c i A 9.5 dm^3
B 16 dm^3 (2 marks)
ii to supply oxygen to clear the oxygen debt (2 marks)
iii release of energy without using oxygen (1 mark)
2 a nucleus (1 mark)
b *Any two from:*
- traps dust *or* dirt *or* stops dust entering lungs
- traps bacteria, viruses,micro-organisms, pathogens, germs
- moistens (inhaled air)
(*Reject:* prevents infection) (2 marks)
c beating action
remove dust, dirt, bacteria, viruses, microorganisms,
pathogens, germs, mucus; (*Reject:* prevent entry/get rid of)
(2 marks)
3 a number of deaths increases as number cigarettes smoked increases;
most marked increase at lower numbers cigarettes/less marked
at higher numbers cigarettes (2 marks)
b i Alveolus/alveoli/air sacs (*Reject:* air) (1 mark)
ii *In table:*
1 less – less
2 thicker – less (4 marks)
c i trap bacteria/germs/dust/cleans the air (1 mark)
ii action of cilia/tiny hairs (1 mark)
iii Award mark for concise and logical account, only if one or
more is correct (1 mark)
Any four from:
- cilia paralysed
- microbes (/germs named e.g.) enter lungs/stick in the
mucus/infection occurs
- irritation causes more mucus secretion
- mucus (/microbes) not removed
- microbes (/germs named e.g.) cause disease/microbes
cause damage;
- blockage of air passages (4 marks)

d (Lung) cancer/heart disease/other circulatory disorder/
thrombosis/hypertension/allow other cancers (e.g. cervix/
bladder)/atherosclerosis/ gangrene (1 mark)
4 a i coats surfaces with tar/dirt
ii nicotine narrows arteries
iii destroys air sacs (3 marks)
b mucus drains into lungs while asleep;
accumulate in breathing passage/named breathing passage;
causes coughing to shift mucus (from lungs) (1 mark)
c i *One of the following:*
- cancer
- emphysema
- bronchitis (1 mark)
ii *Two of the following:*
- praise/encouragement for stopping;
- check for hidden cigarettes;
- buy them cigarette substitutes;
- (accept any sensible suggestion e.g. give up with
them/do not smoke in front of them) (2 marks)
iii addiction (1 mark)

Chapter 5

1 a place a small bone in dilute acid and leave overnight – the
bone becomes flexible and rubbery (soft) (2 marks)
b i yellow bone marrow (1 mark)
ii light (1 mark)
2 a i smooth/strong/rigid (1 mark)
ii lubrication (1 mark)
iii strong/elastic (2 marks)
b i spinal chord (1 mark)
ii muscle and ligament attachment (1 mark)
iii shock absorber/prevents bones rubbing together/
allows slight movement (1 mark)
3 a A = triceps
B = biceps (2 marks)
b contracts *or* shortens
pulls (on ulna)
(*Reject:* tightens/tenses) (2 marks)
4 a back straighter
legs straighter
whole of foot on the ground; neck straight (3 marks)
b i A
ii body held upright (2 marks)
5 a One mark for each correct answer (3 marks)
b e.g. smooth, strong (2 marks)
6 a *Any four from:*
- (diseased) head removed
- femur cut at epiphysial plate
- artificial head attached via titanium strands
- metal cap fixed over new head of femur
- plastic cup fitted into pelvis (4 marks)
b i smooth movement/3D movement/allows rotation (1 mark)
ii hard wearing (1 mark)
7 a *Any two from:*
- too much weight on toe bones
- abnormal bending of metatarsals/bones in toe region
of foot
- abnormal bending in ankle/heel region (2 marks)
b *Any two from:*
- fatigue in leg muscles
- affects posture in trunk causing fatigue
- deform pelvic girdle/deform hip (2 marks)
c allow bones to grow fully/in correct position/shoes should not
slip causing claw toe (1 mark)
8 a humerus (1 mark)
b cartilage (1 mark)
c i lumbar (1 mark)
ii back is straight and supported (1 mark)

Chapter 6

1 a 5 (five) (1 mark)
b heat/cold/pressure/movement (1 mark)
c heat – a sweat gland would produce more sweat (1 mark)
2 a i skin (1 mark)
ii ear (1 mark)

Answers

b A = sclera/sclerotic coat *(1 mark)*
  B = suspensory ligaments *(1 mark)*
c cornea/pupil *(1 mark)*
  cornea/lens *(1 mark)*
d i retina *(1 mark)*
  ii rods/cones/light sensitive cells/electrical signals/impulses *(2 marks)*
e i A = radial muscles
  B = circular muscles *(2 marks)*
  ii iris *(1 mark)*
f i circular muscles (of iris) *(1 mark)*
  ii too much light/a lot of light may enter the eye;
  causes damage to retina/sensitive cells *(2 marks)*

3 a i P = cornea
  Q = lens
  R = ciliary muscle/ciliary body
  (*Reject:* circular/radial) *(3 marks)*
  ii 1 thinner/narrower/flatter/stretched by suspensory ligament *(1 mark)*
  2 relax *(1 mark)*
  iii *Any two from:*
  • adjusts size of pupil/(iris opens and closes)
  • adjusts amount of light entering
  • reduces light scattering (resulting in sharp vision) *(2 marks)*
b i short-sighted/myopic *(1 mark)*
  ii eyeball too long lens too strong/lens too fat/too converging/light rays/image focused in vitreous humour/not on retina/in front of retina/image not focussed/image blurred *(2 marks)*
  iii *On diagram:*
  diverging lens drawn (wider at edges than middle) *(1 mark)*
c **Retina:**
  sensitive to light/has light receptors/has rods and/or cones; generates impulses/electrical signals
  (*Reject:* messages/information) *(2 marks)*
  Optic nerve:
  carries impulses/electrical signals (from retina to brain) *(1 mark)*
  Brain:
  unscrambles/interprets impulses/"sees"/"forms a picture"/ co-ordinates muscle action in eye *(1 mark)*

4 a A = ossicles/named bones
  B = cochlea
  C = ear drum/tympanium/tympanic membrane *(3 marks)*
b cochlea *(1 mark)*
c i external ear/pinna/earflap *(1 mark)*
  ii arrow from external ear canal to ear drum;
  arrow from eardrum through ossicles to cochlea *(2 marks)*
d left ear more stimulated/closer to sound/sound arrives at left ear first;
  brain compares amount of stimulation/time of arrival/input from each ear *(2 marks)*
e i sound waves cannot pass/absorbed by wax (idea of a blockage)
  ii ossicles unable to vibrate properly/fluid absorbs vibration
  iii impulses (from receptors) unable to travel to brain/accept "messages" *(3 marks)*
f ear drum at bottom of external ear may be damaged/broken, may prevent it from vibrating *(2 marks)*

Chapter 7

1 a i both require a stimulus
  both result in a change/response in organs *(2 marks)*
  ii message carried by nerve or blood/no hormones involved in nervous system/hormones involved in endocrine system/no nerves involved in endocrine system. *(1 mark)*
2 a A = (cell surface) membrane
  B = cytoplasm
  C = nucleus
  (*Accept:* nuclear membrane, *Reject:* nucleus) *(3 marks)*
b (Increases) contacts with other cells *or* impulses/signal/messages from (/to) other cells
  (*Accept:* contact more cells) *(1 mark)*
c brain, spinal cord, CNS, grey matter
  (*Reject:* spine/spinal column) *(1 mark)*

d arrow pointing downwards/into cell body from denrites/out of motor end plate *(1 mark)*
3 a response/reaction
  involuntary/sub-conscious/automatic *(2 marks)*
b i A = sensory/afferent neurone
  (/nerve fibre/axon/nerve cell)
  B = motor/efferent neurone
  (/nerve fibre/axon/nerve cell)
  (*Accept:* neurone) *(2 marks)*
  ii 1 in skin (of hand)
  2 muscle (in arm)/correctly named example *(2 marks)*
  iii cerebral hemispheres/cerebrum/forebrain *(1 mark)*
  iv any cerebral reflex
  pupil size change, blinking, salvation, change in size of pupil *(1 mark)*
c i (before) – 140 mm
  (after) – 184 mm *(2 marks)*
  ii appropriate reference to slower response (or application of this)
  e.g. slows reactions/slows braking/difficult to avoid sudden obstacles.
  (*Reject:* "blurred vision"/"can't concentrate"/etc) *(1 mark)*

4 a *On diagram:*
  X on cerebral hemisphere
  Y on cerebellum
  Z on medulla *(3 marks)*
b i automatic action or involuntary action/uncontrolled
  (*Accept:* no thinking. *Reject:* does not involve brain)
  response (to stimulus) or reaction
  (*Reject:* examples of reactions) *(2 marks)*
  ii *In table:*
  (braking) – voluntary
  (blinking) – reflex
  (dropping) – reflex *(3 marks)*
c *Any two from:*
  • stimulant speed up reactions/speeds up brain activity *or* depressant slows
  • stimulant causes wakefulness/alertness/awareness *or* depressant causes drowsiness
  • stimulant increases heart rate *or* depressant slows *(2 marks)*

5 a diagram correctly labelled *(3 marks)*
b receptor at the end of the sensory neurone *(1 mark)*
c i reading/writing/playing the piano *(1 mark)*
  ii involuntary/no control over/automatic *(1 mark)*
  iii message cannot travel out of CNS to effector/ no message reaches effector *(1 mark)*

Chapter 8

1 a i provides energy *(1 mark)*
  ii replace salt lost in sweat *(1 mark)*
b sweat glands increase production
  evaporation of sweat
  cools body *(3 marks)*
  heart rate increases
  more oxygen to muscles
  more glucose to muscles *(3 marks)*
  breathes faster
  more oxygen into blood
  more carbon dioxide out of blood *(3 marks)*
c anaerobic respiration; to provide extra energy *(2 marks)*

2 a i 2.025 m^2 *(1 mark)*
  ii person A because they have a larger surface area (to volume ratio) *(1 mark)*
b vasoconstriction/hairs stand on end/no sweat produced *(1 mark)*

3 a X pituitary
  Y ovaries
  Z adrenal *(3 marks)*
b i 0.1%/1 mg cm^{-3}/100 mg per 199 cm^3/5 mmol per litre *(1 mark)*
  ii increased secretion of insulin and more glucose is converted to glycogen;
  blood sugar levels falls *(2 marks)*
  increased secretion of glucagon and more glycogen is converted into glucose so blood sugar level rises *(2 marks)*

iii if blood sugar level falls or gets above normal;
there is feedback by the blood to glucose detectors in the pancreas;
hormone causing change no longer produced/other hormone secretion increased *(3 marks)*
iv *Graph must show:*
the blood glucose level rising and the axes labelled correctly *(3 marks)*
v The blood glucose level would fall *(1 mark)*

4 a *On diagram:*
X on glomerulus/Bowman's capsule;
Y to artery entering glomerulus (to point where branching);
Z to collecting duct; reject side branches *(3 marks)*
b i 1 protein *(1 mark)*
2 too big *(1 mark)*
ii reabsorption/taken back into blood
by kidney tubule/any named part
glucose 100% AND sodium only partial *(3 marks)*
c i *Any three from:*
- exchange of materials across membrane/ material cross the membrane
- by diffusion/"osmosis" if water
- to give/until same concentration/until balance equilibrium/until correct body concentration/ correct reference homeostasis reference
- prevents loss of glucose/amino acids
- prevents water loss/gain/blood pressure changes *(3 marks)*
ii 1 blood (/platelets) contact with 'foreign' surface *(1 mark)*
2 *Any three from:*
- narrowing/blockage of arterioles/capillaries/any named blood vessel
- hinders/prevents blood flow
- hinders/prevents supply of food/oxygen
- hinders/prevents respiration/energy release
- tissues/cells die/stroke/heart attack/gangrene/ thrombosis if qualified e.g. pulmonary
(*Reject:* heart failure)
(*Give coronary thrombosis = 2 marks*) *(3 marks)*

5 a i A = blood capillary/vessel
B = sweat gland *(2 marks)*
ii on the surface of the skin it absorbs heat from the skin and evaporates/latent heat of vaporisation *(2 marks)*
b i vasoconstriction/blood vessels narrower so less blood flow *(1 mark)*
ii involuntary contraction of muscles (skeletal muscles) *(1 mark)*

Chapter 9

1 a i Swims using energy released in its mitochondria from food (nutrients) in the semen *(2 marks)*
ii 23 *(1 mark)*
b i X
ii Y
iii XY *(3 marks)*
c the zygote divides into two identical cells each develops into a foetus *(2 marks)*
d i after menstruation the lining repairs
an extra layer (enidometrium) develops
controlled by hormones/names of *(3 marks)*
ii prevents implantation of the embryo *(1 mark)*
e i egg cannot reach the uterus *(1 mark)*
ii woman will be treated with hormones to produce eggs which can be collected;
eggs are mixed with semen sample in a petri dish;
fertilisation results in pre-embryos;
pre-embryo transferred into woman's uterus 3 days later *(4 marks)*

2 a i A = ovary
B = vagina
C = uterus/womb
D = oviduct/Fallopian tube *(4 marks)*
ii fusion of gametes/fusion of egg and sperm nucleus *(1 mark)*
On diagram: 'X' on oviduct *(1 mark)*
iii *Any three from:*
- supplies oxygen to foetus
- supplies food (*or named nutrients*) to foetus
- removes waste (urea/carbon dioxide)
- prevents infection acts as immunological barrier *(3 marks)*

iv shock absorber/support/maintains moisture/stabilises temperature *(1 mark)*
v sperm can't reach egg/egg can't reach uterus *(1 mark)*
b i all increase *(1 mark)*
ii growth of baby's bones *(1 mark)*
iii protein in milk
for growth/making cells/repair *(2 marks)*

3 a i fertilisation – the fusion of the gametes/fusion of the egg and sperm nucleus
ii implantation – the embedding of the embryo in the uterus wall *(2 marks)*
iii with progesterone only pill, ovulation still occurs so an egg will be present for fertilisation *(2 marks)*

4 a very young baby is fed on milk – no starch/no starch in milk/enzyme not required – baby does not eat starch *(1 mark)*
b the foetus stores iron during pregnancy/the baby will have a store of iron *(1 mark)*
c babies drink a lot of milk, adults do not *(1 mark)*

5 a i uterus/womb *(1 mark)*
ii *Any two from:*
- thin surface/two blood supplies close together
- large surface area
- good blood supply/capillary network/large number of capillaries/lake of mother's blood *(2 marks)*
b i (*From mother to foetus*): *Any two from:*
- oxygen
- food/correct named e.g. water (*Reject:* "protein")
- antibody; drug/named examples
- virus/named e.g. *(2 marks)*
(*from foetus to mother*) *Any two from:*
- carbon dioxide
- urea
- "waste products" = max 1 mark *(2 marks)*
ii diffusion (*Reject:* osmosis) *(1 mark)*
c i virus is small(er) *(1 mark)*
ii avoid rejection
(*Reject:* "harm"/"kill") *(1 mark)*

6 a i gets wider/dilates *(1 mark)*
ii detaches from uterus *(1 mark)*
iii breaks/bursts *(1 mark)*
b i receives colostrum/antibodies from mother;
closer contact with mother *(2 marks)*
ii convenient/does not require mother's presence *(1 mark)*

7 a i ovary *(1 mark)*
ii nucleus *(1 mark)*
iii contains the chromosomes/female chromosomes *(1 mark)*
iv nutrients for the development of the embryo *(1 mark)*
b can move/swim on its own *(1 mark)*
c i stops eggs reaching the uterus/prevents sperms reaching the egg *(1 mark)*
ii prevents implantation of an embryo *(1 mark)*

8 a i 0.006 mm *(1 mark)*
ii to release energy for swimming/movement *(1 mark)*
b penetration by the egg *(1 mark)*

Chapter 10

1 a i head and/ or neck
ii legs *(2 marks)*
b *Any two from:*
- shorter/small
- (shorter) *legs*
- head looks big (proportion) *(2 marks)*
c *Any two from:*
- facial hair/hair on chest/pubic hair/hair on legs/in armpits
- voice breaking; sperm production
- acne/"spots" increase in testosterone/sex hormone *(2 marks)* *(1 mark)*

2 a 22–24
b steep slope to age 3 – due to rapid infant growth;
curve less steep to age 10 as growth rate slows as child is more active;
steep slope as growth rate increases during the adolescent growth spurt; *(4 marks)*
c 9 months (just less than 1 year) – foetus is growing in the uterus *(2 marks)*

3 a i to hold the testes outside of the body *(1 mark)*

Answers

ii egg passes along this from the ovary to the uterus *(1 mark)*
iii carries semen out of the penis *(1 mark)*
b i growth of body hair/pubic hair *(1 mark)*
   ii breasts develop/facial hair/widening of hips *(1 mark)*
   iii male – 12, female – 11 *(1 mark)*
c i menstruation;
   egg is maturing in the ovary *(2 marks)*
   ii ovulation occurs during this period;
   egg present after ovulation;
   fertilisation most likely;
   sperm released into vagina before ovulation may survive
   long enough to fertilise egg *(4 marks)*
d oestrogen and progesterone continue to be produced;
build-up in the blood;
FSH is not produced/FSH production is inhibited *(3 marks)*

4 a i ovary *(1 mark)*
   ii vagina;
   uterus/cervix;
   Fallopian tube/oviduct *(3 marks)*
b egg and sperm fuse/combine/join *(1 mark)*
c uterus/womb *(1 mark)*
d provides/supplies oxygen/soluble food/named food/removes
urea/carbon dioxide;
reference to mother's and baby's blood *(2 marks)*
e i growth slows down/line falls *(1 mark)*
   ii puberty/adolescence/sexual maturity/ hormones/named
   hormones *(1 mark)*
   iii curve approximately same shape (earlier in time) *(1 mark)*
f i bases in DNA/mRNA;
   order forms a code/mRNA copies code;
   code controls order of amino acids in proteins *(3 marks)*
   ii gene has mutated *(1 mark)*

5 a i 139 cm *(1 mark)*
   ii male *(1 mark)*
   iii selecting and adding the ten figures correctly (1534 cm);
   dividing by 10 (1534/10);
   153.4 cm;
   value inserted into table (accept value calculated) *(4 marks)*
b i *Graph must show:* scale provided (not own scale);
   plotting figures for males accurately;
   plotting figures for females (accept candidate's value);
   joining points accurately;
   identifying curves *(5 marks)*
   ii 13–13.2 years (accept value on graph) *(1 mark)*
   iii 12–14 years *(1 mark)*
c onset of puberty earlier in females *(1 mark)*

Chapter 11

1 a carries oxygen *(1 mark)*
b H listless *(1 mark)*
c Hh, h, h, hh *(3 marks)*
d both have the H gene *(1 mark)*
e 1 in 4 *(1 mark)*
2 a the number of chromosomes/more chromosomes/
46 chromosomes *(1 mark)*
b the daughter cells have the same number of chromosomes as
the parent cell;
the chromosomes are present as pairs/homologons pairs
(2 marks)
3 a i bases, purines *and* pyrimidines *(1 mark)*
   ii replicating, duplicating, multiplying, reproducing
   (Reject: just dividing/splitting/unzipping) *(1 mark)*
   iii *On diagram:*
   A opposite T *and* C opposite G on appropriate bases;
   (Accept: if just given on one side) *(1 mark)*
   iv *Either:*
   sequences of bases/letters (in DNA);
   codes for sequence of amino acids (in protein) *(2 marks)*
   Or: DNA codes for protein *(1 mark)*
4 a i NN, Nn
   ii nn *(3 marks)*
b P genotypes correct – both Nn;
gametes correct P genotypes – e.g. N + n and N + n;
offspring genotypes correctly derived from gametes;
offspring phenotypes correct reference to genotypes
(Accept: points derived correctly from the previous point, even if
previous point is incorrect and allow alternative letters) *(4 marks)*

c 1 in 4 *(1 mark)*
5 a i *Any two from:*
   • distinct types/relatively few types or no in-betweens
   • caused by inheritance of single gene/only a few genes
   • no (/or minimal) environmental influence/remains
    same throughout lifetime *(2 marks)*
   ii change in DNA, in a gene, in a chromosome
   (Reject: examples) *(1 mark)*
   iii (recessive) – idea that allele not expressed in
   heterozygote/only in homozygote
   • characteristic not expressed in heterozygote/only in
    homozygote
   • effect overwhelmed by dominant allele(s)
   • allele whose effect is not visible but may be in later
    generations *(2 marks)*
   iv DNA; codes for a protein, an enzyme, a characteristic;
   (Reject: "genes code for characteristics") *(2 marks)*
b i genotypes of parents – both Nn;
   gametes from P genotypes, (if no P genotypes) – N + n and
   N + n;
   F$_1$ genotypes correctly derived from gametes
   e.g. NN + 2Nn + nn;
   non-PKU correctly identified in F$_1$ genotypes; PKU correctly
   identified in F$_1$ genotypes
   (Accept: any standard form for presentation of argument
   (4 marks)
   ii 1. $\frac{1}{4}$, 0.25, 25%, 1 in 4, 1:3
   (Reject: 3:1)
   2. $\frac{1}{2}$ or 0.5, 50%, 1 in 2, 1:1
   (Reject: 1:2, 50/50) *(2 marks)*
c i enzyme 1 not formed, enzyme 1 non-functional;
   not broken down, myalamine substance not changed to A
   (2 marks)
   ii phenylalanine = amino acid found in proteins or must
   have low phenylalanine in diet or must prevent build-up
   of phenylalanine; *(Reject:* "amino acids") *(1 mark)*

Chapter 12

1 a i fat *(1 mark)*
   ii 73 (72–74) kg *(1 mark)*
   iii person A – reduce intake of fat/carbohydrate/high energy
   foods/other named food *(1 mark)*
   person B – increase intake of energy foods/named food
   (1 mark)
   iv *Any one from:*
   high blood pressure/strain on heart/bad posture/damage
   to joints/unable to take exercise/diabetes/varicose veins/
   built up of fat in arteries/thrombosis/heart attack *(1 mark)*
   v *Any two from:*
   • less fat
   • lower cholesterol
   • more fibre
   • higher carbohydrate
   • more energy from carbohydrate *(2 marks)*
2 a optimum temperature for the enzyme/recreate body
temperature *(1 mark)*
b litmus *(1 mark)*
c Tube A – no acid produced
Tube B – acid produced
Tube C – no acid produced
Tube D – no acid produced *(6 marks)*
d Tooth scrapings contain bacteria;
bacteria ferment sugar to produce acid which causes decay
(2 marks)
3 a 0.14 seconds (0.25 → 0.39) *(2 marks)*
b alcohol slows reaction times and affects judgement so you do
not react as quickly to situations and are more likely to have
an accident *(3 marks)*
c i the drug causes chemical changes in the body/drug
   becomes part of the body chemistry *(1 mark)*
   ii sweating/vomiting/mental confusion/uncontrolled
   muscular spasms/coma *(1 mark)*
d i by sharing needles the virus can be transmitted from an
   infected person *(2 marks)*
   ii liver damage, brain damage, kidney damage, heart
   damage/other sensible answer *(2 marks)*

4 a alcohol is a small molecule and can dissolve in fat *(1 mark)*
b enzyme in men gets rid of/removes some alcohol;
women smaller than men *(2 marks)*
c i alcohol passes out of/excreted by lungs/breathed out
(1 mark)
ii alcohol passes out/excreted by kidney *(1 mark)*
d extra enzymes to break down alcohol;
need more to replace/compensate for that broken down by
enzyme *(2 marks)*
e *Any three from:*
- swelling due to fat
- destruction/damage due to immune response
- jaundice/yellow eyes and skin due to liver unable to
remove broken down blood pigments
- cirrhosis due to fibrous tissue replacing damaged cells
(Reject: blood flow references) *(3 marks)*
f Interferes with brain function/slows down
brain/nerves/depressant;
causes loss of self control/judgement/removes inhibitions
(2 marks)

Chapter 13

1 a tuberculosis – bacterium;
athlete's foot – through contact (skin/appropriate article);
rabies – virus;
– bite of infected animal *(4 marks)*
b i bacterium; *(1 mark)*
ii excessive/lot of/more than normal loss of fluids/fluid loss
so high as 20l per day;
(death) due to dehydration *(2 marks)*
iii replaces body fluids (lost by diarrhoea);
replaces salts/ions *(2 marks)*
iv antibiotics kills bacteria/pathogens *(1 mark)*
c boiled water has been sterilised/tap water may contain
cholera bacteria/boiling kills bacteria/pathogen *(1 mark)*
d 1 Lymphocyte *(1 mark)*
Produces antibodies which react with antigens/disease
organisms/produce antitoxins which
destroy/neutralise/counteract toxins produced by
pathogens/kill pathogens *(1 mark)*
2 Leucocyte/phagocyte *(1 mark)*
engulf/digest/ingest pathogens *(1 mark)*
2 a i correctly labelled
ii correctly labelled *(2 marks)*
b bacteria/microbes use oxygen;
for respiration *(2 marks)*
c bacteria (in tank);
convert ammonium compounds to nitrate *(2 marks)*
d effluent cleaner/can be discharged without further treatment
(1 mark)
e i (microbes) feed on organic material;
microbes increase in number;
more oxygen used/*more* respiration *(3 marks)*
ii solids from sewage/alga growth *(1 mark)*
iii nitrates (formed when sewage) released in water;
acts as fertiliser *(2 marks)*
3 a i number of cases increases (when antibiotics used) or stays
high/stays the same/doesn't drop *(1 mark)*
ii number of cases decreases (when vaccination used)
(1 mark)
b (in range) 1975–1979/late '70s;
when rise in number of cases or when line goes up
(Reject: '80s)
(Accept: if wrong date but line is rising) *(2 marks)*
c *Any four from:*
- use of non-reproducing/non-virulent/harmless/'treated'/dead/
fragments of virus/bacterium/germ/antigen/modified toxin
(Reject: mild, *Accept:* denatured *not* disease)
(Reject: phagocytes)
- reference to white blood cells or lymphocytes
- manufacture of antibodies
- antibodies combine with microbes *or* clump together
microbes *or* destroy/kill microbes *or* destroy antigen
- antibodies are specific
- cells (which make antibodies) multiply
- more rapid or more extensive secdonary reaction

- reference to immunological memory *or* still able to make
antibodies/recognise 'disease' again/antibodies are still
there *(4 marks)*
d *Any two from:*
- (infected person) breathes out, coughs, sneezes (germs into air)
- breathed in by other people
- microbes/germs carried in drops of water *(2 marks)*
4 a *On graph paper:*
orientation of axes correct;
scale: linear and > $\frac{1}{2}$ of each axis for data spread;
axes labelled inc. units;
points correctly plotted; *Accept:* omission of 0–0
line ruled point-to-point
(Reject: if more than $\frac{1}{2}$ square out) *(5 marks)*
b *Any four from:*
- white blood cells make (/release) antibodies
- white blood cells (/lymphocytes/antibodies) react with
antigens (on bacteria)
(Accept: virus, microbes, micro-organisms)
- "activated" (/"more") white blood cells act in secondary
response; secondary response gives more rapid (/greater)
- antibody-production; circulating antibodies (/"activated"
white blood cells) can respond (to infection with live
bacteria);
(Accept: references to other microbes)
reference to specificity of Antibodies or white blood
cells/reference to "recognise" microbes
(Reject: fight bacteria) *(4 marks)*
Award mark for logical sequence linking cause to effect
throughout only if one or more explanations is correct
(1 mark)
5 a i mass of abnormally arranged/mutated cells; multiply
without the need for repair or enlargement of
organism/cell division uncontrolled *(2 marks)*
ii cells from/part of cancer enter blood stream/lymph;
carried to other part of body and colonise/invade/grow
(2 marks)
b increase risk of lung/mouth/throat cancer *(1 mark)*
sunlight contains ultra-violet light;
may cause skin tumours/melanoma *(2 marks)*
c *Any two from:*
- (risk of) leaks greater
- radiation levels in environment higher
- work place has higher exposure and workers live in the
area
- radiation carcinogenic
- damage to gametes causing cancer in children *(2 marks)*
d *Any two from:*
- environmental differences (e.g. food, industrial carcinogens)
- industrialised countries people live longer so more exposure
to carcinogens
- industrialised countries older people with cancer more likely
to die
- different countries have different types of cancer causing
deaths
- developing countries more deaths from infectious disease
higher so fewer old age cancers
- industrialised countries better diagnosis of cancer
(Accept: any other valid comparison related to cancer)
(2 marks)
6 a i *Any four from:*
- reference to pathogen being/having antigens
- reference to white blood cells/lymphocytes
- reference to making antibodies
- reference to antibodies reacting with/destroying
- antigens/pathogens/bacteria
- reference to phagocyte *(4 marks)*
ii *Any two from:*
- reference to phagocytes digesting bacteria;
- reference to memory cells/antibodies being
retained/reference to immunity being due to presence of
memory cells/antibodies;
- reference to response being more rapid *(2 marks)*
iii *Any one from:*
antibodies/memory cells do not recognise the new form;
each form of virus needs a different antibody *(1 mark)*

Answers

Chapter 14

1 a B A D C *(1 mark)*
   b petri dish containing food but not contaminated by
      housefly/same but miss stage C out *(1 mark)*
   c no bacterial or fungal growth on the food medium/no growth
      of micro-organisms *(1 mark)*
2 a i *Any four from:*
   • two chains, helix
   • double helix
   (*Accept:* any of these points from a (labelled) diagram: twisted/
   winding held together by bases/bases drawn down centre/
   4 correctly named bases/purines & pyrimidines/nucleotides)
   • A (always pairs) with T
   • G (always pairs) with C
   • held together with hydrogen bonds
   Further detail e.g. correct reference to sugar *or* phosphate
      (4 marks)
   ii specificity explained – at G–A *or* at same sequence/at same
      place *or* to give same base sequence on ends *or* to give
      TTAA on ends;
      advantage explained – ref complementarity *or* reference
      to human DNA & plasmid can bind to each other/2 types
      of DNA can bind to each other *(2 marks)*
   iii *Any two from:*
   • all formed from same original cell *or* same bacterium
   • by 'mitosis'/asexual reproduction
   • reference to copying of DNA *or* copying of genes *(2 marks)*
   b i *Any two from:*
   • less chance of disease (transmission)
      (*Accept:* BSE or CJD or other e.g. no need to kill animals)
   • product identical to human growth hormone, no
      rejection
   • easy to purify
   • cheap to produce
   • bacteria multiply quickly/ more hGH made
      (*Accept:* quick to produce GH) *(2 marks)*
3 a i *Any five from:*
   • two chains, helix – double helix
   • held together by bases
   • four types of bases, A, T, C, G,
   • A pairs with T, C with G
   • held together by hydrogen bonds
   • chains made from sugar and phosphates
   • molecule is spiral/twisted
      (*Accept:* any on a diagram) *(5 marks)*
   ii DNA molecule unzips/splits into two strands;
      new nucleotides are attached to each strand;
      only complementary bases bond together/
      A bonds with T, C bonds with G *(3 marks)*
   b i Hepatitis B *(1 mark)*
   ii surface antigen;
      micro-organism/yeast/bacteria;
      antigens *(3 marks)*
   c the gene will be replicated when the cell divides; the gene will
      influence development *(2 marks)*
4 a penicillium/fungus *(1 mark)*
   b i sugar goes down as growth goes up;
      sugar being used for the growth/respiration/oxidised (by
      micro-organism) *(2 marks)*
   c 170–200 hours;
      reaches maximum then/very little increase after that *(2 marks)*
   d filtered/suitable method of separating cells from culture
      medium;
      penicillin extracted from filtrate/culture medium *(2 marks)*
   e i cholera;
      TB *(2 marks)*
   ii *Any two from:*
   • viruses
   • live inside cells
   • antibiotics unable to enter cells
   • antibiotics do not kill viruses/only kill bacteria *(2 marks)*
   f i mutation *(1 mark)*
   ii *Any one from:*
   • develop new antibiotics
   • restrict use of antibiotics
   • rotate/change antibiotics used *(1 mark)*

5 a respiration;
      produces carbon dioxide;
      gas bubbles are light and therefore rise *(3 marks)*
   b i amylase *(1 mark)*
   ii breaks down starch to sugar *(1 mark)*

Chapter 15

1 a i rabbit *or* chicken
   ii human
   iii wheat *(3 marks)*
   b i sun *or* light;
      (*Reject:* photosynthesis/respiration/minerals/soil/water
      (1 mark)
   ii pyramid drawn correct shape i.e. 3 blocks, decreasing in
      size going upward;
      correct labels – largest = wheat, middle = rabbit, smallest =
      fox
      (*Reject:* extra correct tier if labelled 'sun'/'light') *(2 marks)*
2 a bacteria;
      fungi *(2 marks)*
   b respiration *(1 mark)*
   c to make amino acids/proteins/nucleic acids/DNA *(1 mark)*
3 a *Correct sequence:*
      third-order consumer
      second-order consumer
      first-order consumer
      producer *(1 mark)*
   b i plant eater *(1 mark)*
   ii $\dfrac{88}{88\,000} \times 100$
      $= 0.1$ *(2 marks)*
   iii *Any two from:*
   • heat
   • movement
   • respiration (*Reject:* "used for" respiration)
   • active transport
   • egestion
   • excretion
   • dead (lost/inedible) parts
   • mating
   • evaporation/sweating/transpiration
      (*Reject:* growth *or* reproduction) *(2 marks)*
4 a radiation from Sun *(1 mark)*
   b i 20000 kJ *(2 marks)*
   ii 3000 kJ *(1 mark)*
   c route A;
      reference to energy losses in cow;
      by wastes;
      maintenance;
      movement;
      to environment *(6 marks)*
5 a i four *(1 mark)*
   ii nitrifying bacteria *(1 mark)*
   iii protein/ammonia/nitrate *(1 mark)*
   iv consumption/eating/consumes *(1 mark)*
   v allows water to drain/prevents water building up;
      reduces the activity of denitrifying bacteria/ reduces the
      number of denitrifying bacteria *(2 marks)*
   vi plants use the nitrates to make proteins;
      more nitrates have to be added in fertilisers *(2 marks)*
6 a i ecosystem *(1 mark)*
   ii community *(1 mark)*
   b pesticides washed/drain into pond/blown by wind;
      kill/harm animals and plans *(2 marks)*
7 a i 45 500 *(1 mark)*
   ii $\dfrac{45\,500}{1\,880\,000} \times 100\%$
      $= 2.4\%$ *(2 marks)*
   b some energy is reflected;
      some is not absorbed;
      some is used in plant respiration;
      some is used to heat the plant *(4 marks)*
   c heat *(1 mark)*

Chapter 16

1 a i 14(%) *(1 mark)*

ii 70–79 years over 90 years *(1 mark)*

b *Any one from:*
- rises
- fewer *children/babies* die/more survive
- more reach reproductive age *(1 mark)*

c *Any two from:*
- (more) use of vaccines
- clean water
- (better) sewage/waste disposal
- better diet/example of better food hygiene
- ante/post natal care/better medical facilities
- reference to an example of improved hygiene *(2 marks)*

d i waste gases/named gases from power stations enter air;
dissolve in/react with/combine with rain water/clouds;
acid rain falls into lakes and rivers *(3 marks)*

ii more carbon dioxide in air (from fuels used);
absorbs energy radiated from Earth;
keeps earth warmer/insulates/prevents heat loss from Earth *(3 marks)*

2 a domestic *(1 mark)*

b i from animal and plant remains, which were buried million of years ago *(2 marks)*

ii produce gases *(1 mark)*
which may cause acid rain;
one effect of acid rain described *(2 marks)*

c i one which will not "run out";
reason e.g. recycled *(2 marks)*

ii e.g. not enough high ground *(1 mark)*

3 a i rainfall, run-off, leaching, wind, spray-drift
(*Accept:* description)
(*Reject:* 'through air/soil') *(1 mark)*

ii removal of waste/one named substance from the body
(*Reject:* faeces/urine)
(*Reject:* one named substance) *(1 mark)*

iii 1 $\dfrac{25\,000\,000;}{5}$

5 million times *(2 marks)*
(*Accept:* equivalent working)
(*Allow:* 1 mark for working if incorrect answer *2 marks for correct answer if no working or incorrect working*)

2 *Any three from:*
- DDT passed along food chain *or* DDT in birds' food/in fish
- one (predator) eats many (prey)
- DDT stored in organisms *or* DDT not excreted
- increase in concentration of DDT
- high concentration is enough to poison birds or to kill birds
(*Accept:* amount) *(3 marks)*

b Aldrin breaks down more quickly/does not remain as long;
less likely to build up in food chain/less likely to be eaten/less will be eaten/less enters food chain/less passes up food chain *(2 marks)*

4 a i air will be unchanged in composition since it was trapped in the snow *(1 mark)*

ii 0/present day;
120 thousands of years; *(2 marks)*
Any two from:
- contain highest levels of carbon dioxide
- carbon dioxide absorbs heat radiated by Earth
- carbon dioxide causes atmosphere to increase in temperature *(2 marks)*

b *Any five from:*
- deforestation
- decreases amount taken up by plants/reference to trees using carbon dioxide
- increases amount by burning of wood
- increases amount due to microbial decomposition of wood
- (increased burning) of fossil fuels
- burning releases carbon dioxide into air *(5 marks)*

c *Any two from:*
- use alternative energy sources/named energy source
- reforestation
- fertilisation of oceans to increase use (by sea plants) *(2 marks)*

5 a built on *(1 mark)*

b i to free land for farming/agriculture/growing crops;
to produce paper/wood for burning/paper products/wood for building *(2 marks)*

ii amount of carbon dioxide is increasing;
less oxygen is being produced;
because of less photosynthesis;
or amount of water vapour is falling;
because of less transpiration *(3 marks)*

c i adds nitrogen to the soil *(1 mark)*

ii reduces competition by destroying pests *(1 mark)*

iii reduces competition by destroying weeds *(1 mark)*

d i the chemicals could leave toxic residues on the food/chemicals in food could accumulate in the body *(1 mark)*

ii more wastage/ more of the crop is spoiled by pests/high labour costs/needs more land *(1 mark)*

e i removes food sources/named food sources;
build up in food chain to levels which are toxic to birds;
accumulate in the bird to toxic dose *(3 marks)*

ii use biodegradable pesticides *(1 mark)*

Index ━━━━━━━━━━━━━━━━━━━━━━━━━━━━

G

gametes 116, 118, 156
  see also ova; sperms
GE see genetic engineering
gene therapy 115, 222–3, 236
genes 140, 154–5, 156, 157, 158–63
  mutations 164–5
  and senescence 146
genetic code 154, 155
genetic engineering (GE) 226, 227, 228–9, 232
  and agriculture 232–3, 258
  and enzyme production 230
genetic predicting 160–61
genetic screening 164
genetically modified (GM) foods 151, 232
genetics, laws of 158
genotype 158, 159
  and health 171
gestation period 126
glands
  of digestive system 24, 25
  endocrine 94–5
  exocrine 94
glaucoma 80
global warming 256, 262, 264, 265
glucagon 102, 103
glucose
  detection in urine 99, 230, 231
  production in photosynthesis 244, 245
glycogen 18, 48, 102
GM foods see genetically modified foods
Graafian follicle 118, 119
greenhouse gases 256, 264, 265
growth and development 136–47
gum disease 174, 175

H

habitats 242
  carrying capacity 254
haemodialysis 106, 107
haemoglobin 36, 38
haemophilia 160, 161, 164, 170
hallucinogenic drugs 184
hazard warning symbols 173
HCG see human chorionic gonadotrophim
health 168–85
health behaviour 170, 171, 174–5
health education 210, 211
health and safety legislation 172
hearing 82–3
heart 42–3
heart bypass surgery 34, 35
heart disease 35-6, 44–5
heat exhaustion 110
heat stroke 110
heavy metals, pollution by 266, 267
heroin 184
HGH see human growth hormone
high blood pressure 35, 44, 168, 169

histamine 38, 188
HIV see human immunodeficiency virus
homeostasis 98–111, 170
  see also osmoregulation
homologous pairs (chromosomes) 156
hormone replacement therapy (HRT) 144
hormones 94, 95
  transport 38
  see also specific hormones
human chorionic gonadotrophim (HCG) 115, 122, 126
human growth hormone (HGH) 126, 140, 144
human immunodeficiency virus (HIV) 192–3
human populations 254–5
Huntington's chorea 164, 165
hybridomas 236, 237
hyperglycaemia 99
hypertension see high blood pressure
hypoglycaemia 99
hypothalamus 87, 92, 94, 95, 100, 101, 107
  and body temperature regulation 108, 110
  and lactation 133
  and puberty 144
hypothermia 110

I

imaging techniques 2, 190
immune response 16, 38, 206
immune system 204, 206, 207
implantation 122, 123
in vitro fertilisation (IVF) 115
infectious diseases 190, 200–1, 208, 209
infertility 114–15
inflammation response 38, 188
influenza virus 190, 191
inheritance 154–65
inhibitors (enzymes) 10, 11
insects, vectors of disease 199, 200
insulin 94, 95, 98–9, 102, 103, 140
  production of human 236
intestinal juice 28, 29
ionising radiation 264
IVF see in vitro fertilisation

J

joints 66–7
  replair and replacement 60–1

K

keyhole surgery 61, 66
kidneys 100, 104–5, 106, 107
knee joint 60–61, 66, 67

L

labour 130–31
lactation 132, 133
lactic acid 48, 49, 50
lactose intolerance 16

land use 256–7
large intestine 28
legume plants 248
LH see luteinising hormone
ligaments 62, 66, 67
limbic system 87
lipase 10, 28, 29
lipids 18, 19
liver 30, 31, 104, 183
  and homeostasis 100, 101, 102, 103
lock and key hypothesis (enzyme action) 8, 9
long sight 80, 81
LSD 184
lung cancer 56, 202
lungs 52, 53, 54, 55
  and homeostasis 100, 101
luteinising hormone (LH) 95, 120, 144, 145
lymphatic system 30, 31, 40, 41
lymphocytes 36, 37, 40, 204, 206
lysozyme 204

M

malaria 198, 199
malnutrition 140
mammary glands 118, 119, 133
medicine, biotechnology in 236–7
medulla (brain) 92, 93
meiosis 156, 157
meninges 92, 93
meningitis 92, 195
menopause 144, 145
menstrual cycle 120–1
mental developmen 142, 143
mental health 180–81
mesothelioma 56
metabolism 8–9
methedrine 184
micro-organisms 190, 191
  in biotechnology 226, 227, 228, 229, 234, 235
  and disease 190–91, 194–7
  and food poisoning 216–17
  growing 224–5
  in sewage treatment 214
micrometre (defined) 4
micropropagation 234
microvilli 30, 31
milk, lactose-free 230, 231
minerals 20, 21, 22, 30
miscarriage 130
mitochondria 4, 5
mitosis 156, 157
monoclonal antibodies 236, 237
monohybrid inheritance 160
morphine 184, 208
motor development 142-3
moulds 196
mouth to mouth resuscitation 54
MRI (magnetic resonance imaging) 3
MRSA (methicillin resistant *Staphylococcus aureus*) 151